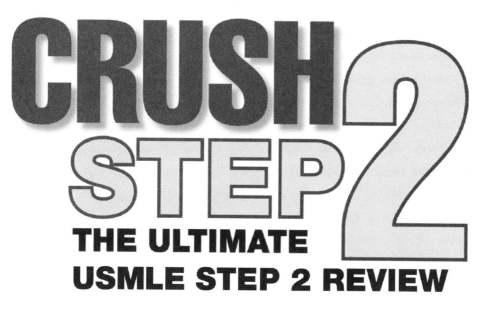

CRUSH STEP 2

THE ULTIMATE
USMLE STEP 2 REVIEW

3rd Edition

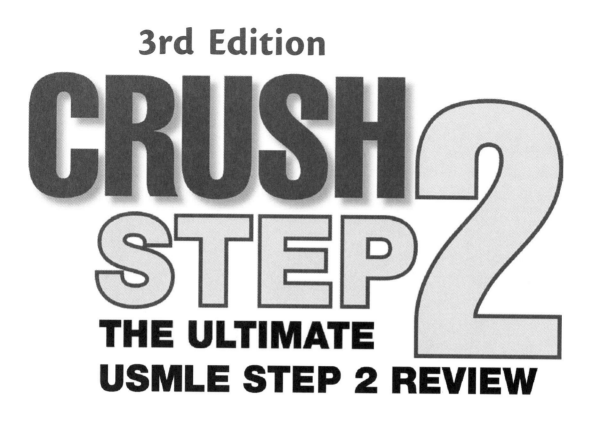

CRUSH STEP 2

THE ULTIMATE
USMLE STEP 2 REVIEW

Adam Brochert, MD

Staff Radiologist
Eisenhower Medical Center
Rancho Mirage, California

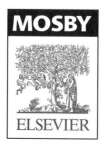

MOSBY

ELSEVIER

1600 John F. Kennedy Blvd.
Ste 1800
Philadelphia, PA 19103-2899

CRUSH STEP 2: The Ultimate USMLE Step 2 Review
Third Edition

ISBN-13: 978-1-4160-2976-2
ISBN-10: 1-4160-2976-1

Notice

Knowledge and best practice in this field are constantly changing. As new research and experience broaden our knowledge, changes in practice, treatment and drug therapy may become necessary or appropriate. Readers are advised to check the most current information provided (i) on procedures featured or (ii) by the manufacturer of each product to be administered, to verify the recommended dose or formula, the method and duration of administration, and contraindications. It is the responsibility of the practitioner, relying on their own experience and knowledge of the patient, to make diagnoses, to determine dosages and the best treatment for each individual patient, and to take all appropriate safety precautions. To the fullest extent of the law, neither the Publisher nor the Author assumes any liability for any injury and/or damage to persons or property arising out or related to any use of the material contained in this book.

The Publisher

Previous editions copyrighted 2003

Library of Congress Cataloging-in-Publication Data

Brochert, Adam, 1971-
    Crush step 2 : the ultimate USMLE step 2 review / Adam Brochert. — 3rd ed
        p. ; cm.
    Includes index.
    ISBN-13: 978-1-4160-2976-2
    ISBN-10: 1-4160-2976-1
    1. Clinical medicine—Examinations, questions, etc.   2. Clinical medicine—United States—Examinations—Study guides.   I. Title.   II. Title: Crush step two.
        [DNLM: 1. Clinical Medicine—Examination Questions. WB 18.2 B863c 2007]
RC58.B755 2007
616.0076—dc22

2006035878

ISBN-13: 978-1-4160-2976-2
ISBN-10: 1-4160-2976-1

Acquisitions Editor: Jim Merritt
Editorial Assistant: Nicole DiCicco
Publishing Services Manager: Linda Van Pelt
Project Manager: Joan Nikelsky
Design Direction: Ellen Zanolle

Printed in the United States of America.

Last digit is the print number: 9   8   7   6   5   4   3

CONTENTS

INTRODUCTION

This book was originally written because I believed there was not a good, comprehensive, high-yield review book for the USMLE Step 2. This third edition attempts to incorporate the many changes that have occurred in medicine and the exam since 2003, as well as suggestions from readers based on material they encountered on their exams. Though the format of the exam is constantly changing, many of the basic concepts you need to know to be a successful house officer have not changed in decades. If you understand the concepts in this book, you should do much better than pass: You should *Crush Step 2!*

Though Step 2 is the same level of difficulty as Step 1, the focus is more clinical and the questions are more relevant to the everyday practice of medicine. Knowing how to recognize, diagnose, manage, and treat common conditions is stressed. The exam tests not just theory but practice—in other words, what you should *do next*. Treatable emergency conditions are also tested, because you will soon be asked to take care of patients in the middle of the night, some of whom may require heroic measures if they are to survive until morning rounds.

Some information from Step 1 is still relevant and high yield for Step 2. Epidemiology and biostatistics, pharmacology, and microbiology are all tested with a slightly more clinical slant. Cardiac physiology and pathophysiology and behavioral science are also retested and are high yield. Overall, though, Step 2 has a different focus, and that focus is clinical. If a patient presented with chest pain, what would you do? What kinds of questions would you ask him or her? Which tests would you order? How would you select medications or treatments?

Here are five general tips to keep you focused while studying for and taking the test:

- Always get more history when it is an option, unless the patient is unstable and you think immediate action is needed.

- Know the cutoff values for the treatment of common conditions (e.g., at what numbers do you treat hypertension, diabetes, and hypercholesterolemia; below what CD4 count should you institute chemoprophylaxis in HIV patients).

- A presentation might be normal, especially in psychiatry and pediatrics, and require no treatment!

- Don't forget to study your subspecialties. Just because you never took an ophthalmology or dermatology rotation doesn't mean there won't be any basic questions on these topics. You don't have to be an expert, but knowing common and life-threatening diseases in the subspecialties can significantly increase your score.

◆ Residency programs generally only see those magic two- and three-digit scores, not the breakdown. Don't skip studying a subject because you know you aren't going into it—you might miss out on easy points.

Studying for Step 2 can seem like an overwhelming task. Given the time constraints of medical students in their clinical years, most need a concise, high-yield review of the tested topics. It is my hope that *Crush Step 2*, third edition, will meet your needs in this regard.

Adam Brochert, MD

Hypertension

SCREENING

Screening for hypertension should be done roughly every 2 years, starting at the age of 3 years. Whenever a patient comes in for any kind of medical visit or hospitalization, it is standard practice to measure the blood pressure. The current accepted cut-off value is 140/90 mm Hg (lower in children). A blood pressure of 145/75 mm Hg is still considered hypertension (isolated systolic hypertension) and should be treated if it persists. Systolic and diastolic hypertension both decrease life expectancy. Hypertension is not diagnosed until *three separate measurements on three separate occasions are* >140/90 mm Hg (except in pregnancy, when waiting for a return visit could be devastating). Also, if hypertension is severe (>210 systolic, >120 diastolic, or end-organ effects), immediate treatment with medication is warranted. Medication for hypertension is listed in Table 1-1.

EVALUATION

Basic studies and evaluation in a new hypertensive patient include urinalysis, chemistry panel 7, electrocardiogram (EKG), and hemoglobin and hematocrit. Do *not* treat hyper-

Table 1-1. INITIAL DRUG TREATMENT FOR HYPERTENSION

Systolic BP (mm Hg)	Diastolic BP (mm Hg)	Classification*	Initial Drug Treatment
<120	<80	Normal	None
120–139	80–89	Prehypertension	None unless compelling indications[†]
140–159	90–99	Stage 1 hypertension	Thiazides preferred. Use other agents for comorbidities or combination treatment.
≥160	≥100	Stage 2 hypertension	Thiazide plus at least one other agent (if tolerated) typically needed.

Note: All patients should make lifestyle modifications.

  *__Classification is based on the worse number__ (e.g., 168/60 mm Hg is considered stage II hypertension even though diastolic pressure is normal).

  [†]Compelling indications are __diabetes__ and __chronic kidney disease__. Such patients should be treated with a goal of <__130/80__ mm Hg. BP, blood pressure.

tension until you have a diagnosis (hypertension on three separate visits)! Once you have a diagnosis, first allow the patient 3 to 4 months of weight reduction, exercise, and other lifestyle modifications (low-salt and low-cholesterol diet, no alcohol, no smoking). If this approach is unsuccessful, only then do you start medication.

TREATMENT

There are five first-line agents for treating hypertension: thiazide diuretics (preferred agent in patients without additional comorbidities or indications), β-blockers, angiotensin-converting enzyme (ACE) inhibitors, angiotensin-receptor blockers (ARBs), and calcium channel blockers. Which one you choose is often based on comorbidities (Table 1-2).

For **pregnant patients,** use hydralazine, labetalol, or α-methyldopa. Remember that in patients with preeclampsia, magnesium sulfate (MgSO$_4$) lowers blood pressure. For side effects of hypertension medications (high yield), see Chapter 29, Pharmacology.

A **hypertensive urgency** or **emergency** occurs when blood pressure is >200/120 mm Hg with (emergency) or without (urgency) acute end-organ damage. Evidence of end-organ damage includes acute left ventricular failure, unstable angina, myocardial infarction, or encephalopathy (e.g., headaches, mental status changes, vomiting, blurred vision, dizziness, papilledema). Hypertensive urgencies and emergencies are an exception to the rule of measuring blood pressure three times before treating! Use nitroprusside, nitroglycerin, or β-blocker (e.g., labetalol) emergently.

Table 1-2. INDICATIONS AND CONTRAINDICATIONS FOR ANTIHYPERTENSIVE MEDICATION

Drug Class	Use in Patients with	Avoid in Patients with
ACE inhibitors	Heart failure, diabetes, acute coronary syndrome or unstable angina, acute or prior myocardial infarction, high risk of coronary artery disease or stroke, chronic kidney disease	Pregnancy, angioedema, renovascular hypertension (can cause renal failure)
Aldosterone receptor blockers (e.g., spironolactone, eplerenone)	Heart failure, prior myocardial infarction	Hyperkalemia, pregnancy
ARBs (e.g., losartan, irbesartan)	Heart failure, diabetes, chronic kidney disease	Pregnancy, renovascular hypertension (can cause renal failure)
β-Blockers	Stable angina, acute coronary syndrome or unstable angina, acute or prior myocardial infarction, high risk of coronary artery disease, atrial tachycardia or fibrilliation, thyrotoxicosis (short term), essential tremor, migraines	Asthma, chronic obstructive pulmonary disease, heart block, sick sinus syndrome
Calcium channel blockers	Raynaud's syndrome, atrial tachyarrhythmias	Heart block, sick sinus syndrome, congestive heart failure (all related to central-acting agents), pregnancy
Thiazides	Heart failure, diabetes, high risk of coronary artery disease or stroke, osteoporosis	Gout, electrolyte disturbances (e.g., hyponatremia), pregnancy

ACE, angiotensin-converting enzyme; ARB, angiotensin-receptor blocker.

Nitroprusside dilates arteries and veins. Nitroglycerin is a venodilator only; other medications are arterial dilators only (hydralazine, α1 antagonists, calcium channel blockers). Venodilators reduce preload, and arterial dilators reduce afterload. Nitroprusside does both.

Lowering blood pressure lowers risk for stroke (hypertension is the most important stroke risk factor), heart disease, myocardial infarction, renal failure, atherosclerosis, and dissecting aortic aneurysm. Coronary disease is the most common cause of death among untreated hypertensive patients. Don't forget to treat isolated systolic or diastolic hypertension if it persists.

SECONDARY HYPERTENSION

Clues to **secondary hypertension** include onset before age 30 years or after age 55 years and other suggestive history or lab values. In a young woman, the most common cause is birth control pills (discontinue them). The next most common cause is renovascular hypertension due to fibrous dysplasia; look for renal bruit, using computed tomography (CT) or magnetic resonance (MR) angiogram for diagnosis (ultrasound and nuclear medicine screening tests for renovascular hypertension are also used), and treat with angioplasty. In a young man, think of excessive alcohol intake or "exotic" conditions (pheochromocytoma, Cushing's syndrome, Conn's syndrome, polycystic kidney disease). In elderly patients with new-onset hypertension, think of renovascular hypertension due to atherosclerosis (look for renal bruit; ACE inhibitors precipitate renal failure). If you suspect secondary hypertension (95% of cases of hypertension are essential, primary, or idiopathic), remember the following hints and tests to order:

- Pheochromocytoma: Urinary catecholamines (vanillylmandelic acid, metanephrine) plus intermittent severe hypertension, dizziness, and diaphoresis
- Polycystic kidney disease: Flank mass, family history, elevated creatinine, and elevated blood urea nitrogen (BUN)
- Cushing's syndrome: Dexamethasone suppression test or 24-hour urine cortisol level
- Renovascular hypertension: MR or CT angiogram, ultrasound, or ACE-inhibitor nuclear renal scan (standard catheter angiogram is too invasive to use for routine diagnosis). If there is a bruit on exam (Fig. 1-1), treat with angioplasty and stenting.

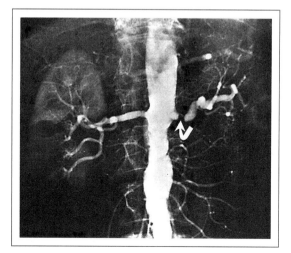

FIGURE 1-1. Conventional renal angiogram revealing a high-grade, proximal left renal artery atherosclerotic-type stenosis (arrow) and associated atherosclerotic irregularity in the abdominal aorta. Fibromuscular dysplasia usually occurs in the mid-renal artery, has a beaded appearance, and usually occurs without other evidence of atherosclerosis (i.e., in young patients).

◆ Conn's syndrome: High aldosterone, **low renin**

◆ Coarctation of the aorta: upper extremity hypertension only, unequal pulses, radio-femoral delay, associated with **Turner's syndrome**, rib notching on x-ray

Diabetes

SCREENING

Universal screening is generally *not recommended*. Screening in patients who are obese, are older than 45 years, have a positive family history, or are members of certain subgroups (black, American Indian, Latin American) is more accepted, but not uniformly.

SIGNS AND SYMPTOMS

Classic signs and symptoms of diabetes mellitus (DM) are polydipsia, polyuria, polyphagia, and weight loss. Diagnosis is made by a fasting plasma glucose of 126 mg/dL (after an overnight fast) or a random glucose (no fasting) of 200 mg/dL. If the patient has classic symptoms, one measurement is enough to confirm a diagnosis, but in an asymptomatic patient, the test should be repeated. Rarely, an oral glucose tolerance test is done, and DM is diagnosed if 200 mg/dL is reached within 2 hours of oral administration of a 75-g glucose load. Differences between type 1 DM (T1DM) and type 2 DM (T2DM) are shown in Table 1-3.

TREATMENT

The **goal of treatment** is to keep postprandial glucose <180 to 200 mg/dL and fasting glucose <130 mg/dL. Stricter control results in too many episodes of hypoglycemia (look for symptoms of sympathetic discharge and mental status changes), which can cause brain damage in the long term. Good glucose control, however, delays or prevents nearly all of the complications of diabetes.

Table 1-3. DIFFERENCES BETWEEN TYPE 1 AND TYPE 2 DIABETES MELLITUS

Feature	Type 1	Type 2
Age at onset	Most commonly <30 y	Most commonly >30 y*
Associated body habitus	Thin	Obese
Develop ketoacidosis	Yes	No
Develop hyperosmolar state	No	Yes
Level of endogenous insulin	Low to none	Low to high (insulin resistance)
Twin concurrence	<50%	>50%
HLA association	Yes	No
Response to oral hypoglycemics	No	Yes
Antibodies to insulin	Yes (at diagnosis)	No
Risk of diabetic complications	Yes	Yes
Islet cell pathology	Insulitis (loss of most beta cells)	Normal number, but with amyloid deposits

*Be aware, however, of the "epidemic" of type 2 diabetes in those younger than 30 years, including children and adolescents, which is due in part to the obesity epidemic.

HLA, human leukocyte antigen.

IMPORTANT POINTS

1 Remember the importance of C peptide in distinguishing between too much exogenous insulin (low C peptide with accidental overdose in a diabetic patient or in a patient with factitious disorder) and an insulinoma (high C peptide).

2 Because IV contrast agents can precipitate acute renal failure in diabetic patients and other renal patients, use iodinated contrast for imaging studies only when absolutely necessary. To prevent renal damage, make sure a patient with kidney disease or diabetes is well hydrated before using contrast agents.

3 Diabetic ketoacidosis is seen in patients with T1DM. Diagnosis of diabetic ketoacidosis requires hyperglycemia, hyperketonemia, and metabolic acidosis. Treatment involves fluids, IV regular insulin, and potassium and phosphorus replacement. Do not use bicarbonate unless the pH is <7. Search for the cause, which often is infection. Death occurs without treatment.

4 Nonketotic hyperglycemic hyperosmolar state is seen in patients with T2DM. Diagnosis of nonketotic hyperglycemic hyperosmolar state requires hyperglycemia and hyperosmolarity without ketonemia. Treatment involves IV fluids (first initial choice), IV insulin, and electrolyte replacement. Mortality rate is high.

COMPLICATIONS

Long-term complications of diabetes mellitus happen in both T1DM and T2DM and include:

◆ Atherosclerosis: Coronary artery disease, peripheral vascular disease (claudication, atrophy), myocardial infarction, stroke

◆ Retinopathy: When proliferative, treat with panretinal laser photocoagulation to prevent progression and blindness. All diabetic patients should be seen once a year (initially) by an ophthalmologist to monitor retinal changes.

◆ Nephropathy: ACE inhibitors help prevent nephropathy; 30% of end-stage renal disease is caused by diabetes.

◆ Infections

◆ Neuropathy (see later)

◆ Foot ulcers, infections, and gangrene: Diabetes is the most common cause of nontrauma amputations. Amputation is usually required because of some mix of diabetes-induced vascular disease (poor blood flow), neuropathy (patient doesn't feel the problem), and immune dysfunction or infection (caused by hyperglycemia). Patients should wear comfortable, properly fitting shoes and should regularly inspect their feet.

Peripheral neuropathy (autonomic and sensory) causes many problems in diabetic patients:

◆ Gastroparesis (early satiety, nausea; treat with metoclopromide)

◆ Charcot's joints (joints deform due to lack of sensation; patient puts too much stress on joints and might not feel injury or stress)

◆ Impotence from autonomic neuropathy as well as peripheral vascular disease

◆ Cranial nerve palsies (especially cranial nerves III, IV, and VI: ocular palsies); these usually resolve spontaneously within a few months.

◆ Orthostatic hypotension due to lack of effective sympathetic innervation; when the patient stands up, the heart rate and vascular tone do not increase appropriately to maintain blood pressure

◆ "Silent" myocardial infarction (because of neuropathy, there is no chest pain)

For the more common T2DM patients, once the patient is stabilized (with inpatient treatment, if needed), remember that the cheapest and most effective treatment is a combination of diet changes, exercise, and weight loss; this cures 90% of T2DM! In the real world, however, this often does not work, so use oral medications, typically a sulfonylurea (e.g., glimepiride, glipizide, glyburide), metformin, and/or a thiazolidinedione (e.g., pioglitazone, rosiglitazone). A combination of an insulin secretagogue–like sulfonylurea and an insulin sensitizer like metformin is common, and insulin is often needed later, if not initially.

INSULIN

Know how to use different preparations of insulin, especially lispro, **regular,** and **neutral protamine Hagedorn** (NPH) insulin (Table 1-4). Patients with T1DM generally require insulin 0.5 to 1.0 U/kg of body weight per day, though initial requirements are often less than this because of a small amount of residual endogenous insulin production. In T2DM,

Table 1-4. INSULIN PREPARATIONS AND USE

Insulin Preparation	Onset (h)	Peak (h)	Duration (h)	When to Use
Ultra Rapid Acting				
Insulin aspart	<0.25	1–3	3–5	Right before meals
Insulin lispro	0.25–0.5	0.5–2.5	3–5	Right before meals
Rapid Acting				
Regular insulin	0.5–1	2–4	5–8	Inpatients (can be given IV), 0.5–1 h before a meal for outpatients
Intermediate Acting				
NPH insulin	2–3	4–12	12–24	Generally part of standard regimens that mix with shorter-acting insulin (e.g., 70/30 or 50/50 of NPH/regular)
Lente insulin	2–3	4–12	12–24	
Long Acting				
Ultralente insulin	6–10	8–16	18–26	Provide basal insulin level; supplement with short-acting insulin
Ultra Long Acting				
Insulin glargine	1.5–4	None	24+	Provide basal insulin level; supplement with short-acting insulin

IV, intravenous; NPH, neutral protamine Hagedorn.

save insulin for inpatients and those who fail oral preparations. Requirements may be greater than 1 U/kg per day due to resistance.

- If the patient has high (low) 7 AM glucose, increase (decrease) NPH insulin at dinner the night before.

- If the patient has high (low) noon glucose, increase (decrease) morning regular insulin or increase (decrease) before-breakfast lispro or aspart insulin.

- If the patient has high (low) 5 PM glucose, increase (decrease) morning NPH or increase (decrease) before-lunch lispro or aspart insulin.

- If the patient has high (low) 9 PM glucose, increase (decrease) dinner-time regular insulin or increase (decrease) before-dinner lispro or aspart insulin.

SOMOGYI EFFECT VERSUS DAWN PHENOMENON

The *Somogyi effect* is the body's reaction to hypoglycemia. If too much NPH or other longer-acting insulin preparation is given the day or night before, the 3 AM glucose will be low (hypoglycemia). The body reacts by releasing stress hormones, which cause the 7 AM glucose to be high. Treatment is to *decrease* insulin. The *dawn phenomenon* is hyperglycemia caused by normal early AM growth hormone secretion. The 7 AM glucose is high, without 4 AM hypoglycemia (glucose is normal or high at 4 AM). Treatment is to *increase* insulin.

COMPLIANCE

Follow compliance by checking the hemoglobin A1c (Hb$_{A1c}$) level, which is an accurate measure of overall control for the previous 3 months. Patients are not afraid to alter their home test numbers to please their doctors, and this is the way to catch them. Strive for a level less than 7%.

SURGERY

For surgery, patients with diabetes (and without diabetes) are allowed nothing by mouth (NPO). Give one third to one half of the normal insulin dose, then monitor glucose closely through surgery and postoperatively, using 5% dextrose in water (D$_5$W) and IV regular insulin to maintain glucose control.

MEDICATIONS

Chlorpropamide (rarely used) can cause the syndrome of inappropriate secretion of antidiuretic hormone (SIADH). Patients with T1DM are not helped by oral medications. Remember that β-blockers can prevent many of the physical manifestations of hypoglycemia (tachycardia, diaphoresis), thereby also preventing early detection, but treatment benefits might outweigh the risks (e.g., following a myocardial infarction).

Cholesterol

Measure a fasting lipoprotein profile (total cholesterol, low-density lipoprotein [LDL] cholesterol, high-density lipoprotein [HDL] cholesterol, and triglycerides) every 5 years (unless abnormal) starting at age 20 years. Consider earlier and more aggressive screening for a strong family history and/or obesity.

Lipoprotein analysis involves measuring total cholesterol, HDL, and triglycerides. LDL can then be calculated from the formula LDL = total cholesterol − HDL − (triglycerides/5).

Total cholesterol goal is <200 mg/dL; >240 mg/dL is considered high. Normal triglyceride level is <150 mg/dL; >200 is considered high. LDL is usually the main player for treatment decisions; interventions at various LDL levels are given in Table 1-5. Look for xanthelasma (Fig. 1-2), corneal arcus (in younger patients), lipemic-looking serum, and obesity as markers of possible **familial hypercholesterolemia.** Family members should be tested. Also, look for pancreatitis with no risk factors (e.g., no alcohol, no gallstones) as a marker for familial hypertriglyceridemia.

Be aware of **secondary causes of hyperlipidemia:** uncontrolled diabetes mellitus, hypothyroidism, uremia, the nephrotic syndrome, obstructive liver disease, excessive alcohol intake (increases triglycerides), and medications (oral contraceptives, glucocorticoids, thiazides, and β-blockers).

Table 1-5. LDL CHOLESTEROL LEVELS AND INTERVENTIONS

No CHD Risk Factors	≥ 2 CHD Risk Factors*	Known CAD or Equivalent[†]	Very High Risk[‡]	Intervention
LDL <160	LDL < 100	LDL < 100	LDL < 70	None (meets goal)
LDL 160–189	LDL 100–129		LDL 70–99	Diet ± medications[§]
LDL ≥190	LDL ≥130	LDL ≥100	LDL ≥100	Medications (+ diet)

*Risk factors for CHD are listed in the text.

[†]CHD equivalents include diabetes mellitus, peripheral arterial atherosclerotic disease, symptomatic carotid artery disease, and abdominal aortic aneurysm.

[‡]"Very" high-risk patients are those with CAD who have a heart attack, diabetes, or other severe and poorly controlled risk factors (e.g., metabolic syndrome, heavy smoking).

[§]"Diet" includes general lifestyle modifications such as eating less and healthier, decreasing alcohol intake, exercising, etc. The trend is toward more aggressive intervention, so you will not be faulted for initiating medications at these gray-area LDL levels, particularly in higher-risk people.

CAD, coronary artery disease. CHD, coronary heart disease.

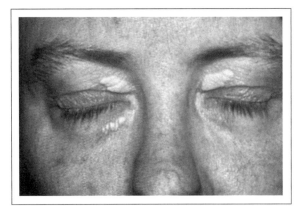

FIGURE 1-2. Patient with xanthelasma in all four lids. (From Tasman W, Jaeger EA: The Wills Eye Hospital Atlas of Clinical Ophthalmology. Philadelphia, Lippincott-Raven, 1996, with permission.)

Atherosclerosis is involved in about one half of all deaths in the United States and one third of deaths between ages 35 and 65 years. Atherosclerosis is the most important cause of permanent disability and accounts for more hospital days than any other illness. (Translation: *Understand atherosclerosis for the boards*).

RISK FACTORS

Risk factors for coronary heart disease include:

◆ Age (men = 45 years, women = 55 years or with premature menopause and no estrogen replacement therapy)

◆ Family history of premature CHD (defined as definite myocardial infarction or sudden death in father or other first-degree male relative younger than 55 years or mother or other first-degree female relative younger than 65 years)

◆ Current cigarette smoking (>10 cigarettes per day)

◆ Hypertension (140/90 mm Hg or on antihypertensive medications)

◆ Low HDL (<40 mg/dL) (note, however, that HDL = 60 mg/dL is considered to be protective and negates one risk factor).

Diabetes is a risk factor but is not used or counted in determining the number of risk factors when deciding cholesterol treatment, because it is considered a CAD equivalent and warrants immediate aggressive treatment by itself.

LDL and total cholesterol are risk factors for CHD, but do not count them in deciding to treat or not to treat high cholesterol. Male sex is also considered a risk factor because men develop coronary heart disease earlier than women (but postmenopausal women quickly catch up with age-matched men). If you give a patient one risk factor for being male, do not give him a second risk factor for age (use one or the other in men).

Obesity is not an independent risk factor for board purposes. Stress, physical inactivity, and type A personality (look for a hard-driving attorney) are controversial (thought to be risk factors by some clinicians). *Hypertriglyceridemia* alone is not considered a risk factor, but when associated with high cholesterol it causes more CHD than high cholesterol alone.

TREATMENT

Give new lower-risk patients 3 to 6 months to try lifestyle modifications (exercise and decreased calories, cholesterol, saturated fats, alcohol, and smoking) before initiating drug therapy.

 High HDL is protective against atherosclerosis and is increased by exercise, estrogens, and moderate alcohol intake (one or two drinks per day) but *not* by high alcohol intake. HDL is decreased by smoking, androgens, progesterone, and hypertriglyceridemia.

First-line agents are niacin (poorly tolerated but effective, particularly to raise HDL), bile acid–binding resins (e.g., cholestyramine, colesevelam), HMG CoA-reductase inhibitors (called "statins," most effective, more expensive, potential liver or muscle damage, almost always the initial agent used in the real world), and ezetimibe (blocks cholesterol absorption and is often combined with a statin).

Smoking

Smoking is the single most significant source of preventable morbidity and premature death in the United States. Whenever you are not sure which risk factor to eliminate, smoking is a safe guess.

IMPORTANT POINTS

1 Smoking is the best risk factor to eliminate to prevent heart disease–related deaths (responsible for 30%–45% of CHD deaths). Risk decreases by 50% within 1 year compared with continuing smokers and decreases to the level of patients who never smoked in 15 years.

2 Smoking also increases the risk of the following cancers: lung (85%–90% of cases), oral cavity (90% of cases), esophagus (at least 50% of cases), larynx, pharynx, bladder (30%–50% of cases), kidney (20%–30% of cases), pancreas (20%–25% of cases), cervix, vulva, penis, and anus. Smoking may also increase stomach cancer risk.

3 Chronic obstructive pulmonary disease is often a result of smoking. Emphysema almost always is due to smoking (unless the patient is very young or has no smoking history, in which case you should consider α_1-antitrypsin deficiency). Although the changes of emphysema are irreversible, risk of death still decreases after smoking cessation.

4 When parents smoke, children are at increased risk for asthma and upper respiratory infections, including otitis media.

5 Smoking retards healing of peptic ulcer disease, and cessation stops Buerger's disease (Raynaud's symptoms in a young male smoker).

6 Smoking by pregnant women increases the risk of low birth weight, prematurity, spontaneous abortion, stillbirth, and infant mortality.

7 Smoking cessation preoperatively is the best way to decrease risk of postoperative pulmonary complications.

8 Do *not* give birth control pills to women older than 35 years who smoke (or heavy smokers at any age).

9 The antidepressant bupropion and nicotine preparations (patch, gum, nasal spray, lozenge, etc.) can help some people quit.

Alcohol

Alcohol is involved in roughly 50% of fatal car accidents, 67% of drownings and homicides, 70% to 80% of deaths in fires, and 35% of suicides. Alcohol abuse is the most common cause of cirrhosis and esophageal varices, and it increases the risk of the following cancers: oral, larynx, pharynx, esophagus, and liver. It can also increase the risk of gastric, colon, pancreatic, and breast cancer.

Wernicke's vs. Korsakoff's syndromes:

- Wernicke's syndrome includes ophthalmoplegia, nystagmus, ataxia, and confusion. It is acute and often reversible and it can be fatal.

- Korsakoff's syndrome includes anterograde amnesia and confabulation; it is chronic and irreversible.

- Both are caused by thiamine deficiency.

- Pathophysiology includes damage to mamillary bodies and thalamic nuclei.

Alcohol withdrawal can be fatal. Treat on an inpatient basis with benzodiazepines (e.g., chlordiazepoxide, lorazepam); barbiturates are rarely used. Gradually taper the dose over days.

Withdrawal stages/symptoms:

1. Acute withdrawal syndrome, 12 to 48 hours after the last drink. Symptoms include tremors, sweating, hyperreflexia, and seizures ("rum fits").

2. Alcoholic hallucinosis, which consists of hallucinations (auditory and/or visual) and illusions without autonomic symptoms.

3. Delirium tremens, usually 2 to 4 days after the last drink; involves hallucinations and illusions plus confusion, poor sleep, and autonomic lability (sweating, increased pulse and temperature). It occasionally is fatal.

Stigmata of chronic liver disease in alcoholics: varices, hemorrhoids, caput medusae, jaundice, ascites, palmar erythema, spider angiomas, gynecomastia, testicular atrophy, encephalopathy, asterixis, prolonged prothrombin time, hyperbilirubinemia, spontaneous bacterial peritonitis, hypoalbuminemia, and anemia.

Conditions commonly caused by alcohol abuse: gastritis, Mallory–Weiss tears, pancreatitis (acute and chronic), peripheral neuropathy (via thiamine deficiency), brain damage (e.g., cerebellar degeneration), and cardiomyopathy (dilated). It also causes testicular atrophy, fatty change in the liver, hepatitis, cirrhosis, hepatocellular carcinoma, Wernicke–Korsakoff syndrome (via thiamine deficiency), and rhabdomyolysis (acute and chronic).

The best treatment for alcoholism is Alcoholics Anonymous or other support group. Disulfiram also may be tried (patients get sick when they drink because of alcohol dehydrogenase enzyme inhibition), and antiopioid naltrexone can help in some.

Alcohol is a definite teratogen. Recognize the **fetal alcohol syndrome:** mental retardation, microcephaly, microphthalmia, short palpebral fissures, midfacial hypoplasia, and cardiac defects. No alcohol is good alcohol during pregnancy. An estimated 1 in 3000 births is affected by fetal alcohol syndrome, which is the *most common cause* of preventable mental retardation.

Incidence. Alcohol abuse is more common in men. Roughly 10% to 15% of the U.S. population abuses alcohol. Alcoholism has a heritable component and is especially passed from fathers to sons.

IMPORTANT POINTS

1 "Skid-row" alcoholics (i.e., homeless) commonly develop aspiration pneumonia with enteric or oral flora bugs such as *Klebsiella* species (currant-jelly sputum), anaerobes, *Escherichia coli*, streptococci, staphylococci.

2 Alcohol can precipitate hypoglycemia (but give thiamine first).

3 Alcoholics develop just about every type of vitamin and mineral deficiency; especially common are deficiencies of folate, magnesium, and thiamine.

4 Give thiamine before glucose in an alcoholic; if you give them in the reverse order, you can precipitate Wernicke's encephalopathy.

5 Bleeding varices are treated with stabilization (IV fluids, blood), then upper endoscopy and sclerotherapy with cauterization, banding, or vasopressin. The mortality rate is high, and rebleeding is common, especially early. Try transjugular intrahepatic portosystemic shunt (TIPS) for intractable cases. Open surgical portacaval shunting procedures are now rarely performed (splenorenal is the most physiologic shunt type).

Acid–Base Status

You must know how to interpret an **arterial blood gas** result when given pH, O_2, CO_2, and bicarbonate. Here are good basic hints:

- pH tells you whether you are dealing with acidosis or alkalosis.
- Look at the CO_2. If it is high, the patient either has respiratory acidosis (pH <7.4) or is compensating for metabolic alkalosis (pH >7.4). If CO_2 is low, the patient either has respiratory alkalosis (pH >7.4) or is compensating for metabolic acidosis (pH <7.4).
- Look at the bicarbonate. If it is high, the patient either has metabolic alkalosis (pH >7.4) or is compensating for respiratory acidosis (pH <7.4). If bicarbonate is low, the patient either has metabolic acidosis (pH <7.4) or is compensating for respiratory alkalosis (pH >7.4).

Clinical correlation: Common causes of different primary disturbances:

- **Respiratory acidosis:** Chronic obstructive pulmonary disease, asthma, drugs (opioids, benzodiazepines, barbiturates, alcohol, and other respiratory depressants), chest wall problems (paralysis, pain), sleep apnea
- **Respiratory alkalosis:** Anxiety or hyperventilation, aspirin or salicylate overdose
- **Metabolic acidosis:** Ethanol, diabetic ketoacidosis, uremia, lactic acidosis (sepsis or shock), methanol or ethylene glycol poisoning, aspirin or salicylate overdose, diarrhea, carbonic anhydrase inhibitors
- **Metabolic alkalosis:** diuretics (except carbonic anhydrase inhibitors), vomiting, volume contraction, antacid abuse or milk-alkali syndrome, hyperaldosteronism
- **Salicylate (aspirin) overdose** causes two primary disturbances: respiratory alkalosis and metabolic acidosis. Look for coexisting tinnitus, hypoglycemia, vomiting, and history of "swallowing several pills." Alkalinization of the urine (with bicarbonate) speeds excretion.
- **In certain patients with chronic lung disease,** pH may be alkaline during the day (classic in patients with sleep apnea) because they breathe better when they are awake or have

just recovered from an episode of bronchitis. The metabolic alkalosis that usually compensates for respiratory acidosis is no longer compensatory and becomes the primary disturbance (elevated pH and bicarbonate).

Treatment. Do *not* use bicarbonate to treat low pH unless the pH is <7 and other measures have failed (always try correction of underlying cause and/or saline first).

 Beware the asthmatic patient whose blood gas goes from alkalotic to normal. The patient might be about to crash and need intubation.

Electrolyte Disturbances

HYPONATREMIA

Signs and symptoms of hyponatremia are confusion, lethargy, mental status changes, anorexia, seizures, disorientation, cramps, and coma. The first step in determining the cause of true hyponatremia is to look at the volume status (Box 1-1).

IMPORTANT POINTS

1 SIADH commonly results from head trauma, surgery, meningitis, small-cell lung cancer, painful states (e.g., trauma, postoperative state), pulmonary infections (pneumonia, tuberculosis), opioids, or chlorpropamide. Treatment is water restriction. Occasionally, when refractive to conservative management, SIADH is treated with demeclocycline (a tetracycline that causes renal diabetes insipidus [DI]).

2 With Addison's disease and hypoaldosteronism, potassium is classically elevated.

3 Treat hypovolemic hyponatremia with saline. Treat euvolemic and hypervolemic hyponatremia with free water restriction and possibly diuretics for hypervolemia.

4 Never correct hyponatremia rapidly, because you can cause brainstem damage (central pontine myelinolysis). Hypertonic saline is used only when the patient has seizures due to hyponatremia and, even then, only briefly and cautiously. *Normal saline is a better choice 99 times out of 100 for board purposes.*

Box 1-1. CAUSES OF HYPONATREMIA BY VOLUME STATUS

Hypovolemic	Euvolemic	Hypervolemic
Dehydration	Syndrome of inappropriate secretion of antidiuretic hormone	Congestive heart failure
Diuretics		Nephrotic syndrome
Diabetic ketoacidosis or diabetes mellitus	Psychogenic polydipsia	Cirrhosis
Addison's disease	Oxytocin use	Toxemia
Hypoaldosteronism		Renal failure

5 "Correct" the spurious hyponatremia of hyperglycemia: Once glucose exceeds 200 mg/dL, sodium decreases by 1.6 mEq/L for each increase of 100 mg/dL in glucose. Hyperlipidemia and severe hyperproteinemia can cause a false (spurious) hyponatremia by their osmotic effect.

6 In a surgical patient, the most common cause of hyponatremia is inappropriate or excessive fluid administration.

7 Oxytocin administration can cause hyponatremia (ADH-like effect) in pregnant women.

HYPERNATREMIA

Signs and symptoms are similar to those of hyponatremia: confusion, mental status changes, hyperreflexia, seizures, and coma.

Common causes:

- Dehydration
- Inability to drink (paralysis, dementia)
- Diuretics
- Diabetes insipidus (pituitary or nephrogenic)
- Diarrhea
- Renal disease (e.g., isosthenuria from sickle cell trait)
- Iatrogenic administration of excessive salt

Hypokalemia and hypercalcemia also cause an impairment in renal concentrating ability that can mimic DI.

Treatment of hypernatremia involves water replacement. Often the patient is so dehydrated that normal saline is initially used until the patient is hydrated and hemodynamically stable. Then the patient may be switched to half-normal saline (0.45% NaCl) if still hypernatremic. Five-percent dextrose in water (D_5W) should *not* be used.

Pituitary vs. nephrogenic diabetes insipidus:

- Pituitary DI responds to vasopressin; nephrogenic DI does not.
- Nephrogenic DI can be caused by medications (lithium, demeclocycline, methoxyflurane, and amphotericin B) and is treated with a thiazide diuretic (paradoxical effect).
- Central DI can be caused by tumor, trauma, or sarcoidosis, although it is often idiopathic.

HYPOKALEMIA

Hypokalemia causes **muscle weakness,** including weakness of smooth muscles. The patient might have an ileus and/or hypotension. Muscle weakness can lead to paralysis and ventilatory failure. EKG findings include loss of T wave, presence of **U waves,** premature ventricular and atrial contractions, and ventricular and atrial tachyarrhythmias.

Changes in pH can cause changes in serum potassium (alkalosis causes hypokalemia; acidosis causes hyperkalemia). For this reason, bicarbonate is given to severely hyperkalemic patients. Normalization of deranged pH most likely will correct the potassium derangement automatically (no need to give or restrict potassium).

IMPORTANT POINTS

1 The heart is particularly sensitive to hypokalemia when the patient is taking digitalis. Potassium should be watched carefully in all patients taking digitalis, especially if they also take diuretics (common).

2 Do *not* replace potassium too quickly! The best method of replacement is oral, but if potassium must be given IV, do not exceed 20 mEq/h. Monitor the EKG if potassium must be given quickly.

3 If hypomagnesemia is present, it is difficult to correct the hypokalemia unless you also correct the hypomagnesemia.

HYPERKALEMIA

If the patient is asymptomatic and the EKG is normal, but the lab result points to hyperkalemia, you should wonder whether the specimen was hemolyzed. Hemolysis causes a **false hyperkalemia.** Repeat the test.

Signs and symptoms can include weakness or paralysis, but the most important (and most tested) effects are cardiac. **EKG changes** (in order of increasing potassium value) include tall, peaked T waves (Fig. 1-3); widening of QRS; PR interval prolongation; loss of P waves; and a sine wave pattern. Arrhythmias include asystole and ventricular fibrillation.

Common causes:

◆ Renal failure (acute or chronic)

◆ Severe tissue destruction

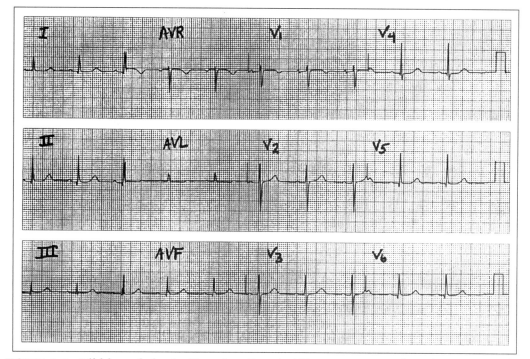

FIGURE 1-3. Mild hyperkalemia. Note the tall, peaked T waves, most prominent in V_2-V_5. No other abnormalities are present.

◆ Hypoaldosteronism (e.g., hyporeninemic hypoaldosteronism in diabetes)
◆ Medications (potassium-sparing diuretics, β-blockers, nonsteroidal antiinflammatory drugs, or ACE inhibitors). Try stopping all implicated medications.
◆ Adrenal insufficiency (associated with low sodium and low blood pressure)

The **best method of therapy** is oral (decreased intake, sodium polystyrene resin). If, however, potassium is very high (>6.5 mEq/L) and/or cardiac toxicity is apparent (more than peaked T waves), immediate IV therapy is needed. First give calcium gluconate, which is cardioprotective, even though it does not change potassium levels. Then give sodium bicarbonate (alkalosis causes potassium to shift inside cells) and glucose with insulin, which also forces potassium inside cells. If the patient has renal failure or initial treatment is ineffective, prepare to institute dialysis emergently.

HYPOCALCEMIA

Hypocalcemia produces **neurologic findings**, the most tested of which is tetany. Tetany is evidenced by tapping on the facial nerve to elicit contraction of the facial muscles (Chvostek's sign) or applying a tourniquet or blood pressure cuff and inflating it to elicit hand muscle (carpopedal) spasms (Trousseau's sign). Other symptoms are depression, encephalopathy, dementia, laryngospasm, and convulsions. EKG shows **QT interval prolongation** (Fig. 1-4).

Common causes:

◆ DiGeorge's syndrome (tetany shortly after birth, absent thymic shadow)
◆ Renal failure (because of the kidney's role in vitamin D metabolism)
◆ Hypoparathyroidism (watch for post-thyroidectomy patients; all four parathyroids might have been accidentally removed)

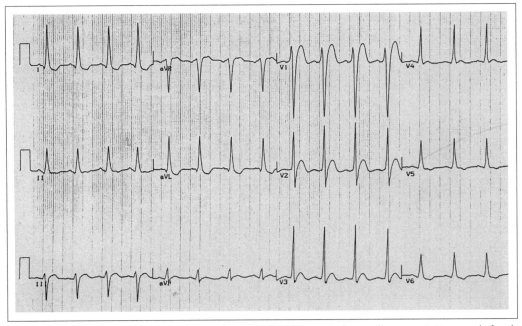

FIGURE 1-4. Hypocalcemia. Note the QT interval of 0.46 seconds (normally up to 0.42 seconds for the heart rate of 65 beats/min). No other EKG abnormalities are present.

- Vitamin D deficiency
- Pseudohypoparathyroidism (short fingers, short stature, mental retardation, and normal levels of parathyroid hormone [PTH] with end-organ unresponsiveness to PTH)
- Acute pancreatitis

IMPORTANT POINTS

1 Hypoproteinemia of any etiology can cause hypocalcemia because the protein-bound fraction of calcium is decreased. In this instance, however, the patient is asymptomatic, because the ionized (unbound) fraction of calcium (which can be ordered and measured as a specific test) is unchanged (no treatment needed).

2 Hypomagnesemia of any cause makes it difficult to correct the hypocalcemia until the hypomagnesemia is also corrected.

3 Rickets and osteomalacia are the skeletal effects of vitamin D deficiency in children and adults, respectively.

4 Alkalosis can cause symptoms similar to hypocalcemia because of effects on the ionized fraction of calcium. Treat by correcting the pH.

5 Phosphorus and calcium levels are usually in opposite directions, and derangements in one can cause problems with the other. In renal failure, therefore, you should not only raise calcium but also restrict phosphorus.

HYPERCALCEMIA

Hypercalcemia is **usually asymptomatic** and discovered by routine labs. *When symptoms are present*, remember "bones, stones, groans, and psychiatric overtones" (bone changes such as osteopenia or pathologic fractures; kidney stones and polyuria; abdominal pain, anorexia, constipation, ileus, nausea, vomiting; depression, psychosis, delirium, and confusion). EKG shows **QT interval shortening** (Fig. 1-5).

Common causes:

- Hyperparathyroidism (most common cause in outpatients)
- Malignancy (most common cause in inpatients)
- Vitamin A or D intoxication
- Sarcoidosis
- Thiazide diuretics
- Familial hypocalciuric hypercalcemia (look for low urinary calcium, which is rare with hypercalcemia)
- Immobilization

Hyperproteinemia of any etiology can cause hypercalcemia because of an increase in the protein-bound fraction of calcium, but the patient is asymptomatic because the ionized (unbound) fraction (which can be measured and ordered directly as a separate test) is unchanged.

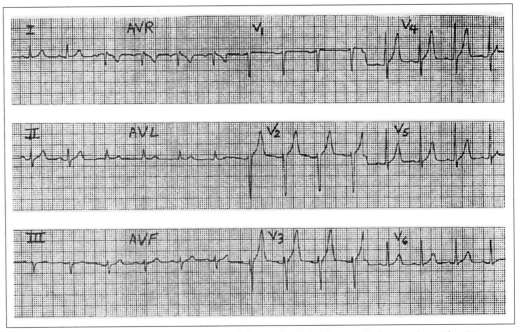

FIGURE 1-5. EKG showing hypercalcemia with marked QT interval shortening. The ST segment is almost absent. (From Carabello BA, Gazes PC: Cardiology Pearls, 2nd ed. Philadelphia, Hanley & Belfus, 2000, with permission.)

Treatment. First, give IV fluids. Once the patient is well hydrated, give furosemide to cause calcium diuresis (thiazides are *contraindicated*). Other treatments include phosphorus administration (oral; IV is rarely used because it is dangerous), calcitonin, diphosphonates (e.g., etidronate, which is also used in Paget's disease), plicamycin, and prednisone (for malignancy-induced hypercalcemia).

 Severe prolonged hypercalcemia can cause nephrocalcinosis, urolithiasis, and renal failure from calcium salt deposits in the kidneys.

OTHER ELECTROLYTE DISTURBANCES AND FLUID ADMINISTRATION

Magnesium Disturbances. Hypomagnesemia is seen most often in alcoholics. Signs and symptoms, which include EKG changes and tetany, are similar to those of hypocalcemia. Hypomagnesemia is notorious because it makes hypokalemia and hypocalcemia difficult to correct. Treat with oral replacement.

Hypermagnesemia is classically iatrogenic (pregnant patients treated with magnesium sulfate for preeclampsia) on boards, but it is often due to renal failure. In patients treated with magnesium sulfate, check for decreased deep-tendon reflexes, hypotension, and respiratory depression.

Treatment includes stopping magnesium sulfate treatment if it is being given (first step) and providing supportive treatment (intubate if necessary), IV hydration, furosemide, and dialysis as a last resort.

Phosphorus Disturbances. Hypophosphatemia is seen primarily in patients with diabetic ketoacidosis and in alcoholics. Signs and symptoms are neuromuscular disturbances (encephalopathy, weakness), rhabdomyolysis (especially in alcoholics), and anemia with white blood cell and platelet dysfunction.

Hyperphosphatemia is seen almost always in patients with renal failure. Treat with phosphate restriction, dialysis, and, possibly, phosphate-binding resins (calcium carbonate [$CaCO_3$]).

Fluid Administration. In trauma patients, the fluid of choice is Ringer's lactate; the second choice is normal saline.

Give hypovolemic patients normal saline or Ringer's lactate, even if they are hypernatremic.

Maintenance fluid in NPO patients is usually 5% dextrose in half-normal saline (0.45% NaCl). In pediatric patients, use 5% dextrose in one-fourth (0.225% NaCl) or one-third (0.3% NaCl) normal saline because of renal differences. Hypokalemia can develop acutely in normal NPO patients if intermittent potassium supplements are not given (e.g., 10 mEq KCl in the first liter of IV fluid each day).

Vitamins and Minerals

Signs and symptoms of vitamin and mineral deficiencies and toxicities are shown in Table 1-6.

IMPORTANT POINTS

1 Deficiency of fat-soluble vitamins (A, D, E, K) is often due to malabsorption (e.g., cystic fibrosis, cirrhosis, celiac disease, celiac sprue, duodenal bypass, bile-duct obstruction, pancreatic insufficiency, chronic giardiasis). In such patients, parenteral supplements may be needed, but try high-dose oral supplements first.

2 Alcoholics can have just about any deficiency, but watch for folate, thiamine, and magnesium.

3 Vitamin B_{12} deficiency is most commonly due to pernicious anemia, in which anti-parietal cell antibodies destroy the ability to secrete intrinsic factor. Conditions associated with pernicious anemia include hypothyroidism and vitiligo. Schilling's test is used to diagnose the cause of B_{12} deficiency. The tapeworm *Diphyllobothrium latum* and removal of the ileum also cause B_{12} deficiency.

4 Isoniazid causes B_6 (pyridoxine) deficiency. Patients taking isoniazid (especially young patients) are often given prophylactic B_6 supplements.

5 Anticonvulsants (especially phenytoin) can cause folate deficiency.

6 Vitamin A is teratogenic and any female patient given one of the vitamin A analogues as treatment for acne (e.g., isotretinoin) *must* have a negative pregnancy test before medication is started and *must* be put on some form of birth control and counseled about the risks of teratogenicity if pregnancy occurs. Offer periodic pregnancy tests.

7 Rickets causes interesting physical findings: craniotabes (poorly mineralized skull and bones that feel like a ping-pong ball), rachitic rosary (costochondral beading with small, round masses on anterior rib cage), delayed fontanelle closure, bossing of the skull, kyphoscoliosis, bowlegs, and knock knees. Bone changes first appear at the lower ends of the radius and ulna (x-rays).

8 *Vitamin K is given to all newborns* as prophylaxis against hemorrhagic disease of the newborn. Vitamin K is needed for the synthesis of factors II, VII, IX, and X as well as proteins C and S. Chronic liver disease (cirrhosis) can cause prolongation of the prothrombin time because of inability to synthesize clotting factors, even in the presence of adequate vitamin K. Treat with fresh frozen plasma in this case, because vitamin K is ineffective.

Table 1-6. SIGNS AND SYMPTOMS OF VITAMIN AND MINERAL DEFICIENCIES AND TOXICITIES

Micronutrient	Signs and Symptoms of Deficiency	Signs and Symptoms of Toxicity
Vitamins		
A	Night blindness, scaly rash, xerophthalmia (dry eyes), Bitot's spots (debris on conjunctiva), increased infections	Pseudotumor cerebri, bone thickening, teratogenicity
D	Rickets, osteomalacia, hypocalcemia	Hypercalcemia, nausea and vomiting, renal effects
E	Anemia, peripheral neuropathy, ataxia	Necrotizing enterocolitis (infants)
K	Hemorrhage, prolonged prothrombin time	Hemolysis (kernicterus)
B_1 (thiamine)	Wet beriberi (high-output cardiac failure), dry beriberi, (peripheral neuropathy), Wernicke's and Korsakoff's syndromes	
B_2 (riboflavin)	Cheilosis, angular stomatitis, dermatitis	
B_3 (niacin)	Pellagra (**d**ementia, **d**ermatitis, **d**iarrhea), stomatitis	
B_6 (pyridoxine)	Peripheral neuropathy, cheilosis, stomatitis, convulsions in infants, microcytic anemia, seborrheic dermatitis	Peripheral neuropathy (only B vitamin with toxicity)
B_{12} (cobalamin)	Megaloblastic anemia plus neurologic symptoms	
Folic acid	Megaloblastic anemia without neurologic symptoms	
C	Scurvy (hemorrhages—skin petechiae, bone, gums; loose teeth; gingivitis), poor wound healing, hyperkeratotic hair follicles, bone pain (from periosteal hemorrhages)	
Minerals		
Iron	Microcytic anemia, koilonychia (spoon-shaped fingernails)	Hemochromatosis
Iodine	Goiter, cretinism, hypothyroidism	Can cause myxedema
Fluorine	Dental caries (cavities)	Fluorosis with mottling of teeth and bone exostoses
Zinc	Hypogeusia (decreased taste), rash, slow wound healing	
Copper	Menke's disease (X-linked, kinky hair, and mental retardation)	Wilson's disease
Selenium	Cardiomyopathy and muscle pain	Loss of hair and nails
Manganese		"Manganese madness" in miners of ore
Chromium	Impaired glucose tolerance	

Shock

Definition: Shock is a state in which blood flow to and perfusion of peripheral tissues is inadequate to sustain life. Although not included in a rigid definition of shock for board purposes, associated findings include hypotension and oliguria or anuria. Tachycardia is also usually present.

Pragmatically speaking, there are four clinical types of shock:

◆ Hypovolemic

◆ Cardiogenic

◆ Septic

◆ Neurogenic

Your job is to figure out why the patient is in shock while keeping him or her alive. Give fluids while you're thinking. If the patient does not respond to a fluid bolus and you are given the choice, use invasive hemodynamic monitoring (Swan–Ganz catheter) to help make diagnostic and therapeutic decisions. Hemodynamic parameters of shock are shown in Table 1-7.

Associated findings help to differentiate the etiology of shock:

◆ **Hypovolemic shock:** History of fluid loss (blood, diarrhea, vomiting, sweating, diuretics, inability to drink water). The patient has cold, clammy skin and looks pale. Fluid loss may be internal, as with a ruptured abdominal aortic aneurysm or spleen, with pancreatitis, or after surgery. Other signs include orthostatic hypotension, tachycardia, sunken eyes, tenting of skin, and sunken fontanel (in babies).

◆ **Cardiogenic shock:** History of myocardial infarction, chest pain, congestive heart failure, or several risk factors for coronary artery disease. The patient has cold, clammy skin and looks pale. Distended neck veins, pulmonary congestion (on exam and x-ray). Patients usually need diuretics—IV fluid can make them worse!

◆ **Neurogenic shock:** History of severe central nervous system trauma or bleed; flushed skin. Heart rate may be normal.

◆ **Septic shock:** Fever, changes in white blood cell count, skin flushed and warm to the touch, extremes of age. Use broad-spectrum antibiotics after "pan-culturing" the patient (get blood, sputum and urine cultures plus others if history dictates).

Table 1-7. HEMODYNAMIC PARAMETERS OF SHOCK

Type of Shock	CO	PCWP	SVR	SVO₂
Hypovolemic*	Low	Low	High	Low
Cardiogenic	Low	High	High	Low
Septic (early)	High	Low	Low	High
Neurogenic	Low	Low	Low	Low

*Also the parameters for late septic shock.

CO, cardiac output; PCWP, pulmonary capillary wedge pressure; Svo_2; systemic venous oxygen saturation; SVR, systemic vascular resistance.

◆ **Anaphylaxis:** Look for bee stings, peanuts, and shellfish and for penicillins, sulfas, and other medications. Treat with epinephrine and fluids, administer O_2, intubate if necessary (do a tracheostomy or cricothyroidotomy if laryngeal edema prevents intubation). Antihistamines help only when the reaction is mild. Use corticosteroids when the reaction is prolonged or severe (not first-line drugs for treatment of anaphylaxis). Monitor all patients for at least 6 hours after the initial reaction.

◆ **Pulmonary embolus:** Look for risk factors for deep vein thrombosis (Virchow's triad: endothelial damage, stasis, hypercoagulable state), history of recent delivery (amniotic fluid embolus), fractures (fat emboli), deep vein thrombosis (positive Homan's sign with painful, swollen leg), and recent surgery (especially orthopedic or pelvic surgery). Patients have chest pain, tachypnea, shortness of breath, parasternal heave, right-axis shift on EKG, and/or positive ventilation–perfusion ($\dot{V}/\dot{Q}$) scan. Heparinize to prevent further clotting and emboli.

◆ **Pericardial tamponade:** Classic is a history of stab wound in left chest, distended neck veins. Do pericardiocentesis emergently.

◆ **Toxic shock syndrome:** Classic patient is woman of reproductive age who leaves tampons in place too long. Look for skin desquamation. Caused by *Staphylococcus aureus* toxin.

ABCs (airway, breathing, circulation) come first. Patients in shock often need heroic measures to survive. Intubate at the drop of a hat, keep NPO, and avoid narcotics if possible (mental status changes are often an important clue to impending doom). Monitor EKG, vital signs, Swan–Ganz parameters, urine output, arterial blood gases (ABGs), chest x-ray, hemoglobin, and hematocrit.

Most patients in shock need fluid. The standard bolus is 10 to 20 mL/kg of normal saline (roughly 1–2 L infused as fast as it will go). After the bolus, reassess the patient to determine whether the bolus helped. Do not be afraid to bolus twice if the first bolus has no effect. Of course, you must watch for fluid overload, which can cause congestive heart failure.

Remember Addison's disease as a cause of shock, especially in a postoperative patient who has taken steroids in the past year and received no extra steroids perioperatively. Give the patient steroids!

Understand IV medications and their use to support blood pressure:

◆ **Dobutamine:** β_1-Agonist used to increase cardiac output by increasing contractility (ICU equivalent of digoxin).

◆ **Dopamine:** Low doses hit dopamine receptors in renal vasculature and keep kidney perfused. Higher doses have β_1-agonist effects to increase contractility. Highest doses have α_1-agonist effects and cause vasoconstriction. Some authorities debate this differential effect, but it might still come up on boards.

- **Norepinephrine:** Used for its α_1-agonist effects; given in hypotension to increase peripheral resistance so that perfusion to vital organs can be maintained. Also has β-agonist effects.
- **Phenylephrine:** Used for its α_1-agonist effects
- **Epinephrine:** Used for cardiac arrest and anaphylaxis
- **Milrinone and amrinone:** Phosphodiesterase inhibitors used in refractory heart failure (*not* first-line agents) because they have a positive inotropic effect.

For shock in the setting of trauma, see trauma section in Chapter 20, General Surgery.

2 CARDIOVASCULAR MEDICINE

Chest Pain, Myocardial Infarction, and Acute Coronary Syndrome

When a patient presents with chest pain, your job is to make sure that the cause is not life-threatening, which usually means that you investigate the possibility of myocardial infarction (MI).

Findings that make MI unlikely:

- **Wrong age:** In the absence of known heart disease, strong family history, or risk factors for coronary artery disease (CAD), a patient younger than 40 years is extremely unlikely to have had an MI.

- **Risk factors:** A 50-year-old marathon runner who eats well and has a high HDL without other risk factors for coronary heart disease (CHD) is unlikely to have had an MI. A long-term smoker with a positive family history and chronic hypertension, diabetes, and hypercholesterolemia has had an MI until you prove otherwise!

- **Physical characteristics of pain:** If the pain is reproducible by palpation, its source is the chest wall, not an MI. Pain should *not* be sharp and well-localized or related to certain foods.

Findings that elevate suspicion of MI:

- **EKG:** After an MI, you should see flipped or flattened T waves, ST segment elevation, and/or Q waves in a segmental distribution (e.g., leads II, III, and aV_F for an inferior infarct) as shown in Figure 2-1.

- **Pain characteristics:** Usually described as crushing, poorly localized substernal pain that might radiate to the shoulder, arm, or jaw; not reproducible on palpation. Pain usually does not resolve with nitroglycerin (as it often does in angina), and generally lasts at least a half-hour.

- **Laboratory values:** A patient with a possible MI should have serial determinations of troponin I or T (usually drawn every 8 hours three times before MI is ruled out). Creatine kinase (the MB isoenzyme) is now less commonly used but also can be positive. *Late patient presentation (>24 hours):* Troponin I or T can be used because both are still elevated several days after MI (creatine kinase might normalize and give a false

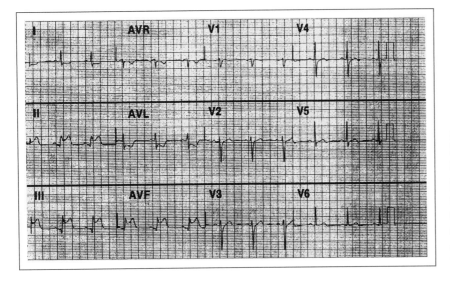

FIGURE 2-1. Acute MI localized to inferior leads (II, III, and aV$_F$). The EKG shows ST elevation with hyperacute peaked T waves and early development of significant Q waves. Reciprocal ST depression is also seen (leads I and aV$_L$). (From Seelig CB: Simplified EKG Analysis. Philadelphia, Hanley & Belfus, 1992, with permission)

negative). Lactate dehydrogenase (LDH) elevation and flip (LDH$_1$ > LDH$_2$) is now rarely used and takes 24 hours to become positive. Aspartate aminotransferase is also elevated in an MI but is not used clinically. X-ray might show cardiomegaly and/or pulmonary congestion; brain natriuretic peptide (BNP) may be elevated; echocardiography might show ventricular wall motion abnormalities.

◆ **Physical exam:** Bilateral pulmonary rales in the absence of other pneumonia-like symptoms, distended neck veins, S$_3$ or S$_4$, new murmurs, hypotension, and/or shock should make you think along the lines of an MI. Patients are often diaphoretic, tachycardic, and pale; nausea and vomiting may be present.

◆ **History:** Patients with MI often have a history of angina or previous chest pain, murmurs, arrhythmias, or risk factors for CAD. Some are taking cardiovascular medications (digoxin, furosemide, antihypertensives, cholesterol medications).

 Twenty-five percent of MIs are silent, meaning that they manifest without chest pain (especially in diabetic patients who have neuropathy). Such patients present with CHF, shock, or confusion and delirium (especially elderly patients).

Treatment for an MI involves hospital admission to the intensive care or cardiac care unit with adherence to several basic principles:

◆ **Early thrombolysis** (usually <6 h after pain onset) is done if the patient meets strict criteria for use. PTCA (percutaneous transluminal coronary angioplasty) may be used if thrombolysis is contraindicated (or in combination with it).

◆ **EKG monitoring:** If ventricular tachycardia develops, use amiodarone or lidocaine (*do not use prophylactically*).

◆ **Give O$_2$** by nasal cannula or face mask (maintain O$_2$ saturation >90%).

◆ **Pain control** with morphine (which can help with pulmonary edema if present)

◆ **Nitroglycerin**

◆ **β-Blocker** (which patient should take for life if no contraindications are present; proven to reduce incidence of second MI)

◆ **Aspirin** (and possibly low-dose heparin or other newer antiplatelet agents)

◆ **Begin anticoagulation** with intravenous (IV) heparin in patients with cardiac thrombus, large area of dyskinetic ventricle, or severe congestive heart failure (CHF).

◆ **Patients with CHF** (ejection fraction <40%) should be started on an angiotensin-converting enzyme (ACE) inhibitor, which has been shown to reduce mortality in this setting.

 Remember that the patient can reinfarct on the same hospital visit, even with adequate medical management.

Other causes of chest pain and clues to diagnosis:

◆ **Gastroesophageal reflux disease (GERD) and peptic ulcer disease:** Relation to certain foods (spicy, chocolate), smoking, caffeine, lying down; relieved by antacids or acid-reducing medications; often positive for *Helicobacter pylori* if caused by peptic ulcer disease.

◆ **Stable angina:** Pain begins with exertion or stress and remits with rest or calming down; relieved by nitroglycerin. EKG shows ST segment depression with pain, then reverts to normal when pain stops; pain lasts less than 20 minutes.

◆ Chest wall pain (costochondritis, bruised or broken ribs): reproducible on palpation and well localized.

◆ Esophageal problems (achalasia, nutcracker esophagus, or esophageal spasm): Difficult differential. Question will probably mention a negative work-up for MI; look for barium swallow (achalasia) or esophageal manometry abnormalities. Treat achalasia with pneumatic dilation; treat nutcracker esophagus or esophageal spasm with calcium channel blockers, then with myotomy if calcium channel blockers are ineffective

◆ **Pericarditis:** Look for viral upper respiratory infection prodrome. EKG (Fig. 2-2) shows diffuse ST segment elevation. Other signs include elevated erythrocyte sedimentation

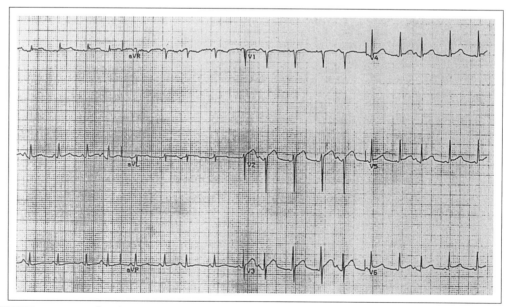

FIGURE 2-2. EKG showing pericarditis with diffuse ST elevation most evident in the precordial leads. (From Silver RM, Smith EA: Rheumatology Pearls. Philadelphia, Hanley & Belfus, 1997, with permission)

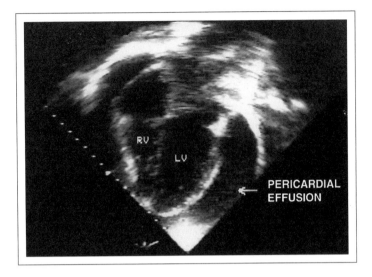

FIGURE 2-3. Echocardiogram revealing a significant pericardial effusion *(arrow)*. LV, left ventricle; RV, right ventricle.

rate and low-grade fever. The most common cause is viral (coxsackievirus); others include tuberculosis, uremia, malignancy, and lupus or other autoimmune diseases. Patients might have a pericardial effusion (Fig. 2-3).

◆ **Pneumonia:** Chest pain due to pleuritis. Patients also have cough, fever, and/or sputum production, with possible sick contacts.

◆ **Unstable angina** classically manifests with normal cardiac enzymes and EKG changes (ST depression) with prolonged chest pain that does not respond to nitroglycerin initially (like MI). Pain often begins at rest. Treat like an MI, but consider IV heparin or low-molecular weight (LMW) heparin to anticoagulate, and consider percutaneous transluminal coronary angioplasty (PTCA) emergently if pain does not resolve. Almost all patients have a history of stable angina and CAD risk factors. In strict terms, **unstable angina is defined** as a change from previous stable angina; thus, if a patient who used to get angina once a week now gets it once a day, he or she has unstable angina.

◆ **Variant (Prinzmetal's) angina** is rare and is associated with anginal pain at rest with **ST elevation;** cardiac enzymes, however, are normal. The cause is coronary artery spasm. Variant angina responds to nitroglycerin; long-term treatment usually is with calcium channel blockers.

Valvular Heart Disease

Characteristics of murmurs are shown in Table 2-1.

An understanding of the pathophysiologic changes associated with long-standing valvular disease (Figs. 2-4 and 2–5) is high yield on Step 2. For example, do you understand why mitral stenosis or regurgitation can cause right heart failure?

Endocarditis prophylaxis is slightly controversial, but consider it for people with known prosthetic valve, prior endocarditis, or valvular heart disease. With mitral valve prolapse, use prophylaxis only if a murmur is heard on physical exam or if the patient has a history of endocarditis. Give standard patients amoxicillin before and after the procedure; use clindamycin, azithromycin, or a cephalosporin in penicillin-allergic patients.

Table 2-1. MURMUR CHARACTERISTICS

Valve Problem	Physical Characteristics (Best Heard Here)	Other Findings
Mitral stenosis	Late-diastolic blowing murmur (at apex)	Opening snap, loud S_1, atrial fibrillation, LAE, PH
Mitral regurgitation	Holosystolic murmur (radiates to axilla)	Soft S_1, LAE, PH, LVH
Aortic stenosis	Harsh systolic ejection murmurs (aortic area, radiates to carotids)	Slow pulse upstroke, S_3/S_4, ejection click, LVH, cardiomegaly, syncope with angina and CHF
Aortic regurgitation	Early-diastolic decrescendo murmur (apex)	Widened pulse pressure, LVH, LV dilation, S_3
Mitral prolapse	Mid-systolic click or late-systolic murmur	Panic disorder

CHF, congestive heart failure; LAE, left atrial enlargement; LV, left ventricle; LVH, left ventricular hypertrophy; PH, pulmonary hypertension.

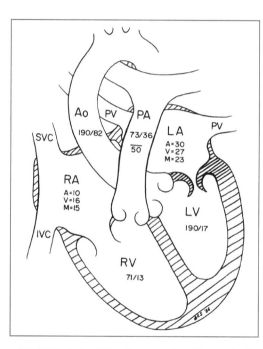

FIGURE 2-4. **Mitral stenosis.** The mitral valve orifice is narrowed, resulting in obstruction to flow out of the atrium and an increase in pressure in the left atrium and pulmonary veins. Pulmonary hypertension develops secondarily. Systolic and diastolic pressures are shown in arteries and ventricles (mm Hg). A, A wave; Ao, aorta; IVC, inferior vena cava; LA, left atrium; LV, left ventricle; M, mean pressure; PA, pulmonary artery; PV, pulmonary vein; RA, right atrium; RV, right ventricle; SVC, superior vena cava; V, V wave. (From James EC, Corry RJ, Perry JF: Principles of Basic Surgical Practice. Philadelphia, Hanley & Belfus, 1987, with permission.)

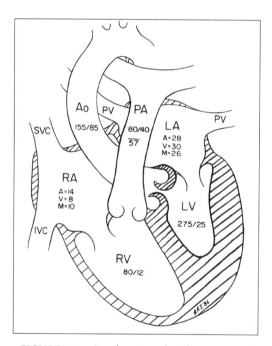

FIGURE 2-5. **Aortic stenosis.** The narrowed aortic valve results in high pressures in the left ventricle, which are transmitted to the left atrium and ultimately result in pulmonary hypertension. The left ventricle is hypertrophied due to the chronic pressure overload. Systolic and diastolic pressures are shown in arteries and ventricles (mm Hg). A, A wave; Ao, aorta; IVC, inferior vena cava; LA, left atrium; LV, left ventricle; M, mean pressure; PA, pulmonary artery; PV, pulmonary vein; RA, right atrium; RV, right ventricle; SVC, superior vena cava; V, V wave. (From James EC, Corry RJ, Perry JF: Principles of Basic Surgical Practice. Philadelphia, Hanley & Belfus, 1987, with permission.)

Deep Vein Thrombosis, Pulmonary Embolism, Anticoagulation

IMPORTANT POINTS

1 Remember Virchow's triad (endothelial damage, stasis, and hypercoagulable state) as a clue to the diagnosis of deep vein thrombosis (DVT).

2 Common causes or situations in which DVT occurs: surgery (especially orthopedic, pelvic, or abdominal), neoplasms, trauma, immobilization, pregnancy, oral contraceptives, disseminated intravascular coagulation (DIC), lupus anticoagulant, factor V Leiden, thrombin variant, or deficiency of antithrombin III, protein C, or protein S.

3 DVTs commonly manifest with unilateral leg swelling, pain or tenderness, and/or Homan's sign (present in 30% of patients and unreliable, but classic).

4 The best way to diagnose DVT is Doppler ultrasound. Other acceptable tests include impedance plethysmography or computed tomography (CT) or magnetic resonance (MR) venography. Traditional venography is invasive and reserved for settings in which the diagnosis is not clear.

5 Superficial thrombophlebitis (erythema, tenderness, edema, and palpable clot or cord in the distribution of a superficial vein) is *not* a risk factor for pulmonary embolism (PE) and generally is considered a benign condition. Treat with nonsteroidal antiinflammatory drugs (NSAIDs) or aspirin.

6 In patients with DVT or PE, systemic anticoagulation is necessary. Use parenteral heparin or LMW heparin, followed by gradual crossover to oral warfarin. Patients are maintained on warfarin for at least 3 to 6 months, possibly permanently if they experience more than one episode. If clots recur on anticoagulation or the patient has contraindications to anticoagulation, use an inferior vena cava filter (e.g., Greenfield filter).

7 The best DVT prophylaxis for surgery is pneumatic compression boots and early ambulation; also consider LMW heparin if ambulation is not possible or in a high-risk situation. Warfarin is an alternative, especially for orthopedic hip or knee surgery.

8 Pulmonary embolus follows DVT, delivery (amniotic fluid embolus), or fractures (fat emboli). Symptoms include tachypnea, dyspnea, chest pain, hemoptysis (with a lung infarct), and hypotension, syncope, and death in severe cases. Rarely, on a chest x-ray you will see a wedge-shaped defect due to a pulmonary infarct.

9 Left-sided heart clots (from atrial fibrillation, ventricular wall aneurysm, severe congestive heart failure, or endocarditis) that embolize cause arterial-sided infarcts (stroke and renal, GI, and extremity infarcts), *not* PEs. Right-sided clots that embolize (DVTs) cause PEs, *not* arterial emboli. The exception is a patent foramen ovale or other abnormal right-to-left shunt, in which the clot can cross over to the left side of the circulation and cause an arterial "paradoxical" infarct.

10 Use CT scan of the chest with contrast to screen for PE (nuclear medicine $\dot{V}/\dot{Q}$ scan if contrast is contraindicated). Invasive traditional pulmonary angiogram is reserved for unclear cases and treatment of massive PE (i.e., catheter-based thrombolysis).

Table 2-2. OTHER FACTORS AFFECTING COAGULATION TESTS

Disease	Prolonged Test	Other Aids to Diagnosis
Hemophilia A	PTT	Low levels of factor VIII; normal PT and bleeding time; X-linked
Hemophilia B	PTT	Low levels of factor IX; normal PT and bleeding time; X-linked
vWF deficiency	Bleeding time *and* PTT	Normal levels of factor VIII; normal PT; autosomal dominant
DIC	PT, PTT, bleeding time	Positive D-dimer or FDPs; postpartum, infection, malignancy; schistocytes, fragmented cells on peripheral smear
Liver disease	PT	PTT normal or prolonged; all factors but factor VIII are low; stigmata of liver disease, no correction with vitamin K
Vitamin K deficiency	PT, PTT (slight)	Normal bleeding time; low levels of factors II, VII, IX, and X, proteins C and S; look for neonate (who did not receive prophylactic vitamin K), malabsorption, alcoholism, or prolonged antibiotics (which kill vitamin K-producing bowel flora)

DIC, disseminated intravascular coagulation; FDPs, fibrin degradation products; PT, prothrombin time; PTT, partial thromboplastin time; vWF, von Willebrand's factor.

11 Heparin causes thrombocytopenia and arterial thrombosis in some unlucky patients. *Discontinue heparin immediately!*

12 Heparin is followed by determining partial thromboplastin time (PTT) (internal pathway), warfarin is followed by determining prothrombin time (PT) (external pathway), and aspirin affects the bleeding time. In emergencies, reverse heparin with protamine, reverse warfarin with fresh frozen plasma and/or vitamin K, and reverse aspirin with platelet transfusion. LMW heparins are *not followed by testing except in rare circumstances*, when an anti–factor Xa assay can be measured (PT, PTT, and bleeding time all unaffected). Table 2-2 lists other factors that affect coagulation tests.

 Note Uremia causes a qualitative platelet defect. Vitamin C deficiency and chronic corticosteroid therapy can cause a bleeding tendency with normal coagulation tests.

Congestive Heart Failure and Arrhythmias

Symptoms and signs of CHF are shown in Table 2-3.

Elevated brain natriuretic peptide (BNP) levels have made the diagnosis easier in many cases. If the BNP level is less than 100 pg/mL, heart failure is highly unlikely; if BNP is 100 to 500, the results are uncertain but suspicious; if BNP is greater than 500, heart failure (or another acute and serious cardiovascular disorder) is highly likely. False positives for CHF diagnosis include other diseases that cause right or left ventricular stretching, such as pulmonary embolism, pulmonary hypertension, cor pulmonale, renal failure, acute coronary syndrome, and cirrhosis.

Table 2-3. SYMPTOMS AND SIGNS OF CONGESTIVE HEART FAILURE

Left-Sided Failure	Right-Sided Failure
Fatigue, dyspnea, cardiomegaly	Fatigue, dyspnea, cardiomegaly
Left-sided S_3/S_4	Right-sided S_3/S_4
Chest x-ray abnormalities (cardiomegaly, Kerley B lines, pulmonary vascular congestion, and bilateral pleural effusions)	Chest x-ray abnormalities (cardiomegaly)
Pulmonary congestion, rales	Pulmonary congestion
Orthopnea	Peripheral edema
Paroxysmal nocturnal dyspnea	Jugular venous distention
	Hepatomegaly, ascites

Treatment:

- Sodium restriction
- ACE inhibitor (first-line agents; proved to reduce mortality in CHF)
- β-Blockers (also reduce mortality; give only in stable CHF)
- Diuretics
- Digoxin (not in hypertrophic obstructive cardiomyopathy or atrioventricular conduction blocks; usually reserved for moderate-to-severe CHF with low ejection fraction)
- Vasodilators (arterial and venous)
- IV sympathomimetics (dobutamine, dopamine, amrinone) or nesiritide (recombinant BNP) for inpatients with severe CHF

IMPORTANT POINTS

1 Many factors can precipitate **exacerbation of CHF** in a previously stable cardiac patient. Common causes are noncompliance, myocardial infarction, hypertension, arrhythmias, infections or fever, pulmonary embolism, anemia, thyrotoxicosis, and myocarditis.

2 **Cor pulmonale** is right ventricular enlargement, hypertrophy, or failure due to primary lung disease. Common causes are chronic obstructive pulmonary disease (COPD) and pulmonary embolism. In a young woman (ages 20–40 years) with no other medical history or risk factors, think of primary pulmonary hypertension (after excluding PE and other more common causes). Treat with pulmonary vasodilators such as prostacyclins (parenteral epoprostenol), antiendothelins (bosentant), and/or calcium channel blockers while awaiting heart–lung transplant. Sleep apnea also can cause cor pulmonale (e.g., an obese snorer who is sleepy during the day). Patients with cor pulmonale have tachypnea, cyanosis, clubbing, parasternal heave, loud P_2, and right-sided S_4 in addition to signs and symptoms of pulmonary disease.

3 **Restrictive cardiomyopathy** usually results from amyloidosis, sarcoidosis, hemochromatosis, or myocardial fibroelastosis (ventricular biopsy is abnormal in all of these conditions). Constrictive pericarditis acts similarly clinically but has a pericardial knock on exam, calcification of the pericardium, and a normal ventricular biopsy; it can be treated by removing the pericardium.

4 **Dilated cardiomyopathy** commonly is due to alcohol abuse, myocarditis, or doxorubicin.

5 The most common cause of right heart failure is left heart failure.

Table 2-4 shows treatments and warnings for various arrhythmias.

IMPORTANT POINTS

1 Sinus tachycardia and atrial fibrillation are common presentations for hyperthyroidism. Check level of thyroid-stimulating hormone.

2 Wolff–Parkinson–White syndrome commonly appears in childhood. The patient becomes dizzy or dyspneic or passes out after playing and then recovers with no other symptoms (transient arrhythmias via accessory pathway). Look for the infamous delta wave.

Table 2-4. TREATMENT OF ARRHYTHMIA

Arrhythmia	Treatment	Warnings	Illustration
Heart Block			
First degree	None	Avoid β-blockers and calcium channel blockers (both slow conduction)	
Second degree	Pacemaker or atropine only if symptomatic in Mobitz type I		
Third degree	Use pacemaker for all Mobitz type II		
Other Causes			
AFib	Anticoagulation (prevent embolic phenomenon); control rate: β-blocker, calcium channel blocker. Medical/electric cardioversion if unstable		

Table continued on following page

Table 2-4. TREATMENT OF ARRHYTHMIA (Continued)

Arrhythmia	Treatment	Warnings	Illustration
PVCs	Usually not treated; if severe and symptomatic, consider lidocaine		
Sinus bradycardia	Usually not treated; use atropine if severe and symptomatic (post-MI)	Avoid β-blockers, calcium channel blockers, and other conduction slowers	
Sinus tachycardia	Usually none; correct underlying cause; use β-blocker if symptomatic		
VFib	Immediate defibrillation		
VTach	Amiodarone or lidocaine		
WPW syndrome	Use procainamide or quinidine	Avoid digoxin and verapamil	

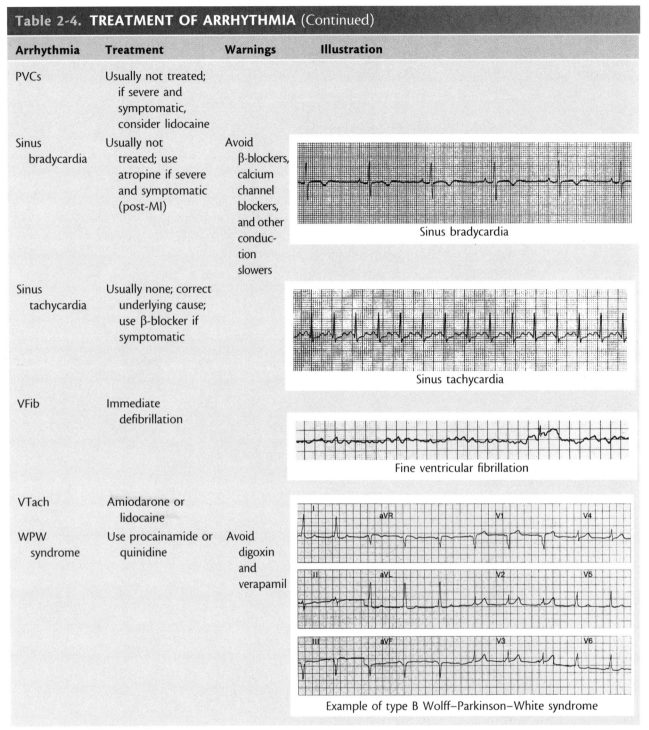

Sinus bradycardia

Sinus tachycardia

Fine ventricular fibrillation

Example of type B Wolff–Parkinson–White syndrome

AFib, atrial fibrillation; PVCs, premature ventricular contractions; VFib, ventricular fibrillation; VTach, ventricular tachycardia; WPW, Wolff–Parkinson–White syndrome.

Pediatric Cardiology

Table 2-5 lists congenital heart defects.

IMPORTANT POINTS

1 A heart rate >100 beats/min may be normal in young children.

2 In the presence of a ventricular septal defect, think about the possibility of fetal alcohol syndrome, TORCH syndrome (toxoplasmosis, other agents, rubella, cyotmegalovirus, herpes simplex virus), or Down's syndrome.

3 Hypertrophic obstructive cardiomyopathy classically appears in a boy who passes out on exertion (watch for collapse or sudden death in an athlete) and often is associated with a family history of sudden death. This disorder is considered a diastolic dysfunction and thus is treated with β-blockers to give the heart more time to fill. Positive inotropic agents (e.g., digoxin), diuretics, and vasodilators are *contraindicated*, because they make the condition worse.

4 Oxygen content in the fetal circulation is highest in the umbilical vein and lowest in the umbilical arteries; oxygen content is higher in blood going to upper extremities than in blood going to lower extremities.

5 Understand the changes in the circulation from intra- to extrauterine life. First breaths inflate the lungs and cause decreased pulmonary vascular resistance, which increases blood flow to the pulmonary arteries. This and the clamping of the cord increase left-sided heart pressures, which functionally close the foramen ovale. Increased oxygen concentration shuts off prostaglandin production in the ductus arteriosus, causing gradual closure.

Table 2-5. CONGENITAL HEART DEFECTS

Defect	Symptoms	Treatment	Other Information
Patent ductus arteriosus	Constant, machine-like murmur in upper left sternal border; dyspnea and possible CHF	Close with indomethacin (or surgery if indomethacin fails); keep open with prostaglandin E_1	Associated with congenital rubella and high altitudes
Ventricular septal defect	Holosystolic murmur next to sternum	Most cases resolve on their own	*Most common congenital heart defect*
Atrial septal defect	Asymptomatic until adulthood; fixed, split S_2 and palpitations	Most defects do not need correction (unless very large)	Secundum type is most common (80%)
Tetralogy of Fallot	Ventricular septal defect, right ventricular hypertrophy, pulmonary stenosis, and overriding aorta	Surgery	*Most common cyanotic congenital heart defect;* look for "tet" spells (squatting after exertion)
Coarctation of aorta	Upper extremity hypertension only; radiofemoral delay; systolic murmur heard over mid-upper back; rib notching on x-ray	Surgery	Associated with Turner's syndrome

Note: Endocarditis prophylaxis is required for all of these cardiac defects except asymptomatic secundum-type atrial septal defect.

PULMONOLOGY

Chronic Obstructive Pulmonary Disease

In chronic obstructive pulmonary disease (COPD), the ratio of the forced expiratory volume in 1 second to the forced expiratory volume (FEV_1/FEV ratio) is less than normal (<0.75), whereas in restrictive lung disease, the FEV_1/FEV ratio is often normal. FEV_1 may be low in both conditions; it is the FEV_1/FEV ratio that is different.

 A patient with COPD can live normally at a higher CO_2 and lower O_2; *treat the patient, not the lab value!* If the patient is asymptomatic and talking to you, the lab value should not make you panic.

 As a rough rule, you should prepare to intubate any patient whose CO_2 is >50 mm Hg or whose O_2 is <50 mm Hg, especially if the pH in either case is <7.30 while the patient is breathing room air. Usually, unless the patient is crashing rapidly, a trial of O_2 by nasal cannula (or face mask or other noninvasive means) is given first. If this approach does not work or if the patient becomes too tired (use of accessory muscles is a good clue to the work of breathing), consider intubation.

Emphysema

Emphysema almost always is due to smoking (even if secondhand). In a young person with minimal smoke exposure (<5 years of smoking), think of α_1 antitrypsin deficiency.

Physical exam findings: barrel chest (increased AP chest diameter), pursed lip breathing, prolonged expiratory phase, clubbing of the digits, end-expiratory wheezing, decreased heart and breath sounds, scattered rhonchi.

Treat with smoking cessation (can't reverse emphysema but slows progression and reduces risk of death), bronchodilator (e.g., β_2-agonists like albuterol) and anticholinergic (e.g., ipratropium) metered dose inhalers, antibiotics for infections, supplemental oxygen if pulse oximetry is <90% on room air, immunizations for influenza and pneumococcus, and as-needed corticosteroids (controversial benefit but commonly used).

Asthma

Look for wheezing in children. Treat with β_2-agonists in the emergency department. As needed β_2-agonists (e.g., albuterol) are first-line agents and all that is needed for mild asthma. Use steroids (acutely or chronically) if asthma is severe and/or does not respond to β_2-agonists. Cromolyn, nedocromil, and leukotriene inhibitors (zafirlukast, zileuton) are sometimes used in asthma maintenance, not for acute attacks. Phosphodiesterase inhibitors (theophylline, aminophylline) are older, second-line agents.

Wheezing in children under age 2 is often due to **respiratory syncytial virus,** especially in the winter. Look for coexisting fever.

 Do *not* put patients with asthma or COPD on β-blockers, which block the β_2-receptors needed to open the airways.

 Beware the acute asthmatic who no longer hyperventilates or whose CO_2 is normal or rising (the patient should hyperventilate, which causes low CO_2). Do *not* think that patients who seem calm or sleepy are okay. They are probably crashing and need an immediate arterial blood gas analysis and possible intubation. Fatigue alone is enough reason to intubate an asthmatic patient.

Pulmonary Nodules

If a **solitary pulmonary nodule** (round, <3 cm) is seen on a chest x-ray, the first step is to check for old films. If the lesion has not changed in more than 2 years, it is likely benign. If there are no old films, get computed tomography (CT) of chest for further characterization. If the nodule is densely calcified, it is benign. Many nodules remain indeterminate after this first assessment, however. Certain clues point to the etiology:

- Immigrant: think tuberculosis (do a skin test).
- Southwestern United States: think *Coccidioides immitis.*
- Cave explorer, person exposed to bird droppings, or someone living in Ohio or Mississippi River valleys: think histoplasmosis.
- Smoker older than 40 years: think lung cancer (PET scan, bronchoscopy and biopsy).
- Person younger than 40 years with none of the above: think hamartoma.

Perform PET scan for initial noninvasive assessment of nodules that remain indeterminate after history, chest x-ray, and CT scan. If PET is positive, think biopsy. If PET is negative, do short interval follow-up CT scans for 2 years and think biopsy if lesion grows.

Acute Respiratory Distress Syndrome

The **definition** of ARDS is acute lung injury that results in noncardiogenic pulmonary edema, respiratory distress, and hypoxemia. Common causes are sepsis, major trauma, pancreatitis, shock, near drowning, and drug overdose. Look for ARDS to develop within 24 to 48 hours of the initial insult. Classic symptoms include mottled or cyanotic skin, intercostal retractions, rales and rhonchi, and no improvement of hypoxia with O_2 administration. X-ray shows patchy pulmonary edema or air space disease, classically with a normal heart size (i.e., makes congestive heart failure much less likely). Treat with intubation, mechanical ventilation with high percentage of O_2, and positive end-expiratory pressure (PEEP). High mortality.

Pneumonia

The diagnosis of pneumonia is usually based on clinical findings plus elevated white blood cell count and chest x-ray abnormalities. On physical exam, look to differentiate between typical (*Streptococcus pneumoniae*) and atypical (other bugs) pneumonia (Table 3-1), although the distinction is not always clear-cut.

Certain clinical clues should make you think of certain bugs:

- **College student:** Think *Mycoplasma* spp. (look for cold agglutinins) or *Chlamydia* spp.
- **Alcoholic:** Think *Klebsiella* spp. ("currant jelly" sputum), *Staphylococcus aureus*, other enteric bugs (aspiration).
- **Cystic fibrosis:** Think *Pseudomonas* spp. or *Staphylococcus aureus*.
- **Immigrant:** Think tuberculosis.
- **COPD:** Think *Haemophilus influenzae*, *Moraxella* spp.
- **Patient with known tuberculosis and pulmonary cavitation:** Think *Aspergillus* sp.
- **Patient with silicosis (metal, granite, pottery workers):** Think tuberculosis.
- **Exposure to air conditioner or aerosolized water:** Think *Legionella* sp.
- **HIV/AIDS:** Think *Pneumocystis jiroveci* or cytomegalovirus (if shown a picture of koilocytosis).
- **Exposure to bird droppings:** Think *Chlamydia psittaci* or *Histoplasma* spp.
- **Child younger than 1 year:** Think respiratory syncytial virus.
- **Child 2 to 5 years:** Think parainfluenza (croup) or epiglottitis.

Recurrent pediatric pneumonia in the same lung segment is classically due to **foreign body aspiration**, especially when in the right middle or lower lobe (a foreign body is more

Table 3-1. CHARACTERISTICS OF TYPICAL AND ATYPICAL PNEUMONIA

Characteristic	Typical Pneumonia	Atypical Pneumonia
Prodrome	Short (<2 days)	Long (>3 days): headache, malaise, other aches
Fever	High (>102° F)	Low (<102° F)
Age	>40 y	<40 y
Chest x-ray	One distinct lobe involved	Diffuse or multilobe involvement
Infective agent	*S. pneumoniae*	Many (e.g., *Haemophilus influenzae*, *Mycoplasma* spp., *Chlamydia* spp.)
Medications*	Third-generation cephalosporin or broad-spectrum fluoroquinolone	Azithromycin

*Avoid the temptation to pull out the "big gun" antibiotics (very wide spectrum) unless the patient is crashing or unstable.

likely to go down the right bronchus). Other possibilities include reflux with aspiration, congenital lung malformation, and immunodeficiency. Patients with immunodeficiency have other signs (e.g., other types of infections, cystic fibrosis symptoms, should not always be the same lung segment involved).

Sinusitis

Sinusitis is usually due to *S. pneumoniae* or *Haemophilus* spp. Look for purulent (green or yellow) nasal discharge with tenderness over the involved sinus. Associated symptoms are headache and/or toothache (maxillary sinusitis). You cannot transilluminate the sinuses, and an x-ray or CT scan shows opacification of the frontal or maxillary sinuses (consider ordering a sinus x-ray or CT to confirm the diagnosis if it has not already been done). Empiric treatment choices include amoxicillin or second-generation cephalosporin for 10 to 14 days.

 The most common cause of epistaxis in children is nose-picking (i.e., trauma). Do *not* assume low or defective platelets without evidence.

Neonatal Respiratory Disorders

RESPIRATORY DISTRESS SYNDROME

Respiratory distress syndrome, which is due to atelectasis from deficiency of surfactant, almost always occurs in premature infants and/or infants of diabetic mothers. Look for rapid, labored respirations; substernal retractions; cyanosis; grunting; and/or nasal flaring. Arterial blood gases show hypoxemia and hypercarbia. X-ray shows a diffuse granular pattern in the lungs (Fig. 3-1). Treat with O_2, give surfactant, and intubate if needed (often). Complications include pneumothorax or **bronchopulmonary dysplasia** (acute or chronic mechanical ventilation complications) and intraventricular hemorrhage.

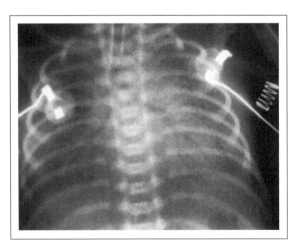

FIGURE 3-1. Respiratory distress syndrome. Chest radiograph in a premature infant shows fine, uniform granularity distributed symmetrically throughout both lung fields. The baby is intubated.

DIAPHRAGMATIC HERNIA

Diaphragmatic hernia commonly causes respiratory problems right after birth because bowel herniates into the chest in utero, pushing on the developing lung and causing lung hypoplasia on the affected side. Look for a scaphoid abdomen and bowel sounds in the chest. Herniated bowel also may be seen in the chest on x-ray. Ninety percent of hernias are *left-sided*, and they are more common in boys.

 Look for meconium aspiration if the infant is covered with meconium when delivered. Suction secretions first from the mouth (oropharynx) and then from the nose with a bulb syringe or catheter immediately after the head is delivered. Intubate if necessary.

TRACHEOESOPHAGEAL FISTULA

The most common type (85%) of tracheoesophageal fistula is an esophagus with a blind pouch proximally (i.e., esophageal atresia) and a fistula between a bronchus or the carina and the distal esophagus. Look for a neonate with excessive oral secretions, coughing and cyanosis with attempted feedings, abdominal distention (because breaths transmit air to the gastrointestinal [GI] tract), and aspiration pneumonia. Diagnosis is made by inability to pass a nasogastric tube; air-contrast x-ray shows the proximal esophagus only. Treatment is early surgical correction.

Cystic Fibrosis

Cystic fibrosis (CF) occurs via autosomal recessive inheritance. It is the most common lethal genetic disease in white children. Always suspect it in children when mom says child tastes salty, or with recurrent pulmonary infections, rectal prolapse, meconium ileus, esophageal varices, and/or failure to thrive. Some states perform routine neonatal screening. The **diagnosis** can be made by an abnormal increase in sweat electrolytes (sodium and chloride), immunoreactive trypsinogen assay, and the confirmatory DNA probe test.

Treatment includes chest physiotherapy (to loosen viscous mucus), immunizations including influenza and pneumococcus, treatment for pancreatic insufficiency (give pancreatic enzyme replacements and fat-soluble vitamin supplements), and as-needed antibiotics and bronchodilators. In addition, 98% of male and many female patients are infertile; those who aren't need genetic counseling. Many eventually develop cor pulmonale (right heart failure). Look for *S. aureus* and *Pseudomonas* spp. to cause respiratory infections.

Treat with chest physical therapy, annual influenza vaccine, fat-soluble vitamin supplements, pancreatic enzyme replacement, and aggressive treatment of infections with antibiotics.

Pleural Effusion

Physical exam shows dull percussion note and decreased breath sounds in area of effusion. Confirm with chest x-ray. If you do not know the cause after chest x-ray (and possibly CT scan), always consider thoracentesis to examine the fluid using Gram stain, culture and sensitivity (including tuberculosis culture), cell count with differential, cytology (if malignancy is a possibility), glucose (low in infection), LDH, and protein (high in infection). A pleural effusion is common in the setting of **pneumonia** and often goes away with the pneumonia, but watch for progression to empyema (infected, loculated pleural fluid), which requires chest tube drainage. Common and classic causes include infection (including tuberculosis in appropriate setting), malignancy, congestive heart failure (often bilateral), abdominal inflammation (e.g., pancreatitis, subphrenic abscess), and collagen vascular disease (e.g., rheumatoid arthritis).

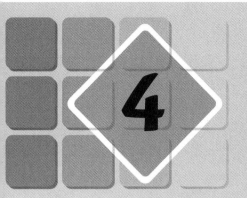

4 GASTROENTEROLOGY

Gastroesophageal Reflux Disease

Gastroesophageal reflux disease (GERD) is due to inappropriate, intermittent lower esophageal sphincter (LES) relaxation. It classically presents as heartburn, often related to eating and lying supine. However, GERD can also manifest as chest pain, regurgitation, cough or asthma, sore throat, dysphagia, laryngitis or hoarseness, or recurrent pneumonia.

IMPORTANT POINTS

1 Incidence of GERD is increased in those with a sliding-type hiatal hernia and obesity.

2 Symptoms include heartburn, chest pain, painful swallowing, and asthma-type symptoms. Initial treatment is to lose weight, elevate the head of the bed, and avoid coffee, alcohol, tobacco, chocolate, spicy and fatty foods, and medications with anticholinergic properties. If this fails, antacids, H_2-blockers, or proton-pump inhibitors may be tried; often these are started empirically at initial presentation.

3 Surgery (e.g., Nissen fundoplication) is reserved for severe or resistant cases.

4 Sequelae include esophagitis, esophageal stricture (can mimic esophageal cancer), esophageal ulcer, hemorrhage, Barrett's metaplasia, and esophageal adenocarcinoma (adenocarcinoma has become the leading type of esophageal cancer and incidence has rapidly increased, paralleling the rapid rise in obesity).

5 In cases that are atypical or do not respond to medical therapy, consider endoscopy. The gold standard for diagnosis is 24-hour esophageal pH monitoring (probe inserted into the esophagus).

Hiatal Hernia

This term, when used without a qualifier, implies a sliding hiatal hernia; that is, the entire gastroesophageal junction moves above the diaphragm, pulling the stomach with it—a common and benign finding that is associated with GERD. A *paraesophageal hiatal hernia* means that the gastroesophageal junction stays below the diaphragm, but the

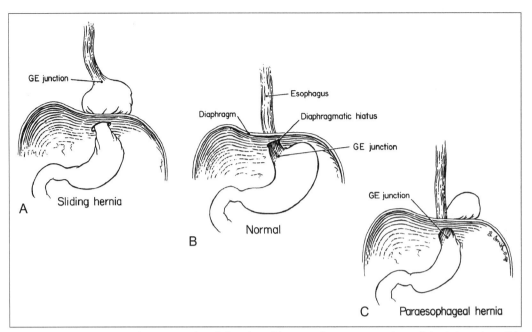

FIGURE 4-1. Hiatal hernias. A, In the sliding hiatal hernia, the gastroesophageal (GE) junction slides freely above and below the diaphragmatic hiatus. **B,** Normal GE junction. **C,** In a paraesophageal hernia, the GE junction is fixed below the diaphragm, allowing part of the stomach to herniate into the chest. (From Crapo JD, Hamilton MA, Edgman S: Medicine and Pediatrics. Philadelphia, Hanley & Belfus, 1988, with permission.)

stomach herniates through the diaphragm into the thorax. This is an uncommon, more serious type of hernia that can become strangulated and should be repaired surgically when found. Hiatal hernias are illustrated in Figure 4-1.

Peptic Ulcer Disease

Peptic ulcer disease manifests with chronic, intermittent, epigastric pain—burning, gnawing, or aching—that is localized and often relieved by antacids or milk. Look for epigastric tenderness. Patients may have occult blood in stool and nausea or vomiting. Peptic ulcer disease is more common in male patients. There are two types: gastric and duodenal (Table 4-1.)

Table 4-1. CHARACTERISTICS OF DUODENAL AND GASTRIC ULCERS

Characteristic	Duodenal	Gastric
% of cases	75	25
Acid secretion	Normal to high	Normal to low
Main etiology	*Helicobacter pylori*	Nonsteroidal antiinflammatory drugs
Peak age	40s	50s
Eating food	Pain improves, then worsens 2–3 h later	Pain not relieved or made worse

IMPORTANT POINTS

1 Endoscopy is becoming the first-line diagnostic study (upper GI barium x-ray study was classically done first) and is more sensitive (but more expensive) than x-ray.

2 Always biopsy any gastric ulcer to exclude malignancy (duodenal ulcers do not have to be biopsied initially).

3 The feared complication is perforation. Look for peritoneal signs, history of peptic ulcer disease, or free air on abdominal x-ray. Treat with antibiotics and laparotomy with repair of perforation. Can also get obstruction due to inflammation and/or stricture.

4 If ulcers are severe, atypical, or nonhealing, think about Zollinger–Ellison syndrome (get gastrin level) or stomach cancer.

5 Diet changes *are not* thought to help heal ulcers (but reduced alcohol and/or tobacco probably help).

6 Start treatment with H_2 blockers or proton pump inhibitors (latter favored), as well as antibiotics to eliminate *H. pylori*. Triple or quadruple drug therapy (e.g., amoxicillin, clarithromycin, and a proton pump inhibitor such as lansoprazole) for 2 weeks is generally given, and many regimens are in use.

7 Surgical options are considered only after failure of medical treatment or in patients with complications (perforation, bleeding). Common procedures include antrectomy, vagotomy, and Billroth I and II. After surgery (especially Billroth procedures) watch for dumping syndrome (weakness, dizziness, sweating, nausea or vomiting after eating). The following also may develop: hypoglycemia 2 to 3 hours after the meal (causes recurrence of dumping symptoms), afferent loop syndrome (bilious vomiting after a meal relieves abdominal pain), bacterial overgrowth, and vitamin deficiencies (B_{12} and/or iron, causing anemia).

8 Gastric acid seems to be necessary, but not sufficient, to cause ulcers. Patients with achlorhydria (e.g., pernicious anemia, which results in destruction of parietal cells) generally don't get ulcers, but patients with ulcers may have normal or even low gastric acid secretion.

Upper versus Lower Gastrointestinal Bleeding

Table 4-2 compares upper and lower GI bleeding.

Table 4-2. UPPER VERSUS LOWER GASTROINTESTINAL BLEEDING

Characteristic	Upper	Lower
Location	Proximal to ligament of Treitz	Distal to ligament of Treitz
Common causes	Gastritis, peptic ulcer disease, varices	Vascular ectasia, diverticulosis, colon cancer, colitis or inflammatory bowel disease, hemorrhoids
Stool	Tarry, black stool (melena)	Red blood seen in stool (hematochezia)
Nasogastric tube aspirate	Positive for blood	Negative for blood

IMPORTANT POINTS

1 The first step is to make sure that the patient is stable (ABCs, IV fluids, and blood if needed); then get a diagnosis.

2 Endoscopy is usually the first test performed (upper or lower, depending on symptoms).
- Endoscopically treatable lesions include polyps, vascular ectasias, and varices.
- Radionuclide or nuclear medicine scan can detect slow or intermittent bleeding if source cannot be found with endoscopy. Angiography can detect more rapid bleeding, and embolization of bleeding vessels can be done with this procedure.

3 Surgery is reserved for severe or resistant bleeding and usually involves resection of affected bowel (often the colon).

Diverticulosis

Diverticulosis (Figs. 4-2 and 4-3) is extremely common (roughly half of 50-year-olds in the United States have it), and the incidence increases with age. It is thought to be partially caused by a low-fiber, high-fat diet. Complications are lower GI bleeding (common cause) and diverticulitis (inflammation of a diverticula). Diverticulitis causes lower left quadrant pain and tenderness, fever, diarrhea or constipation, and leukocytosis. CT scan confirms diagnosis and excludes complications requiring intervention (e.g., abscess, perforation, malignancy).

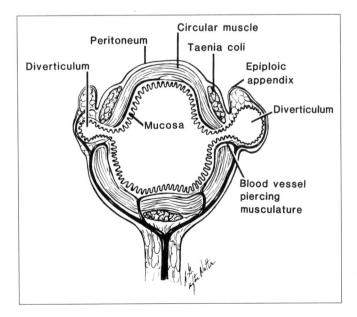

FIGURE 4-2. Diverticulosis. Herniation of mucosa between two taeniae. Note the point of weakness where the main blood vessel passes into the mucosa. (From James EC, Corry RJ, Perry JF: Principles of Basic Surgical Practice. Philadelphia, Hanley & Belfus, 1987, with permission.)

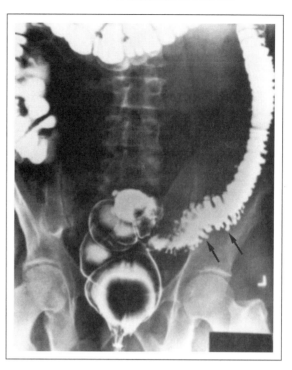

FIGURE 4-3. Simple diverticulosis (arrows) without muscle thickening.

Diarrhea

Diarrhea has multiple etiologies and is best broken down into categories:

- **Systemic causes:** Any illness can cause diarrhea as a systemic symptom, particularly in children (e.g., hyperthyroidism, infection).

- **Osmotic diarrhea:** Nonabsorbable solutes remain in the bowel, where they retain water (e.g., lactose or other sugar intolerances). When the patient stops ingesting the substance (e.g., no more milk or a trial of NPO), the diarrhea stops—an easy diagnosis.

- **Secretory diarrhea:** Bowel secretes fluid. Causes include bacterial toxins (cholera, some strains of *Escherichia coli*), vasoactive intestinal peptide-secreting tumor (pancreatic islet cell tumor), or bile acids (after ileal resection). Diarrhea continues with NPO status.

- **Malabsorption:** Causes include celiac sprue (look for dermatitis herpetiformis, and stop gluten in the diet), Crohn's disease, gastroenteritis, and exocrine pancreatic insufficiency. Diarrhea stops with NPO status.

- **Infectious causes:** Look for fever, white blood cells in stool (not with toxigenic bacteria; only with invasive bacteria such as *Shigella*, *Salmonella*, *Yersinia*, and *Campylobacter* spp.), and travel (Montezuma's revenge caused by *E. coli*). Hikers and stream drinkers can get *Giardia* spp., which manifests with steatorrhea (fatty, greasy, malodorous stools that float) from small bowel involvement and unique protozoal cysts in the stool. Treat with metronidazole.

◆ **Exudative diarrhea:** Inflammation in bowel mucosa causes seepage of fluid. Due to inflammatory bowel disease (Crohn's disease or ulcerative colitis) or cancer.

◆ **Altered intestinal transit:** After bowel resections or medications that interfere with bowel function.

IMPORTANT POINTS

1 With all diarrhea, watch for dehydration and electrolyte disturbances (e.g., metabolic acidosis, hypokalemia), a common and preventable cause of death in underdeveloped areas.

2 Do a rectal exam, look for occult blood in stool, and examine stool for ova or parasites, fat content (steatorrhea), and white blood cells.

3 If the patient has a history of antibiotic use, think of *Clostridium difficile* and test the stool for C. *difficile* toxin. If the test is positive, treat with oral metronidazole (if it fails or is not a choice, use oral vancomycin).

4 Do not forget about factitious diarrhea (surreptitious laxative abuse, usually by medical personnel), hyperthyroidism, colorectal cancer, and diabetes as causes of diarrhea.

5 **Irritable bowel syndrome** (IBS) is a common cause of GI complaints. Patients are anxious or neurotic and have a history of diarrhea aggravated by stress; bloating; abdominal pain relieved by defecation; and/or mucus in the stool. Look for psychosocial stressors in the history and normal physical findings and diagnostic tests. This diagnosis of exclusion requires basic lab tests, rectal and stool examination, and sigmoidoscopy, but because it is *very common*, it is the most likely diagnosis in the absence of positive findings, especially in young adults. IBS is three times more common in women than men. Treat with reassurance and try increased dietary fiber. Avoid treating with medications on boards.

6 After bacterial diarrhea (especially *E. coli* or *Shigella* spp.) in children, watch for hemolytic uremic syndrome: thrombocytopenia, hemolytic anemia (schistocytes, helmet cells, fragmented red blood cells), and acute renal failure. Treat supportively. Patients might need dialysis and/or transfusions.

Inflammatory Bowel Disease

Crohn's disease and ulcerative colitis are compared in Table 4-3.

Both Crohn's disease (Fig. 4-4) and ulcerative colitis can cause uveitis, arthritis, ankylosing spondylitis, erythema nodosum or multiforme, primary sclerosing cholangitis, failure to thrive or grow in children, toxic megacolon, anemia of chronic disease, and fever. Both are treated with 5-ASA with or without a sulfa drug (e.g., sulfasalazine). Corticosteroids and other immunosuppressants (e.g., infliximab, azathioprine) are used for more severe disease and flare-ups. Avoid antidiarrheal medications, which can precipitate toxic megacolon.

Toxic megacolon (Fig. 4-5) is classically seen with inflammatory bowel disease (more common in ulcerative colitis) and infectious colitis (especially C. *difficile*). It may

Table 4-3. COMPARISON OF CROHN'S DISEASE AND ULCERATIVE COLITIS

Characteristic	Crohn's Disease	Ulcerative Colitis
Site of origin	Distal ileum, proximal colon	Rectum
Thickness of pathology	Transmural	Mucosa and submucosa only
Progression	Irregular (skip-lesions)	Proximal, continuous from rectum; no skipped areas
Location	From mouth to anus	Involves colon and rectum; rarely extends to ileum
Change in bowel habits	Obstruction, abdominal pain	Bloody diarrhea
Classic lesions	Fistulas/abscesses, cobblestoning, string sign on barium x-ray	Pseudopolyps, lead-pipe colon on barium x-ray, toxic megacolon
Colon cancer risk	Slightly increased	Markedly increased
Surgery cures bowel disease?	No (can worsen it)	Yes (proctocolectomy with ileoanal anastomosis)

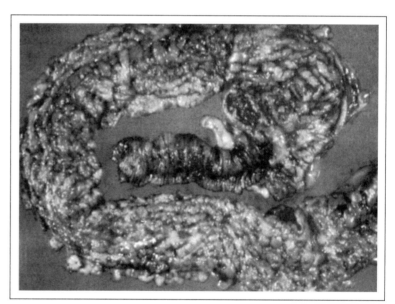

FIGURE 4-4. Cobblestone appearance of Crohn's colitis.

be precipitated by antidiarrhea medications. Symptoms include high fever, leukocytosis, abdominal pain, rebound tenderness, and a markedly dilated colon on abdominal x-ray. Toxic megacolon is an *emergency.* Start treatment by discontinuing all antidiarrhea medications; then place the patient on NPO status, insert a nasogastric tube, and administer IV fluids, antibiotics to cover bowel flora (e.g., ampicillin or cefazolin), and steroids if the cause is inflammatory bowel disease. Go to surgery if perforation occurs (free air on abdominal x-ray).

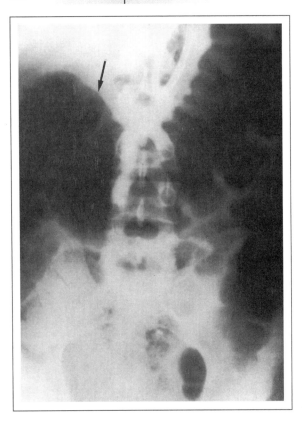

FIGURE 4-5. Dilated transverse colon with air *(arrow)* in toxic megacolon.

Liver Disease

ACUTE LIVER DISEASE

Signs of acute liver disease include elevated liver function tests, jaundice, nausea and vomiting, right upper quadrant pain or tenderness, and/or hepatomegaly

IMPORTANT POINTS

1 **Alcoholic hepatitis:** Elevated liver function tests; aspartate aminotransferase (AST) levels are more than twice as high as alanine aminotransferase (ALT) levels in many cases (fairly specific).

2 **Hepatitis A:** Look for outbreaks from food-borne source; no long-term sequelae. **Serology:** positive IgM antibody to hepatitis A virus during jaundice or shortly thereafter.

3 **Hepatitis B:** Prevention is best treatment (vaccination); acquired through needles, sex, or perinatally. Transfused blood is now screened for hepatitis B, but a history of transfusion years ago is still a risk factor. Use **hepatitis B immunoglobulin** for exposed neonates and health care workers. **Serology:** HBsAg-positive with unresolved infection (acute or chronic). HBeAg is a marker for infectivity (HBeAb-positive patients have low likelihood of spreading disease). The first antibody to appear is IgM anti-HBc, during the window phase, when both HBsAg and HBsAb are negative. Positive HBsAb means that the patient is immune (due either to recovery from infection or vaccination) and never appears if the patient develops chronic hepatitis. Sequelae are cirrhosis and hepatocellular cancer (only with chronic infection). Interferon-α can help slow liver damage and progression.

4 **Hepatitis C:** The new king of chronic hepatitis (causes two thirds of cases); usually transmitted through shared IV needles (rarely if ever transmitted sexually; donated blood is now screened). Like hepatitis B, it can also progress to chronic hepatitis (roughly 75% of cases), cirrhosis, and cancer. **Serology:** antibody to hepatitis C virus shows evidence of prior exposure, but not immunity, as most have chronic, active infection. A test for HCV RNA detects virus directly and allows better determination of infection status and prognosis. Treatment is not curative but can help slow progression to cirrhosis (e.g., interferon-α, ribavarin).

5 **Hepatitis D:** Seen only in patients with hepatitis B; can become chronic with hepatitis B coinfection. Acquired in same ways as hepatitis B. IgM antibodies to hepatitis D antigen show recent resolution of infection; presence of hepatitis D antigen means chronicity.

6 **Hepatitis E:** similar to hepatitis A (food- and waterborne, no chronic state). Often fatal in pregnant women.

7 **Drug-induced:** Look for acetaminophen, isoniazid (other tuberculosis drugs), halothane, carbon tetrachloride, tetracycline. *Stop the drug!*

8 **Reye's syndrome:** Develops in a child given aspirin for fever.

9 **Acute fatty liver of pregnancy:** Develops in third trimester. Treat with immediate delivery.

10 **Ischemia or shock:** History of shock.

11 **Idiopathic autoimmune hepatitis:** 20- to 40-year-old women with anti–smooth muscle or antinuclear antibodies and no risk factors or lab markers of other causes for hepatitis. Treat with steroids.

12 **Biliary tract disease:** See later section; look for markedly elevated alkaline phosphatase.

CHRONIC LIVER DISEASE

Often due to alcohol, hepatitis, or metabolic diseases (hemochromatosis, Wilson's disease, α_1 antitrypsin deficiency). Stigmata of chronic liver disease include gynecomastia, testicular atrophy, palmar erythema, spider angiomas on skin, and ascites.

IMPORTANT POINTS

1 **Alcoholism:** Positive history, Mallory bodies on histology (not specific).

2 **Hepatitis B or C:** Positive history and serology.

3 **Hemochromatosis:** Primary form is autosomal recessive disease (look for family history) caused by excessive iron absorption that is deposited in liver (cirrhosis, hepatocellular carcinoma), pancreas (diabetes), heart (dilated cardiomyopathy), skin (pigmentation, classically called "bronze diabetes"), and joints (arthritis). Impotence, amenorrhea, loss of libido, hair loss, and koilonychia ("spooning" of the fingernails) also occur. Most common inherited disorder in whites. Men are symptomatic earlier and three times more often in part because women lose iron with menstruation. Suspect diagnosis based on elevated serum iron, transferrin saturation, and ferritin levels. Confirm with DNA testing. Treat with phlebotomy and genetic counseling. Secondary iron overload can cause a hemochromatosis-like picture, usually seen with anemia from ineffective erythropoiesis (e.g., thalassemia) or excessive iron intake.

4 **Wilson's disease:** Autosomal recessive disease that results in excessive copper accumulation. Serum ceruloplasmin is low and urinary copper is high. Serum copper usually low; liver biopsy shows excessive copper and confirms diagnosis. Patients also have central nervous system or psychiatric manifestations (copper deposits in basal ganglia and lentiform nucleus; another name for this disease is hepatolenticular degeneration) and Kayser–Fleischer rings in the eye (nearly pathognomonic). Treat with penicillamine (copper chelator); zinc and trientine are other agents used.

5 **α-1 Antitrypsin deficiency:** Younger adult who develops cirrhosis and emphysema without risk factors for either; autosomal recessive inheritance. Confirm diagnosis with low blood levels of α-1 antitrypsin or DNA testing. Replacement therapy can be given to slow progression and delay complications.

Metabolic derangements that accompany liver failure:

- **Coagulopathy:** Prolonged prothrombin time (PT); in severe cases, partial thromboplastin time (PTT) may be prolonged. Because the damaged liver cannot use vitamin K, patients must be treated with fresh frozen plasma.

- **Jaundice and hyperbilirubinemia:** Elevated conjugated and unconjugated bilirubin with hepatic damage (vs. biliary tract disease).

- **Hypoalbuminemia:** Liver synthesizes albumin.

- **Ascites:** Due to portal hypertension and/or hypoalbuminemia. Ascites can be detected on physical exam by shifting dullness or a positive fluid wave. Possible complication is **spontaneous bacterial peritonitis**—infected ascitic fluid that can lead to sepsis. Look for fever and/or change in mental status in a patient with known ascites. Do a paracentesis, and examine the ascitic fluid for white blood cells (elevated neutrophil count), Gram stain, culture and sensitivity, glucose (low with infection), and protein (high with infection). Usually caused by *E. coli*, *S. pneumoniae*, or other enteric bugs. Treat with broad-spectrum antibiotics.

- **Portal hypertension:** Seen with cirrhosis (chronic liver disease); causes hemorrhoids, esophageal varices, caput medusae.

- **Hyperammonemia:** Liver clears ammonia. Treat with decreased protein intake (source of NH_3) and lactulose (prevents absorption of NH_3). Second choice is neomycin (stops bowel flora from making NH_3).

- **Hepatic encephalopathy:** At least partly due to hyperammonemia; often precipitated by protein, GI bleed, or infection.

- **Hepatorenal syndrome:** Liver failure causes kidney failure (idiopathic).

- **Hypoglycemia:** Liver stores glycogen.

- **Disseminated intravascular coagulation:** Activated clotting factors are usually cleared by liver.

Biliary Tract Disease

Jaundice may be caused by bile duct obstruction. Look for markedly elevated alkaline phosphatase, conjugated bilirubin that is more elevated than unconjugated bilirubin, pruritus, clay-colored stools, and dark urine that is strongly bilirubin-positive. Unconjugated bilirubin is not excreted in the urine because it is tightly bound to albumin.

Causes:

- **Cholestasis:** Often from medications (oral contraceptives, phenothiazines, androgens) or pregnancy.

- **Common bile duct obstruction with gallstone:** Look for history of gallstones or the four Fs (female, forty, fertile, fat). Ultrasound can sometimes image the stone; if not, use endoscopic retrograde cholangiopancreatography (ERCP) or MRCP (MR "virtual ERCP"). Can lead to **cholangitis:** Charcot's triad = fever, right upper quadrant pain, and jaundice. Treat with antibiotics, then later remove stones surgically or endoscopically.

- **Common bile duct obstruction from cancer:** Usually pancreatic cancer, sometimes cholangiocarcinoma or bowel cancer.

- **Primary biliary cirrhosis:** Middle-aged woman with no risk factors for liver or biliary disease, marked pruritus, jaundice, and positive **antimitochondrial antibodies**; rest of work-up is negative. Cholestyramine helps with symptoms, but no treatment (other than liver transplantation) is very effective.

- **Primary sclerosing cholangitis:** Classically seen in young adults with inflammatory bowel disease (usually ulcerative colitis); manifests like cholangitis. Highly irregular biliary tree on imaging.

Esophageal Disorders

Dysphagia and odynophagia are the classic esophageal complaints. Patients can present with atypical chest pain.

Causes:

- **Achalasia:** Hypertensive lower esophageal sphincter (LES), incomplete relaxation of LES, and loss or derangement of peristalsis. Achalasia is usually idiopathic but may be secondary to Chagas' disease (South America). Patients have intermittent dysphagia for solids and liquids classically *without heartburn*. Barium swallow reveals dilated esophagus with distal "bird-beak" narrowing. Diagnosis can be made with esophageal manometry. Treat with pneumatic balloon dilation, local botulinum toxin injection, calcium channel blockers, or, as a last resort, surgery (myotomy).

- **Barrett's esophagus:** Columnar metaplasia due to acid reflux; must be followed with periodic endoscopy and biopsies to rule out progression to adenocarcinoma.

- **Boerhaave's tears:** Full-thickness esophageal ruptures; if not iatrogenic (from endoscopy), they are usually due to vomiting or retching (alcoholics and bulimics). Diagnose with chest x-ray (pleural effusion with or without pneumothorax, both usually and classically on the left, and/or pneumomediastinum), water-soluble contrast esophagram, and/or CT scan and treat with immediate surgical repair and drainage.

- **Diffuse esophageal spasm or nutcracker esophagus:** Both have irregular, forceful, painful esophageal contractions that cause intermittent chest pain. Diagnose with esophageal manometry. Treat with calcium channel blockers, nitroglycerin as needed, and, if needed, surgery (myotomy).

- **Mallory–Weiss tears:** Superficial esophageal erosions that can cause a GI bleed. They usually are seen with vomiting and retching (alcoholics and bulimics) or are iatrogenic (from endoscopy). Diagnosis and treatment are done endoscopically (sclerose any bleeding vessels).

- **Scleroderma:** Can cause aperistalsis due to fibrosis and atrophy of smooth muscle. Lower esophageal sphincter, i.e., LES, becomes incompetent, and patients often develop GERD symptoms. Look for positive antinuclear antibody (anticentromere antibody specific for CREST and antitopoisomerase antibody specific for scleroderma), masklike facies, and other autoimmune symptoms (**CREST** = **c**alcinosis, **R**aynaud's phenomenon, **e**sophageal dysmotility, **s**clerodactyly, **t**elangiectasias).

 With suspected GI perforation, use water-soluble contrast (e.g., Gastrografin) first instead of barium (which can cause chemical peritonitis or mediastinitis). If aspiration is a concern, remember that the lungs tolerate barium well, but they can develop chemical pneumonitis from water-soluble contrast.

Pancreatitis

More than 80% of cases are due to alcohol or gallstones. Other causes include hypertriglyceridemia, viral infections (mumps, coxsackievirus), trauma, and medications (steroids, azathioprine). Patients have abdominal pain radiating to the back, nausea and vomiting that does not relieve the pain, leukocytosis, and elevated amylase and lipase. Perforated peptic ulcer disease also may have elevated amylase and manifests similarly, but patients have free air on abdominal x-ray and history of peptic ulcer disease.

Treatment: NPO, nasogastric tube, IV fluids, narcotics (meperidine, not morphine). Treat chronic pancreatitis with alcohol abstinence, oral pancreatic enzyme replacement, and fat-soluble vitamin supplements.

Severe pancreatitis: Grey Turner's sign = blue-black flanks; Cullen's sign = blue-black umbilicus. Both are due to hemorrhagic exudate.

Complications include pseudocyst (Fig. 4-6) (drain surgically if chronic and symptomatic), abscess or infection (antibiotics and surgical abscess drainage), and diabetes (with chronic pancreatitis).

Pediatric Gastroenterology

Pediatric gastrointestinal malformations are listed in Table 4-4. Esophageal atresia is shown in Figure 4-7. Other pediatric gastrointestinal conditions are shown in Table 4-5.

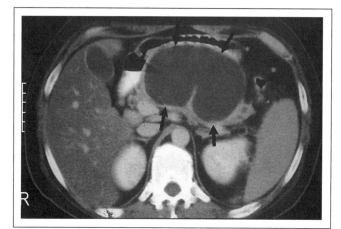

FIGURE 4-6. Large pancreatic pseudocyst *(arrows)* demonstrated on CT.

Table 4-4. GASTROINTESTINAL MALFORMATIONS SEEN IN CHILDREN

Name	Presenting Age	Vomit Description	Findings and Key Words
Pyloric stenosis	0–2 mo	Nonbilious, projectile	M ≫ F; palpable olive-shaped mass in epigastrium, low potassium, metabolic alkalosis
Intestinal atresia	0–1 wk	Bilious	Double-bubble sign, Down's syndrome
Tracheoesophageal fistula	0–2 wk	Food regurgitation	Respiratory compromise with feeding, aspiration pneumonia, inability to pass nasogastric tube, gastric distention (air)
Hirschsprung's disease	0–1 y	Feculent	Abdominal distention, obstipation, no ganglia seen on rectal biopsy, M ≫ F
Anal atresia	0–1 wk	Late, feculent	Detected by initial exam in nursery, M > F
Choanal atresia	0–1 wk	—	Cyanosis with feeding, relieved by crying; inability to pass nasogastric tube

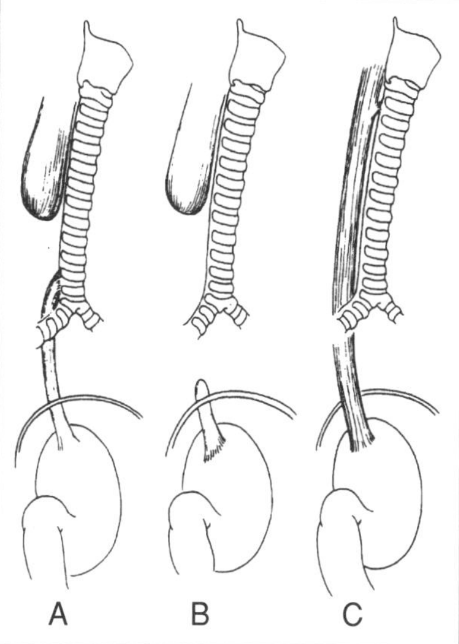

FIGURE 4-7. Esophageal atresia. A, The most common from of esophageal atresia (85%) consists of a dilated proximal esophageal pouch and a connection of the distal esophagus to the carina of the trachea. **B,** Pure esophageal atresia. **C,** Fistula of the H-type without atresia. (From Coran AG (ed): Surgery of the Neonate. Boston, Little, Brown, 1978, p 46, with permission.)

Table 4-5. OTHER GASTROINTESTINAL CONDITIONS SEEN IN CHILDREN

Name	Presenting Age	Vomit Description	Findings and Key Words
Intussusception	4 mo–2 y	Bilious	Currant-jelly stools (blood and mucus), palpable sausage-shaped mass; diagnose and treat with air-contrast x-ray enema
Necrotizing enterocolitis	0–2 mo	Bilious	Premature babies, fever, rectal bleeding, air in bowel wall; treat with NPO, orogastric tube, IV fluids, antibiotics
Meconium ileus	0–2 wk	Feculent, late	Cystic fibrosis manifestation (as is rectal prolapse)
Midgut volvulus	0–2 y	Bilious	Due to malrotation; sudden onset of pain and vomiting; diagnose with upper GI series, and treat with immediate surgery
Meckel's diverticulum	0–2 y	Varies	Rule of 2s*; GI ulceration or bleeding; use Meckel's scan to detect; treat with surgery
Strangulated hernia	Any age	Bilious	Physical exam detects bowel loops in inguinal canal

*Rule of 2s for Meckel's diverticulum: **2% of population** affected (most common GI tract abnormality—remnant of the omphalomesenteric duct), roughly **2 inches long, within 2 feet of ileocolic junction,** and manifests in **first 2 years of life.** Meckel's diverticulum can cause intussusception, obstruction, or volvulus.

Omphalocele versus gastroschisis:

◆ **Omphalocele** is in the midline. Sac contains multiple abdominal organs; the umbilical ring is absent; and other anomalies are common.

◆ **Gastroschisis** is to the right of the midline. Only small bowel is exposed (no true hernia sac); the umbilical ring is present; and other anomalies are rare.

Henoch-Schönlein purpura: Patient can present with GI bleeding and abdominal pain. Look for history of upper respiratory infection, characteristic rash on lower extremities and buttocks, swelling in hands and feet, arthritis, and/or hematuria or proteinuria. Treat supportively.

 Children (more than adults) can develop nausea and vomiting and/or diarrhea with any systemic illness. They also can develop inflammatory bowel disease or irritable bowel syndrome and often have GI complaints with anxiety or psychiatric problems (separation anxiety, reluctance to go to school, depression, child abuse).

Neonatal Jaundice

◆ **Neonatal jaundice:** May be physiologic or pathologic. The first step is to measure total, direct, and indirect bilirubin. The main concern is kernicterus, which is due to high levels of unconjugated bilirubin and subsequent deposit into the basal ganglia. Look for poor feeding, seizures, flaccidity, opisthotonos, and/or apnea to accompany severe jaundice.

- **Physiologic jaundice:** Present in 50% of normal infants; even more common in premature infants. Bilirubin is mostly unconjugated. In *preterm* infants, bilirubin is <15 mg/dL, peaks at 3 to 5 days and may be elevated for up to 3 weeks. In *full-term* infants, bilirubin is <12 mg/dL, peaks at 2 to 4 days, and returns to normal by 2 weeks.

- **Pathologic jaundice:** Levels rise higher than normal and continue to rise or fail to decrease appropriately. *Any jaundice present at birth is pathologic.*

- **Breast milk jaundice:** Breast-fed infants with peak bilirubin of 10 to 20 mg/dL occurring at 2 to 3 weeks of age. Treat with temporary cessation of breast-feeding (switch to bottle) until jaundice resolves.

- **Illness:** Infection or sepsis, hypothyroidism, liver insult, cystic fibrosis, and other illnesses can prolong neonatal jaundice and lower the threshold for kernicterus. The youngest, sickest infants are at greatest risk for hyperbilirubinemia and kernicterus.

- **Hemolysis:** From Rh incompatibility or congenital red cell diseases that cause hemolysis in the neonatal period. Look for anemia, peripheral smear abnormalities, family history, and higher level of unconjugated bilirubin.

- **Metabolic:** Crigler–Najjar syndrome causes severe unconjugated hyperbilirubinemia; Gilbert's disease causes mild unconjugated hyperbilirubinemia; and Rotor and Dubin–Johnson syndromes cause conjugated hyperbilirubinemia.

- **Biliary atresia:** Usually term infants with clay- or gray-colored stools and high levels of conjugated bilirubin. Treat with surgery.

- **Medications:** Avoid sulfa drugs in neonates (displaces bilirubin from albumin and can precipitate kernicterus).

Treatment for unconjugated hyperbilirubinemia that persists, rises higher than 15 mg/dL, or rises rapidly is phototherapy to convert the unconjugated bilirubin to a water-soluble form that can be excreted. The last resort is exchange transfusion (don't even *think* about it unless the level of unconjugated bilirubin is >20 mg/dL).

 Any infant born to a mother with active hepatitis B should get the first immunization shot and hepatitis B immunoglobulin at birth.

5 ENDOCRINOLOGY

It is important to understand the **hypothalamic–pituitary axis** so that you can distinguish primary from secondary disorders. In primary endocrine disturbances, the gland itself is malfunctioning (e.g., from tumor, inflammation, enzyme deficiency), but the pituitary and hypothalamus are functioning normally and exhibit the appropriate response to the gland's action. For example, thyroid-stimulating hormone (TSH) is low in Graves' disease, because the thyroid (or actually, in this case, the immune system) is malfunctioning and overproduces thyroid hormone. The appropriate response is for the pituitary to secrete less TSH because of feedback inhibition. In a secondary endocrine disturbance, the gland is perfectly normal, but the pituitary or hypothalamus is malfunctioning. For example, if the pituitary secretes low levels of TSH or the hypothalamus secretes low levels of thyrotropin-releasing hormone (TRH) in patients with hypothyroidism, the pituitary or hypothalamus is malfunctioning, because it should be secreting *high* levels of TSH or TRH when the level of thyroid hormone is inadequate.

Hypothyroidism

Look for classic symptoms of fatigue, bradycardia, menstrual disturbances (usually menorrhagia), slow speech, cold intolerance, constipation, carpal tunnel syndrome, decreased reflexes, anemia of chronic disease, and/or coarse hair. Hypothyroidism may be associated with hypercholesterolemia, which resolves with treatment. Check thyroid function tests (TSH, thyroxine [T_4], free thyroxine index). Hypothyroidism is usually a primary problem; thus TSH is high and T_4 is low. Treat with thyroid hormone (synthetic T_4).

Causes of hypothyroidism:

◆ **Hashimoto's thyroiditis:** Most common cause; associated with other autoimmune diseases (e.g., pernicious anemia, vitiligo, lupus). Look for positive **antimicrosomal antibodies.** Histology shows lymphocyte infiltration of the gland.

◆ **Subacute thyroiditis:** Acute viral inflammation with fever and enlarged, *tender* (unique symptom usually seen only in acute or subacute thyroiditis) thyroid gland. History of upper respiratory infection is common. Give nonsteroidal antiinflammatory drugs (NSAIDs) for symptom relief. Patients often recover without treatment.

- **Iatrogenic hypothyroidism:** Frequently occurs after treatment for hyperthyroidism (second most common cause in the United States).

- **Sick-euthyroid syndrome:** Any illness can decrease T_4 and/or triiodothyronine (T_3), but TSH is *normal*. The condition is self-limiting, and no treatment is necessary except for the underlying disorder.

- **Iodine deficiency:** Rare in the United States. Can cause cretinism in children (stunted growth and mental retardation).

Hyperthyroidism

Signs and symptoms include nervousness, anxiety, insomnia, tachycardia, palpitations, atrial fibrillation, heat intolerance, weight loss, diarrhea, menstrual irregularities (hypomenorrhea), increased appetite, and thyroid stare. Check thyroid function tests. Hyperthyroidism is usually a primary disturbance; thus TSH is low and T_4 is high.

Treatment begins with antithyroid drugs (propylthiouracil or methimazole). Most patients eventually require further therapy. Consider surgery for patients younger than 25 years or pregnant women and radioactive iodine for other patients. Propranolol is used to control symptoms from thyroid storm (the patient decompensates, physically and mentally, from very high thyroid hormone levels) and symptomatic tachycardia, palpitations, and arrhythmias.

Causes of hyperthyroidism:

- **Graves' disease:** The most common cause, by far. Exophthalmos (Fig. 5-1) and pretibial myxedema (Fig. 5-2) are unique to Graves' disease. Patients have positive thyroid-stimulating immunoglobulins and thyroid-stimulating antibodies, which activate the TSH receptor. Nontender, diffuse goiter also is present. The whole gland takes up excessive radioactive iodine.

- **Plummer's disease (toxic multinodular goiter):** Hyperfunctioning nodules cause a lumpy goiter without positive antibodies or exophthalmos and pretibial myxedema. Radioactive iodine uptake is high in nodules but decreased in the rest of the gland.

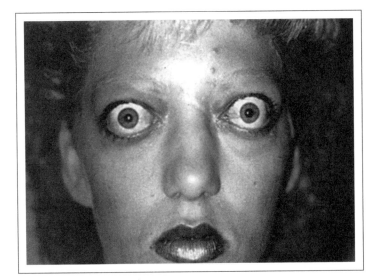

FIGURE 5-1. Thyroid-related ophthalmology with proptosis and lid retraction.

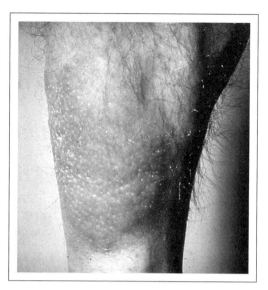

FIGURE 5-2. Example of pretibial myxedema.

- ◆ **Toxic adenoma:** One nodule is palpable and has high radioactive iodine uptake; the rest of the gland shows decreased uptake (thyroid cancer is rarely hyperfunctional).
- ◆ **Thyroiditis:** Hashimoto's or subacute thyroiditis can produce a transient hyperthyroidism due to inflammation before converting to hypothyroidism.

 In pregnancy and other states (administration of oral contraceptives or estrogens; infections), thyroid-binding globulin (TBG) may be elevated. Although this causes elevation of total thyroid hormone levels, free thyroid hormone is not elevated, and *TSH is normal.* Do *not* treat. The nephrotic syndrome, large protein losses of any kind, and anabolic steroids can decrease TBG and, thus, decrease total thyroid hormone levels (again, TSH is normal and you should not treat).

Hypoadrenalism

Addison's disease (*primary* adrenal insufficiency) is most commonly idiopathic (probably autoimmune). Look for increased skin pigmentation, weight loss, dehydration, anorexia, nausea and vomiting, dizziness and syncope, hyponatremia, and hyperkalemia. Under metabolic stress (infection, surgery), patients might have an adrenal crisis: abdominal pain, hypotension or cardiovascular collapse, renal shutdown, and death. Treat with hydrocortisone and IV fluids to avoid adrenal crisis.

The diagnosis of hypoadrenalism, when not obvious, is done by administering adrenocorticotropic hormone (ACTH) and seeing whether levels of plasma cortisol increase over baseline. *Do not delay* giving steroids while you do this test if the patient is doing poorly; the patient can die while you wait for the results.

Secondary adrenal insufficiency is a commonly tested disorder and is most often due to previous use of corticosteroids. Once patients take steroids for more than 1 month, they might not be able to mount an appropriate increase in ACTH when needed for *up to 1 year!* The classic setting is the patient on steroids who stops taking all medications before surgery, then develops refractory hypotension and electrolyte disturbances after surgery. Give corticosteroids!

Other secondary causes of adrenal insufficiency are Sheehan's syndrome (pituitary apoplexy; history of postpartum hypotension, inability to breast-feed, and other endocrine insufficiencies) and neoplasms (pituitary adenomas and craniopharyngiomas). In secondary hypoadrenalism, mineralocorticoid (aldosterone) secretion is not affected because it is not directly under pituitary control; thus, the electrolyte disturbance is not as severe, and there is *no* skin hyperpigmentation. ACTH is decreased, as is melanocyte-stimulating hormone (MSH), which is thought to cause the skin hyperpigmentation in *primary* adrenal insufficiency.

Hyperadrenalism (Cushing's Syndrome)

Cushing's syndrome is usually due to prescribed steroids in the United States. Look for moon facies, truncal obesity, buffalo hump, striae, poor wound healing, hypertension, osteoporosis, secondary diabetes or glucose intolerance, menstrual abnormalities, and psychiatric disturbances (depression, psychosis).

Cushing's *disease* is Cushing's syndrome caused by pituitary overproduction of ACTH, which usually is due to a pituitary adenoma. Get an MRI (magnetic resonance image) of the brain if levels of ACTH and cortisol are high. Other causes are adrenal neoplasms that produce steroids and small cell cancer of the lung, which can produce ACTH (treat by treating the neoplasm).

Diagnosis of noniatrogenic cases is made by first doing a screening test. The best choice is usually a 24-hour urine test for free cortisol; plasma cortisol is not a good test because of wide inter- and intrapatient fluctuation. Second choice is a dexamethasone suppression test.

Hyperaldosteronism

Primary hyperaldosteronism is known as *Conn's syndrome* and is due to an adrenal adenoma. Look for hypertension, hypernatremia, hypokalemia, and **low** renin. Get a CT scan of the abdomen to find the adrenal tumor.

Secondary hyperaldosteronism is much more common; it is related to hypertension (especially with renal artery stenosis) and edematous disorders (congestive heart failure, cirrhosis, the nephrotic syndrome). Look for hypertension, edema, renal bruit, variable sodium and potassium, and *high* renin. Treat the underlying cause.

Pheochromocytoma

Popular on the boards and wards despite rarity in real life. Look for intermittent hypertension that is very high, wild swings in blood pressure, tachycardia, postural hypotension, headaches, sweating, dizziness, mental status changes, and/or feeling of impending doom. Patients also may have glucose intolerance due to high catecholamines.

If you are suspicious, first screen with a 24-hour urine test to look for catecholamines and their breakdown products (vanillylmandelic acid, homovanillic acid, or metanephrines). If the screen is positive, do an abdominal CT, and remove the tumor after stabilizing the patient with α-sympathetic blockers followed by β-sympathetic blockers.

Diabetes Insipidus

Symptoms of diabetes insipidus (DI) include severe polydipsia and polyuria (patients can urinate 25 L/day). When access to water is restricted, patients rapidly develop dehydration and hypernatremia, which can cause death. Giving antidiuretic hormone (ADH) determines whether the cause is central or nephrogenic. Central disease responds to ADH, whereas nephrogenic disease does not.

- **Nephrogenic DI:** Look for medications as cause (lithium, methoxyflurane, demeclocycline). Treat with thiazide diuretics (paradoxical effect; ADH does not help).
- **Central DI:** May be idiopathic or result from trauma, neoplasm, or sarcoidosis. Treat with ADH/vasopressin and treat any possible underlying cause.

Syndrome of Inappropriate Secretion of Antidiuretic Hormone

Signs include hyponatremia as well as low levels of every other electrolyte (and lab values) because of dilution from excessive water retention. Look for medications (morphine, chlorpropamide, oxytocin—be careful in pregnant patients), small cell lung cancer, *postoperative status* (watch for all electrolytes to fall after surgery), trauma, lung infections, and pain. Treat with **water restriction.** For board purposes, *do not* give hypertonic saline, and *do not* try to correct hyponatremia aggressively or quickly. Rapid correction can cause brainstem damage (osmotic myelinolysis, also known as central pontine myelinolysis).

IMPORTANT POINTS

Obesity increases the risk of:

1. Overall mortality (at any age)
2. Cancer, especially endometrial cancer
3. Gallstones (cholesterol stones)
4. Gastroesophageal reflux disease, Barrett's esophagus, and esophageal adenocarcinoma
5. Heart disease and coronary artery disease
6. Hypertension
7. Hypertriglyceridemia (also weakly associated with hypercholesterolemia)
8. Hypoventilation, pickwickian syndrome, sleep apnea
9. Insulin resistance and diabetes mellitus
10. Osteoarthritis
11. Thromboembolism
12. Varicose veins

6 ◇ NEPHROLOGY

Acute Renal Failure

Signs of acute renal failure (ARF) include progressive rise in creatinine and blood urea nitrogen (BUN), metabolic acidosis, hyperkalemia, and hypervolemia. Symptoms include rales, elevated jugular venous pressure, and dilutional hyponatremia. There are three categories: prerenal, postrenal, and renal.

PRERENAL

The most common example is hypovolemia (dehydration, hemorrhage). Look for BUN-to-creatinine ratio higher than 15 or 20. Patients have signs of hypovolemia (e.g., tachycardia, weak pulse, depressed fontanelle). Give intravenous (IV) fluids and/or blood. Other prerenal causes are sepsis (treat the sepsis and give IV fluids), heart failure (give inotropes and diuretics), and liver failure (hepatorenal syndrome; treat supportively).

POSTRENAL

The most common example is benign prostatic hypertrophy (BPH). The patient is a man older than 50 years with BPH symptoms (e.g., hesitancy, dribbling), and ultrasound reveals bilateral hydronephrosis. Treat with catheterization (suprapubic catheterization if necessary) to relieve obstruction and prevent further renal damage; then consider surgery (transurethral prostatectomy [TURP]). Malignancy of the bladder, cervix, or bowel is another cause. Nephrolithiasis is a *rare* cause, because stones have to be bilateral to cause renal failure.

RENAL

Acute tubular necrosis is the most common type.

Examples of renal causes:

◆ **Glomerulonephritis:** Prototype is post-streptococcal syndrome, which is usually seen in children with a history of upper respiratory infection or strep throat 1 to 3 weeks earlier; they present with edema, hypervolemia, hypertension, hematuria, and oliguria. Red blood cell casts on urinalysis clinch the diagnosis. Treat supportively.

◆ **Goodpasture's syndrome:** Due to antiglomerular basement membrane antibodies (linear immunofluorescence pattern on renal biopsy), which also react with the lungs.

Look for a young male patient with hemoptysis, dyspnea, and renal failure. Treat with steroids and/or cyclophosphamide.

- **IV contrast:** Do *not* give to diabetic patients or renal patients if you can avoid it; you can precipitate acute renal failure. If you must give it, give *lots* of hydration.
- **Lupus erythematosus:** Look for malar rash and arthritis. Renal failure is a major cause of morbidity and mortality.
- **Myoglobinuria/rhabdomyolysis:** From strenuous exercise (e.g., marathon), alcohol, burns, muscle trauma, heat stroke, or neuroleptic malignant syndrome. Muscle breaks down and plugs up the renal filtration system. Look for very high levels of creatine phosphokinase (CPK). Treat with hydration and diuretics.
- **Toxins and medications:** Chronic NSAID use (papillary necrosis), cyclosporine, aminoglycosides, methicillin, chemotherapeutic agents (e.g., cisplatin).
- **Wegener's granulomatosis:** Also has lung and kidney involvement, but patients typically present after age 40 years. Look for nasal involvement (bloody nose, nasal perforation) or hemoptysis and pleurisy as presenting symptoms. Patients have positive antineutrophil cytoplasm antibody (ANCA) titer. Treat with cyclophosphamide.

 In all cases of ARF, dialysis may be required. Indications for dialysis include uremic encephalopathy, pericarditis, severe metabolic acidosis (roughly, pH <7.25), heart failure, and hyperkalemia severe enough to cause arrhythmia.

Nephrotic Syndrome

Signs include proteinuria (>3.5 g/day), hypoalbuminemia, edema (classic example is morning periorbital edema), and hyperlipidemia and lipiduria. In children, the nephrotic syndrome is usually due to minimal change disease (also called lipoid nephrosis; effaced podocyte foot processes on electron microscopy), often after an infection. Measure 24-hour urine protein to clinch the diagnosis, and treat with steroids. Causes in adults include diabetes mellitus, hepatitis B, amyloidosis, lupus, and drugs (gold, penicillamine, captopril).

Nephritic Syndrome

Signs include oliguria, azotemia (rising BUN and creatinine), hypertension, and hematuria. Patients might have some proteinuria, but not in the nephrotic range. The classic cause is post-streptococcal glomerulonephritis. Red cell casts are classic on urinalysis.

Chronic Renal Failure

Any of the causes of ARF can cause chronic renal failure (CRF) if the insult is severe or prolonged. The majority of cases of CRF are due to diabetes mellitus (number one cause of CRF) and hypertension. Another classic cause is polycystic kidney disease (multiple cysts in kidney): look for positive family history (usually autosomal dominant; autosomal recessive form occurs in children), hypertension, hematuria, palpable renal masses, berry aneurysms in the circle of Willis, and cysts in liver and other organs.

Metabolic derangements due to CRF:

- **Anemia:** From lack of erythropoietin (synthetic erythropoietin can correct)
- **Anorexia, nausea, vomiting:** From build-up of toxins
- **Azotemia:** High BUN and creatinine
- **Bleeding:** Due to disordered platelet function; patients can have prolonged bleeding time test
- **Central nervous system disturbances:** Mental status changes and even convulsions or coma from toxin build-up
- **Fluid retention:** Can cause hypertension, edema, congestive heart failure, and pulmonary edema
- **Hyperkalemia:** Watch for EKG changes
- **Hypocalcemia or hyperphosphatemia:** Vitamin D production is impaired; bone loss leads to renal osteodystrophy
- **Increased susceptibility to infection:** Due to decreased cellular immunity
- **Metabolic acidosis**
- **Skin pigmentation and pruritus:** Skin turns yellowish-brown and itches due to metabolic byproducts
- **Uremic pericarditis:** Classically causes an audible friction rub

Treatment: Regular dialysis, water-soluble vitamins (removed during dialysis), phosphate restriction or binders (e.g., calcium carbonate), erythropoietin, and hypertension control. The only cure is renal transplant.

Urinary Tract Infection

Urinary tract infections (UTIs) are much more common in female patients, except in the neonatal and early pediatric period. They are usually caused by *Escherichia coli* (less often by other enteric organisms). Look for urgency, dysuria, suprapubic or low back pain, and low-grade fever. The gold standard for diagnosis is urine culture (at the least, get a midstream sample; best is a catheterized sample or suprapubic tap). Urinalysis shows white blood cells, bacteria, positive leukocyte esterase, and/or positive nitrite. Treat with trimethoprim-sulfamethoxazole, amoxicillin, nitrofurantoin, or first-generation cephalosporin for about 1 week.

IMPORTANT POINTS

1 In pediatric patients, UTI is a cause for concern because it may be the presenting symptom of a genitourinary malformation. The most common examples are vesicoureteral reflux (VUR) and posterior urethral valves. Get an ultrasound and a voiding cystourethrogram to evaluate any boy younger than 6 years with a UTI and any girl younger than 6 years with recurrent UTIs or pyelonephritis.

2 Conditions that promote urinary stasis (prostate hypertrophy, pregnancy, stones, neurogenic bladder, VUR) or bacterial colonization (indwelling catheter, fecal incontinence, surgical instrumentation) predispose to UTI. They also predispose to ascending UTI (pyelonephritis) and to bacteremia and sepsis.

3 Asymptomatic bacteriuria is treated in pregnancy (high risk of progression to pyelonephritis).

Pyelonephritis

Pyelonephritis usually results from an ascending UTI and is caused by *E. coli* (>80% of cases). Patients present with high fever, shaking chills, **costovertebral angle tenderness** or flank pain, and/or UTI symptoms. Urinalysis and urine and blood cultures establish the diagnosis. Computed tomography (CT) can detect complications such as abscess. Treat on an inpatient basis with IV antibiotics while awaiting culture results (e.g., fluoroquinolone or extended-spectrum penicillin or cephalosporin).

Kidney and Hematologic Disorders in Children

Table 6-1 shows the differential diagnosis of pediatric kidney and hematologic disorders.

Table 6-1. KIDNEY AND HEMATOLOGIC DISORDERS IN CHILDREN				
Characteristic	HUS	HSP	TTP	ITP
Most common age	Children	Children	Young adults	Children or adults
Previous infection	Diarrhea (*E. coli*)	URI	None	Viral (especially in children)
Red blood cell count	Low	Normal	Low	Normal
Platelet count	Low	Normal	Low	Low
Peripheral smear	Hemolysis	Normal	Hemolysis	Normal
Treatment	Supportive*	Supportive*	Plasmapheresis, NSAIDs, no platelets†	Steroids, splenectomy if medications fail‡
Kidney manifestations	ARF, hematuria	Hematuria	ARF, proteinuria	None
Key differential points	Age, diarrhea	Rash, abdominal pain, arthritis, melena	CNS changes, age	Antiplatelet antibodies

*In HUS and HSP, patients might need dialysis and transfusions.
  †Do not give platelet transfusions to patients with TTP (can form clots).
  ‡Give steroids only if the patient is symptomatic (bleeding) or platelets <20,000/mm³.
  ARF, acute renal failure; CNS, central nervous system; HSP, Henoch–Schönlein purpura; HUS, hemolytic uremic syndrome; ITP, idiopathic thrombocytopenic purpura; NSAIDs, nonsteroidal antiinflammatory drugs; TTP, thrombotic thrombocytopenic purpura; URI, upper respiratory infection.

Renal Stones

Renal stones manifest with severe, intermittent, unilateral flank and/or groin pain. Most stones (85%) show up on abdominal x-ray and are composed of calcium, but CT is now the standard diagnostic method (detects >95% of stones and more accurately localizes them; avoids contrast as needed with intravenous pyelography). Most cases are idiopathic and should be treated with *lots* of hydration and pain control (to see if stone will pass). If stone does not pass, it needs to be removed surgically (preferably endoscopically) or by lithotripsy.

Underlying causes of stones:

◆ **Hypercalcemia:** Due to hyperparathyroidism or malignancy (metastases or squamous cell lung cancer secreting parathyroid hormone).

◆ **Infection:** From ammonia-producing bugs (*Proteus, Staphylococcus* spp). Look for **Staghorn calculi** (Fig. 6-1).

◆ **Hyperuricemia:** Associated with gout and leukemia treatment (allopurinol and IV fluids can be given before chemotherapy as preventive measures).

◆ **Cystinuria and aminoaciduria:** Suspect this hereditary cause if the stone is made of cystine and/or in repetitive stone-forming patients.

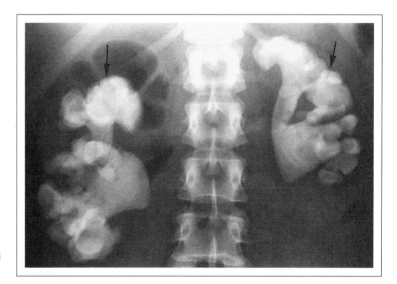

FIGURE 6-1. X-ray of bilateral Staghorn calculi (*arrows*).

Arthritis

The large majority of arthritis cases are due to osteoarthritis (OA). When in doubt, or if you suspect something other than OA, aspirate any fluid from the affected joint for examination. Examine the fluid for cell count and differential, glucose, bacteria (Gram stain and culture), and crystals. The characteristics of the arthritides are shown in Table 7-1.

OSTEOARTHRITIS

Few signs of inflammation on exam (lacks hot, red, tender joints seen in all the others of this group). Symptoms include Heberden's (distal interphalangeal [DIP] joint) nodes (Fig. 7-1) and Bouchard's (proximal interphalangeal [PIP] joint) nodes in the fingers

Table 7-1. CHARACTERISTICS OF ARTHRITIS

Characteristic	Osteoarthritis	Rheumatoid Arthritis	Gout	Pseudogout	Septic Arthritis
Usual age and sex	Older adults	Women 20–45 y	Older men	Older adults	Any age
Classic joints	DIP, PIP, hip, knee	PIP, MCP, wrist	Big toe	Knees, elbows	Knee
Joint fluid WBC count	<2000	>2000	>2000	>2000	>50,000
% Neutrophils	<25	>50	>50	>50	>75

DIP, distal interphalangeal; MCP, metacarpophalangeal; PIP, proximal interphalangeal; WBC, white blood cell.

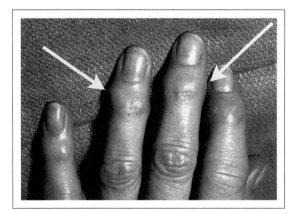

FIGURE 7-1. Patients with degenerative joint disease of the hands can present with Heberden's nodes (*arrows*). These nodules represent osteophytes at the distal interphalangeal (DIP) joint.

and worsening of symptoms in the evening and after use. X-ray shows osteophytes (bone spurs around joints) and joint-space narrowing. Incidence increases with age. Treat with weight reduction and nonsteroidal antiinflammatory drugs (NSAIDs) as needed.

RHEUMATOID ARTHRITIS

Positive rheumatoid factor clinches the diagnosis of rheumatoid arthritis (RA) in most adult patients. Look for systemic symptoms (fever, malaise, subcutaneous nodules, pericarditis or pleural effusion, uveitis), prolonged morning stiffness, and swan neck and boutonnière deformities. One buzzword is **pannus** (articular cartilage looks like granulation tissue due to chronic inflammation). Treat with NSAIDs for symptom relief and disease-modifying agents such as methotrexate, hydroxychloroquine, etanercept, and infliximab. Corticosteroids are used for bad flare-ups. End-stage deformity is shown in Figure 7-2.

With *juvenile* RA, rheumatoid factor is often negative. Watch for uveitis as a presenting symptom, especially in the pauciarticular (few joints affected) form.

GOUT

Gout classically starts with podagra (gout in the big toe). Look for tophi (subcutaneous uric acid deposits, punched-out lesions in bone x-ray) (Fig. 7-3) and needle-shaped crystals (often inside leukocytes) with *negative* birefringence in a joint fluid sample. Gout is more common in men than women. Patients should avoid alcohol (can precipitate an attack). Use colchicine or NSAIDs (*not* aspirin, which causes decreased excretion of uric acid by the kidney) for acute attacks. Maintenance therapy includes high fluid intake, alkalinization of the urine, and/or probenicid or allopurinol (neither for acute attacks).

PSEUDOGOUT

Look for rhomboid-shaped crystals with weakly *positive* birefringence due to calcium pyrophosphate crystal deposition (CPPD). Acute attacks are like gout clinically, thus the name, but pseudogout is a completely different disorder.

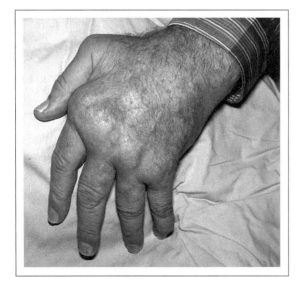

FIGURE 7-2. Classic end-stage rheumatoid hand deformity. This patient has volar subluxation of the metacarpophalangeal (MCP) joints; ulnar deviation of the digits; and hypertrophic, boggy synovium along the dorsum of the hand, particularly over the MCP joints.

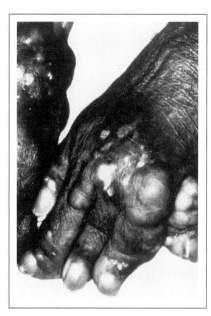

FIGURE 7-3. Gouty tophi. Tophaceous deposits of gout overlying digits of this patient's hand.

SEPTIC ARTHRITIS

Synovial fluid has bacteria on Gram stain. *Staphylococcus aureus* is the most common organism, except in sexually active young adults (*Neisseria gonorrhoeae* is most common in this group). Do blood cultures in addition to joint cultures, because the bug usually reaches the joint via the hematogenous route. Do urethral swabs and cultures in appropriate patients.

Other causes of arthritis:

◆ **Psoriasis:** In the presence of skin lesions, diagnosis is easy. Arthritis usually affects hands and feet, and the arthritis resembles RA but the rheumatoid factor is negative. Treat like RA with NSAIDs, methotrexate, etanercept, infliximab, or corticosteroids.

◆ **Lupus erythematosus or inflammatory bowel disease:** Other symptoms of the primary disease help make the diagnosis.

◆ **Ankylosing spondylitis:** Associated with HLA-B27. Most often a 20- to 40-year-old man with a positive family history presents with back pain and morning stiffness; the patient sometimes assumes a bent-over posture. Sacroiliac joints are primarily affected, and x-rays might reveal a bamboo spine. Patients have other autoimmune-type symptoms, such as fever, elevated erythrocyte sedimentation rate (ESR), and anemia; some develop uveitis. Treatment is exercise, NSAIDs, and RA agents such as methotrexate, etanercept, and infliximab.

◆ **Reiter's syndrome:** Also associated with human leukocyte antigen (HLA)-B27. The classic triad is urethritis (due to *Chlamydia* spp.), conjunctivitis, and arthritis ("can't pee, can't see, can't climb a tree"), but Reiter's syndrome also can follow enteric bacterial infections. Superficial oral and penis ulcers also are common. Diagnose and treat the sexually transmitted disease, and treat sexual partners. NSAIDs are used for arthritis; methotrexate and sulfasalazine for treatment of more severe arthritis symptoms.

◆ **Hemophilia:** Recurrent hemarthroses can cause debilitating arthritis. Treat with acetaminophen (avoid aspirin).

- **Lyme disease:** Look for tick bite, erythema chronicum migrans, and migratory arthritis later. Treat with doxycycline (amoxicillin in pregnant women); use parenteral ceftriaxone for cases with carditis or other serious complications.

- **Rheumatic fever:** Look for previous streptococcal pharyngitis. Migratory polyarthritis is one of the major Jones criteria.

- **Sickle cell disease:** Patients often develop arthralgias and can get avascular necrosis of the femoral or humeral head or other bone infarcts.

- **Trauma:** can lead to arthritis later in life.

- **Childhood orthopedic problem:** Slipped capital femoral epiphysis, congenital hip dysplasia, and Legg–Calvé–Perthes disease can cause arthritis in adulthood. Use history (age of onset) and x-rays to determine which disease the patient had as a child.

- **Charcot joint:** Most commonly seen in diabetes mellitus; also in other neuropathies. Lack of sensation causes patient to overuse or misuse joints, which become deformed and painful. The best treatment is prevention. After even seemingly mild trauma, patients with neuropathy in the area of the trauma need x-rays to rule out fractures.

- **Hemochromatosis and Wilson's disease:** Both may be associated with arthritis due to deposition of iron or copper.

Autoimmune Diseases

Autoimmune diseases affect women of reproductive age unless otherwise specified. For board purposes, classic disease findings differentiate one condition from the other. Almost all patients have systemic signs of inflammation (elevated ESR and C-reactive protein, fever, anemia of chronic disease, fatigue, weight loss).

BEHÇET'S SYNDROME

The classic patient is a 20-something man with painful oral and genital ulcers. Patients can also have uveitis, arthritis, and other skin lesions (especially erythema nodosum). Steroids might help.

DERMATOMYOSITIS

Polymyositis (see Table 7-2) plus skin involvement (heliotrope rash around the eyes with associated periorbital edema is classic). Patients classically have trouble rising out of a chair or climbing steps (proximal muscles affected). Muscle enzymes are elevated, and electromyography is irregular. Muscle biopsy establishes the diagnosis. Patients might have increased incidence of malignancy.

KAWASAKI'S SYNDROME

Kawasaki's syndrome affects children younger than 5 years old (more common in Japanese and female patients). Patients present with truncal rash, high fever (lasts >5 days), conjunctival injection, cervical lymphadenopathy, strawberry tongue, late skin desquamation of palms and soles, and/or arthritis. Patients develop coronary vessel vasculitis and subsequent aneurysms, which can thrombose and cause a myocardial infarction (suspect Kawasaki's disease in any child who has a myocardial infarction). Treat during acute stage with aspirin (one of few pediatric diseases where aspirin is indicated) and intravenous immunoglobulin to reduce the risk of coronary aneurysm development.

POLYARTERITIS NODOSA

Polyarteritis nodosa is associated with hepatitis B infection and cryoglobulinemia. Patients present with fever, abdominal pain, weight loss, renal disturbances, and/or peripheral neuropathies. Lab abnormalities include high ESR, leukocytosis, anemia, and hematuria or proteinuria. Vasculitis involves medium-sized vessels. Biopsy is the gold standard for diagnosis.

SCLERODERMA AND PROGRESSIVE SYSTEMIC SCLEROSIS

Look for **CREST** symptoms (**c**alcinosis, **R**aynaud's phenomenon, **e**sophageal dysmotility, **s**clerodactyly, **t**elangiectasia), heartburn, and mask-like, leathery facies. Screening test is ANA; confirmatory tests are anticentromere antibody (for CREST) and antitopoisomerase (for scleroderma). Steroids might help.

SJÖGREN'S SYNDROME

Look for dry eyes (keratoconjunctivitis sicca) and dry mouth (xerostomia), often associated with other autoimmune disease. Treat with eyedrops and good oral hygiene.

SYSTEMIC LUPUS ERYTHEMATOSUS

Malar rash, discoid rash, photosensitivity, kidney damage, arthritis, pericarditis and pleuritis, positive antinuclear antibody (ANA), positive anti-Smith antibody, positive Venereal Disease Research Laboratory (VDRL) or rapid plasma reagin test for syphilis, positive lupus anticoagulant, -cytopenias (thrombocytopenia, leukopenia, anemia, or pancytopenia), neurologic disturbances (depression, psychosis, seizures) and oral ulcers can all be presenting symptoms. Use ANA titer as a screening test and anti-Smith antibody to confirm. Treat with NSAIDs, hydroxychloroquine, and corticosteroids or other immunosuppressants (e.g., azathioprine).

TAKAYASU'S ARTERITIS

Takayasu's arteritis tends to affect East Asian women between 15 and 30 years old. It is called "pulseless disease" because you might not be able to feel the patient's pulse or measure blood pressure on one or both arms. Vasculitis affects the aortic arch and the branches that arise from it. Carotid involvement can cause neurologic signs or stroke, and congestive heart failure is not uncommon. Computed tomography (CT) or magnetic resonance (MR) angiogram shows the characteristic lesions. Treat with corticosteroids and/or cyclophosphamide.

WEGENER'S GRANULOMATOSIS

Wegener's granulomatosis resembles Goodpasture's syndrome, but older patients are affected and instead of antiglomerular antibody, there is a positive antineutrophil cytoplasmic antibody (ANCA) titer. Look for nasal (nose bleeds, nasal perforation), lung (hemoptysis, dyspnea), and kidney (hematuria, acute renal failure) involvement. Treat with cyclophosphamide.

Table 7-2. DIFFERENTIAL DIAGNOSIS OF FIBROMYALGIA, POLYMYOSITIS, AND POLYMYALGIA RHEUMATICA

Characteristic	Fibromyalgia	Polymyositis	Polymyalgia Rheumatica
Classic age and sex	Young women	40- to 60-year-old women	Women >50 years
Location	Various	Proximal muscles	Pectoral and pelvic girdles, neck
ESR	Normal	Elevated	Markedly elevated (often >100 mm/h)
Muscle biopsy or EMG	Normal	Abnormal	Normal
Classic findings	Anxiety, stress, insomnia, point tenderness over affected muscles, negative work-up	Elevated CPK; abnormal EMG and biopsy	Temporal arteritis, great response to steroids, very high ESR, elderly
Treatment	Antidepressants, NSAIDs, rest	Steroids	Steroids

CPK, creatine phosphokinase; EMG, electromyography; ESR, erythrocyte sedimentation rate; NSAIDs, nonsteroidal antiinflammatory drugs.

Fibromyalgia, Polymyositis, and Polymyalgia Rheumatica

The differential diagnosis of fibromyalgia, polymyositis, and polymyalgia rheumatica is given in Table 7-2.

Paget's Disease

Paget's disease is a disease of bone in which bone is broken down and regenerated, often simultaneously. It is seen in patients older than 40 years and is more common in men. It is often discovered in an asymptomatic patient via x-ray. Classic sites of involvement are the pelvis (Fig. 7-4) and skull.

Watch for a person who has had to buy larger-size hats. Patients might complain of bone pain, osteoarthritis, or, rarely, nerve deafness or paraplegia. Alkaline phosphatase is **markedly elevated** in the presence of normal calcium and phosphorus. The risk of osteosarcoma is increased in affected bones.

Treat with NSAIDs and possibly etidronate or calcitonin for severe disease.

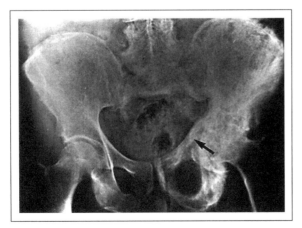

FIGURE 7-4. Paget's disease of the pelvis. The entire left hemi-pelvis is involved, and there are arthritic changes of the left hip. Note the classic thickening of the iliopectineal line (*arrow*).

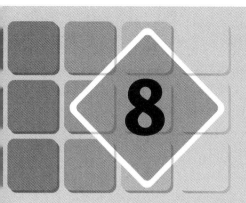

8 ◇ HEMATOLOGY

Anemia

Definition: Hemoglobin <12 mg/dL in women or <14 mg/dL in men.

Symptoms include fatigue, dyspnea on exertion, light-headedness, dizziness, syncope, palpitations, angina, and claudication. **Signs** include tachycardia, pallor (especially of the sclera and mucous membranes), systolic ejection murmurs (from high flow), and signs of the underlying cause (e.g., jaundice in hemolytic anemia, positive stool guaiac in gastrointestinal [GI] bleed).

Important clues in the history:

◆ **Medications:** Many medications can cause anemia through various mechanisms. The classic example is methyldopa, which causes red blood cell (RBC) antibodies and hemolysis. Chloroquine and sulfa drugs cause hemolysis in glucose–6-phosphate dehydrogenase (G6PD) deficiency. Phenytoin causes megaloblastic anemia. Chloramphenicol causes aplastic anemia.

◆ **Blood loss:** Trauma, surgery, melena, hematemesis

◆ **Chronic diseases:** Anemia of chronic disease, especially inflammatory and debilitating conditions, such as autoimmune diseases, infections, and cancer. Chronic conditions such as migraine headaches and osteoarthritis do not cause anemia of chronic disease (must be ongoing significant systemic inflammation).

◆ **Family history:** Hemophilia, thalassemia, G6PD deficiency, etc.

◆ **Alcoholism:** Patients tend to have iron, folate, and B_{12} deficiencies as well as GI bleeds.

Steps to diagnosing the cause of anemia:

1. Complete blood count (CBC) with differential and RBC indices. First and foremost, hemoglobin and hematocrit must be below normal. The mean corpuscular volume (MCV) tells you whether the anemia is microcytic (MCV <80), normocytic (MCV 80–100), or macrocytic (MCV >100).

2. Peripheral smear. Classic findings (Table 8-1) can make for an easy diagnosis.

3. Reticulocyte index (RI). RI should be >2% with anemia; otherwise, the marrow is not responding properly. If the index is very high, think of hemolysis as the cause (the marrow is responding properly, so it is not the problem).

With these three parameters, you can make a reasonable differential diagnosis if the cause is not obvious (Box 8-1).

Table 8-1. CLASSIC FINDINGS OF ANEMIA ON PERIPHERAL SMEAR

Smear Finding	Usual Cause
Acanthocytes, spur cells	Abetalipoproteinemia
Basophilic stippling	Lead poisoning
Bite cells	Hemolytic anemias
Echinocytes, burr cells	Uremia
Heinz bodies	G6PD deficiency
Howell–Jolly bodies	Asplenia, splenic dysfunction
Hypersegmented neutrophils	Folate or vitamin B_{12} deficiency
Iron inclusions in RBCs of bone marrow	Sideroblastic anemia
Parasites inside RBCs	Malaria, babesiosis
Polychromasia	Reticulocytosis (consider hemolysis)
Rouleaux formation	Multiple myeloma
Schistocytes, helmet cells, fragmented RBCs	Intravascular hemolysis
Sickled cells	Sickle cell anemia
Spherocytes, elliptocytes	Hereditary spherocytosis or elliptocytosis
Target cells	Thalassemia, liver disease
Teardrop-shaped RBCs	Myelofibrosis

G6PD, glucose 6 phosphate dehydrogenase; RBC, red blood cell

Box 8-1. RETICULOCYTE INDEXING IN THE DIAGNOSIS OF ANEMIA

Microcytic	Normocytic	Macrocytic
Normal to Elevated Reticulocyte Index		
Hemoglobinopathy	Acute blood loss	None; all forms have low RI
Thalassemia	Hemolytic (multiple causes)	
	Medications (antibody-causing)	
Low Reticulocyte Index		
Anemia of chronic disease (some)	Anemia of chronic disease (some)	B_{12} deficiency
Iron deficiency	Aplastic anemia	Cirrhosis, liver disease
Lead poisoning	Cancer, dysplasia (e.g., myelophthisic anemia)	Folate deficiency
Sideroblastic anemia	Endocrine failure (thyroid, pituitary)	Medications (methotrexate, phenytoin)
	Renal failure	

RI, reticulocyte index.

Clues to the presence of hemolytic anemia:

- ◆ Elevated lactate dehydrogenase (LDH)
- ◆ Elevated bilirubin (unconjugated as well as conjugated if the liver is working)
- ◆ Jaundice
- ◆ Low or absent haptoglobin (with intravascular hemolysis)
- ◆ Positive urobilinogen, bilirubin, or hemoglobin in the urine

Only conjugated bilirubin appears in the urine, and hemoglobin appears only when haptoglobin has been saturated, as in brisk intravascular hemolysis.

MICROCYTIC ANEMIAS

Iron Deficiency Anemia. Iron deficiency (Fig. 8-1) is the most common cause of anemia in the United States. Look for low iron and ferritin levels, elevated total iron-binding capacity (TIBC; also known as transferrin), and low TIBC saturation. Rarely, patients have a craving for ice or dirt (pica) or Plummer–Vinson syndrome (esophageal web producing dysphagia, iron deficiency anemia, and glossitis). In a patient older than 40 years, rule out colon cancer as a cause of chronic blood loss. Iron deficiency anemia is common in women of reproductive age because of menstrual irregularities.

Give iron supplements to all infants except full-term infants who are exclusively breast-fed; giving cow's milk before 1 year of age can cause anemia through GI bleeding. Start iron supplementation at 4 to 6 months for full-term infants and at 2 months for pre-term infants. Iron supplements also are commonly given during pregnancy and lactation because of increased demand.

Treat iron deficiency anemia by correcting the underlying cause, if possible, and prescribe oral iron supplementation for roughly 3 to 6 months.

Thalassemia. Thalassemia must be differentiated from iron deficiency. Iron levels are normal in thalassemia; *iron is contraindicated* because it can cause overload. Look for **elevated hemoglobin A_2** (β-thalassemia only) or hemoglobin F (β-thalassemia only), target cells, nucleated RBCs, diffuse basophilia on peripheral smears, x-ray of the skull showing a "crew-cut" appearance, splenomegaly, and positive family history (more common in blacks, Mediterraneans, Asians).

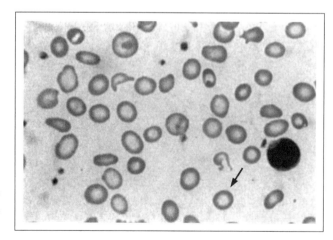

FIGURE 8-1. Peripheral blood smear showing iron deficiency anemia: hypochromia (*arrow*), microcytosis, and poikilocytosis.

Diagnosis is made by hemoglobin electrophoresis. There are four gene loci for α-chain and only two for β-chain thalassemia. α-Thalassemia is symptomatic at birth, or the fetus dies in utero (hydrops); β-thalassemia is not symptomatic until 6 months of age.

No treatment is required for minor thalassemia; patients often are asymptomatic because they are used to living at a lower level of hemoglobin and hematocrit. Thalassemia major is more dramatic and severe. Treat with as-needed transfusions and iron chelation therapy to prevent secondary hemochromatosis.

Lead Poisoning. Lead poisoning is classically seen in children. With acute poisoning, look for vomiting, ataxia, colicky abdominal pain, irritability (aggressive behavior, behavioral regression), and encephalopathy, cerebral edema, or seizures. Usually, however, poisoning is chronic and low-level; look for pica (especially paint chips and dust in old buildings, which often still have lead paint); residence in an old or neglected building; basophilic stippling; and elevated free erythrocyte protoporphyrin. See Chapter 28, Pediatrics, for information on screening for lead poisoning.

Sideroblastic Anemia. Test results show increased or normal iron, ferritin, and TIBC saturation (which distinguishes it from iron deficiency); polychromatophilic stippling; and the classic ringed sideroblast cell in the bone marrow. Sideroblastic anemia may be related to myelodysplasia or future blood dyscrasia. Manage supportively; in rare cases the anemia responds to pyridoxine. *Do not give iron!*

Anemia of Chronic Disease. Anemia of chronic disease can be normocytic. Look for diseases that cause chronic inflammation (rheumatoid arthritis, lupus erythematosus, cancer, tuberculosis). Serum iron is low, but so is TIBC (thus, the percent saturation may be nearly normal). Serum ferritin is elevated (because ferritin is an acute-phase reactant, the level should be increased). Treat the underlying disorder to correct the anemia. *Do not give iron!*

NORMOCYTIC ANEMIAS

Acute Blood Loss. Remember that immediately after blood loss, hemoglobin may be normal (takes a few hours to re-equilibrate). Look for pale cold skin, tachycardia, and hypotension. Transfuse if indicated, even with a normal hemoglobin in the appropriate acute setting.

Autoimmune Hemolytic Anemia. Autoimmune hemolytic anemia has several etiologies: lupus (or medications that cause lupus, such as procainamide, hydralazine, and isoniazid); drugs (classic is methyldopa; also penicillins, cephalosporins, sulfas, and quinidine); leukemia, lymphoma, or infection (classic is *Mycoplasma*, also Epstein-Barr virus). **Coombs test is positive,** and smear might reveal spherocytes due to incomplete macrophage destruction.

Sickle Cell Anemia. Smear gives it away (Fig. 8-2). Look for very high percentage of reticulocytes. Sickle cell anemia is almost always seen in blacks (8% are heterozygotes in the United States).

Watch for classic manifestations of sickle cell disease:

◆ Acute chest syndrome (mimics pneumonia)

◆ Aplastic crises (due to parvovirus B19 infection)

◆ Autosplenectomy (increased infections with encapsulated bugs)

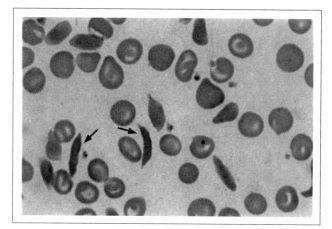

FIGURE 8-2. Sickle cell anemia. Sickled erythrocytes are prominent (*arrows*). Functional hyposplenia is indicated by the presence of a Howell–Jolly body (nuclear remnant in erythrocyte [*center*]).

- ◆ Bone pain (due to bone infarcts; the classic example is avascular necrosis of the femoral or humeral head)
- ◆ Dactylitis (hand–foot syndrome; classic initial manifestation in infants)
- ◆ Renal papillary necrosis
- ◆ Pigment cholelithiasis
- ◆ Priapism
- ◆ Splenic sequestration crisis
- ◆ Stroke

Diagnosis is made by hemoglobin electrophoresis. Screening is done at birth, but symptoms usually do not appear until around 6 months of age because of lack of adult hemoglobin production. Treat with prophylactic penicillin (start as soon as the diagnosis is made), proper vaccination (including pneumococcal vaccine), folate supplementation, early treatment of infections, and proper hydration.

A sickle crisis is characterized by severe pain in various sites due to RBC sickling. Treat with oxygen, lots of intravenous (IV) fluids, and analgesics (including narcotics). Consider transfusions if symptoms and/or findings are severe.

Spherocytosis. Diagnosis is made from peripheral smear (Fig. 8-3), family history (autosomal dominant), splenomegaly, *positive osmotic fragility test*, and an *increased mean corpuscular hemoglobin concentration*. Treatment often involves splenectomy. Remember that

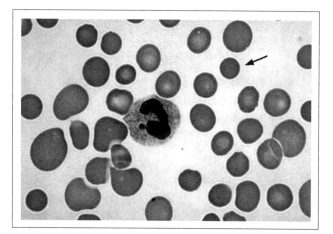

FIGURE 8-3. Hereditary spherocytosis. The peripheral smear reveals multiple fairly small red blood cells with intense staining and absent central pallor (*arrow*), which are called spherocytes. (From Bonner H, Bagg A, Cossman J: The blood and the lymphoid organs. In Rubin E, Farber JL (eds): Pathology, 3rd ed. Philadelphia, Lippincott-Raven, 1999, pp 1050–1151; with permission.)

spherocytes may be seen in extravascular hemolysis (but the osmotic fragility test is normal).

End-Stage Renal Disease. The kidneys make erythropoietin, so give erythropoietin in end-stage renal disease to correct the anemia.

Aplastic Anemia. Aplastic anemia is usually idiopathic. It may be caused by chemotherapy or radiation, malignancy (especially acute leukemias), benzene, and medications (chloramphenicol, carbamazepine, phenylbutazone, sulfa drugs, zidovudine [AZT]). Look for decreased white blood cells and platelets. Treat by stopping any possible causative medication. Patient might need antithymocyte globulin (ATG) or bone marrow transplant.

Myelophthisic Anemia. Myelophthisic (or myeloplastic) anemia is usually due to myelodysplasia, myelofibrosis, or malignant invasion and destruction of bone marrow (most common cause). Look for marked anisocytosis (different size), poikilocytosis (different shape), nucleated RBCs, giant and/or bizarre-looking platelets, and *teardrop-shaped* RBCs on the peripheral smear. A bone marrow biopsy is usually done and might reveal no cells (dry tap from fibrotic marrow in myelofibrosis) or malignant-looking cells.

Glucose–6-Phosphate Dehydrogenase Deficiency. X-linked recessive (males affected); most common in blacks and Mediterraneans. Look for sudden hemolysis or anemia after fava bean or drug exposure (antimalarials, salicylates, sulfa drugs) or after infection. Diagnosis is with RBC enzyme assay (done when the patient is asymptomatic to avoid a false-negative result). Treat by avoiding precipitating foods and drugs (discontinue the triggering medication first).

MACROCYTIC ANEMIAS

Folate Deficiency. Folate deficiency (Fig. 8-4) is commonly seen in alcoholics and pregnant women. Rare causes include poor diet (e.g., tea and toast), methotrexate, prolonged trimethoprim-sulfamethoxazole therapy, phenytoin, and malabsorption. Check folate level (serum or RBC). Treat with oral folate.

Vitamin B_{12} Deficiency. Vitamin B_{12} deficiency (see Fig. 8-4) is most commonly due to pernicious anemia (antiparietal cell antibodies; see Fig. 8-4), but can also result from gastrectomy, terminal ileum resection, diet (strict vegan), chronic pancreatitis, and *Diphyllobothrium latum* (fish tapeworm) infection. Look for neurologic deficiencies (loss

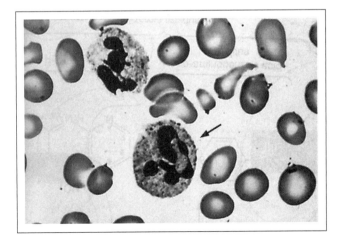

FIGURE 8-4. Hypersegmented neutrophils (*arrow*) and large oval erythrocytes with poikilocytosis (irregular shape of red blood cells), seen in both folate and vitamin B_{12} deficiencies. (From Bonner H, Bagg A, Cossman J: The blood and the lymphoid organs. In Rubin E, Farber JL (eds): Pathology, 3rd ed. Philadelphia, Lippincott-Raven, 1999, pp 1050–1151; with permission.)

of sensation, loss of position sense, paresthesias, ataxia, spasticity, hyperreflexia, positive Babinski sign, dementia) and achlorhydria (no stomach acid secretion, elevated stomach pH). Check serum B_{12}. Antiparietal cell or anti-intrinsic factor antibodies and an elevated gastrin level generally confirm pernicious anemia as the cause of B_{12} deficiency. A nuclear medicine Schilling test can be helpful in cases with uncertain etiology.

Miscellaneous rare causes of anemia:

- *Clostridium perfringens*, malaria, or babesiosis infection
- Endocrine failure (especially pituitary, liver, or thyroid)
- Hemolysis due to microangiopathy (disseminated intravascular coagulation, thrombotic thrombocytopenic purpura, hemolytic uremic syndrome). Look for schistocytes and red blood cell fragments.
- Hypersplenism (always has splenomegaly and often low platelets and white blood cells)
- Mechanical heart valves (which hemolyze red blood cells)

Transfusions

Transfusions are always based on clinical grounds. Treat the patient, not the lab value; there is no such thing as a trigger value for transfusion. Different blood components have different indications:

- **Whole blood:** Used only for rapid, massive blood loss or exchange transfusions (poisoning, thrombotic thrombocytopenic purpura)
- **Packed RBCs:** Used instead of whole blood when the patient needs a transfusion
- **Washed RBCs:** Free of traces of plasma, white blood cells, and platelets; good for IgA deficiency and allergic or previously sensitized patients
- **Platelets:** Given for symptomatic thrombocytopenia (usually $<10,000/\mu L$)
- **Granulocytes:** Rarely used for neutropenia with sepsis caused by chemotherapy (colony-stimulating factors such as filgrastim preferred).
- **Fresh frozen plasma:** Contains all clotting factors; used for bleeding diathesis when one cannot wait for vitamin K to take effect (disseminated intravascular coagulation [DIC], severe warfarin poisoning) or when vitamin K will not work (liver failure).
- **Cryoprecipitate:** Contains fibrinogen and factor VIII; used in von Willebrand's disease and DIC

The most common cause of **blood transfusion reaction** is lab error. Type O negative can be used when you cannot wait for blood typing or the blood bank does not have the patient's type. If a transfusion reaction occurs, the first step is to *stop the transfusion!* Patients with associated oliguria should be treated with IV fluids and diuresis (mannitol or furosemide). Massive transfusions can lead to bleeding diathesis from thrombocytopenia (look for oozing from puncture or IV sites) and citrate (calcium chelator). Hyperkalemia can also develop.

Types of transfusion reactions:

- Allergic reaction (urticaria, edema, dizziness, dyspnea, wheezing, anaphylaxis) from reaction to a (usually unknown) component in donor serum.

◆ Febrile reaction (chills, fever, headache, back pain) from antibodies to white blood cells

◆ Hemolytic reaction (anxiety or discomfort, dyspnea, chest pain, shock, jaundice) from antibodies to red blood cells

Disseminated Intravascular Coagulation

DIC is most commonly due to pregnancy and obstetric complications (50%), malignancy (30%), sepsis, and trauma (especially head trauma, prostate surgery, and snake bites). DIC usually manifests as bleeding diathesis. Look for the classic oozing or bleeding from puncture or IV sites, but patients might have thrombotic tendencies. Labs reveal prolonged prothrombin time (PT), partial thromboplastin time (PTT), and bleeding time; positive D dimer and increased **fibrin degradation products;** thrombocytopenia; and decreases in fibrin and clotting factors (including factor VIII, which is normal in hepatic necrosis).

Treat the underlying cause (evacuate uterus, give antibiotics). Patients might need transfusions, fresh frozen plasma, or, rarely, heparin (only in the presence of thrombosis).

Eosinophilia and Basophilia

Causes of *eosinophilia* or increased eosinophil counts include:

◆ Idiopathic etiology

◆ Adrenal insufficiency

◆ Allergy

◆ Angioedema

◆ Atopy

◆ Autoimmune diseases (e.g., lupus)

◆ Blood dyscrasias (especially lymphoma)

◆ Drug reactions

◆ Eczema

◆ IgA deficiency

◆ Loffler's syndrome (pulmonary eosinophilia)

◆ Parasitic infections

With *basophilia*, or an increased basophil count, think of allergies, neoplasm, or blood dyscrasia.

Coagulopathies

The lupus anticoagulant can cause a prolonged PTT, but the patient has a tendency toward thrombosis. Look for associated lupus, positive VDRL (Venereal Disease Research Laboratory) or rapid plasma reagin test for syphilis, and/or history of miscarriages. Factor V Leiden, thrombin variant, and deficiencies in protein C, protein S, or

Table 8-2. DIFFERENTIAL DIAGNOSIS OF THE COAGULOPATHIES

Disease	PT	PTT	BT	Platelet Count	RBC Count	Other
DIC	High	High	High	Low	Normal/ low	Appropriate history, low factor VIII level
Hemophilia A or B	Normal	High	Normal	Normal	Normal	X-linked recessive; A = low factor VIII, B = low factor IX
Heparin	Normal	High	Normal	Normal or low	Normal	Watch for thrombocytopenia and thrombosis
ITP	Normal	Normal	High	Low	Normal	Watch for preceding URI
TTP	Normal	Normal	High	Low	Low	Hemolysis, CNS symptoms; treat with plasmapheresis; do not give platelets
Liver failure	High	Normal or high	Normal	Normal or low	Normal or low	Jaundice, normal factor VIII level; do not give vitamin K (ineffective)
Scurvy	Normal	Normal	Normal	Normal	Normal	Fingernail and gum hemorrhages, bone hemorrhages
von Willebrand's disease	Normal	High	High	Normal	Normal	Autosomal dominant (look for family history)
Warfarin	High	Normal	Normal	Normal	Normal	Vitamin K antagonist (factors II, VII, IX, and X)

BT, bleeding time; CNS, central nervous system; DIC, disseminated intravascular coagulation; ITP, idiopathic thombocytopenic purpura; PT, prothombin time; PTT, partial thromboplastin time; RBC, red blood cell; TTP, thrombotic thrombocytopenic purpura; URI, upper respiratory infection.

antithrombin III can also cause an increased tendency toward thrombosis. Patients are treated with anticoagulant therapy to prevent deep venous thrombosis, pulmonary embolism, and other complications. The differential diagnosis of the coagulopathies is given in Table 8-2.

Clotting tests: Use prothrombin time for extrinsic system (prolonged by warfarin), partial thromboplastin time for intrinsic system (prolonged by heparin but not affected by low-molecular weight heparins), and bleeding time for platelet function.

Causes of thrombocytopenia include:

◆ Alcohol

◆ Autoimmune disease

◆ Disseminated intravascular coagulation

◆ Hemolytic uremic syndrome

◆ Heparin (treat by first stopping heparin)

◆ Human immunodeficiency virus (HIV) infection

◆ Idiopathic thrombocytopenic purpura

◆ Medications (especially quinidine and sulfa drugs)

- Pancytopenia of any cause
- Splenic sequestration
- Thrombotic thrombocytopenic purpura

Bleeding from thrombocytopenia is in the form of petechiae, nose bleeds, and easy bruising.

 Do *not* give platelets to a patient with thrombotic thrombocytopenic purpura or heparin-associated thrombocytopenia, because you can cause thrombosis.

Vitamin C deficiency (scurvy) can cause bleeding similar to that seen with low platelets (splinter and gum hemorrhages, petechiae); perifollicular and subperiosteal hemorrhages are unique to scurvy. Patients have a poor diet history (classic examples are hot dogs and soda or tea and toast diets), myalgias and arthralgias, and capillary fragility. Bleeding is due to collagen dysfunction in vessels. Treat with oral vitamin C. Chronic steroid use can also cause easy bruising.

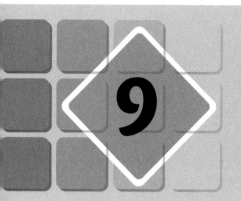

9 ONCOLOGY

General

Blood dyscrasias are listed in Table 9-1. Types of cancer are ranked by incidence and mortality in Table 9-2.

IMPORTANT POINTS

1 In children and younger adults, leukemia is the most common cancer. Remember, however, that *age* has the most significant impact on the incidence and mortality rate of cancer. The incidence of cancer in the United States roughly doubles every 5 years after age 25; therefore, cancer most commonly affects older adults.

2 In most organs, the most common malignancy is *metastatic*. On Step 2, don't be fooled into saying that hepatocellular cancer is the most common malignancy of the liver if metastatic cancer is a choice.

3 Metastases to the spine can cause cord compression (local spinal pain, reflex changes, weakness, sensory loss, paralysis). Cord compression is an emergency, and the first step is to start high-dose corticosteroids. Magnetic resonance imaging (MRI) confirms the diagnosis. The next step is to treat with radiation. Surgical decompression is used if radiation fails or the tumor is known not to be radiosensitive. Prompt treatment is essential, because outcome is closely linked to pretreatment function.

Table 9-3 lists genetic predispositions to cancer. Other diseases with increased incidence of cancer are immunodeficiency syndromes, Bloom syndrome, and Fanconi anemia. Breast, ovarian, and colon cancer have well-known familial tendencies (along with some other types of cancer), but only rarely can a Mendelian inheritance pattern be demonstrated (e.g., BRCA1 gene for breast cancer). Table 9-4 lists avoidable risk factors for cancer. Table 9-5 lists tumor markers for various kinds of cancer.

Lung Cancer

Lung cancer is the number-one cause of overall cancer mortality in the United States. The incidence is rising in women (due to increased smoking). Look for change in a chronic

Table 9-1. BLOOD DYSCRASIAS

Type	Age	What to Look for in Case Description; Buzz Words
Acute lymphoblastic leukemia (ALL)	Children (peak at 3–5 y)	Pancytopenia (bleeding, fever, anemia), radiation therapy, Down's syndrome
Acute myelogenous leukemia (AML)	>30 y	Pancytopenia (bleeding, fever, anemia), Auer rods, disseminated intravascular coagulation
Chronic myelogenous leukemia (CML)	30–50 y	WBC count >50,000, Philadelphia chromosome, blast crisis, splenomegly
Chronic lymphocytic leukemia (CLL)	>50 y	Male gender, lymphadenopathy, lymphocytosis, infections, smudge cells, splenomegaly
Hairy cell leukemia	Adults	Blood smear with hairlike projections (Fig. 9-1), splenomegaly
Mycosis fungoides, Sézary syndrome	>50 y	Plaque-like, itchy skin rash that does not improve with treatment, blood smear with cerebriform nuclei ("butt cells"), Pautrier abscesses in epidermis
Burkitt's lymphoma	Children	Associated with Epstein–Barr virus (in Africa)
CNS B-cell lymphoma	Adults	HIV–AIDS
T-cell leukemia	Adults	HTLV-1 is one cause
Hodgkin's disease	15–34 y	Reed-Sternberg cells (Fig. 9-2), cervical lymphadenopathy, night sweats
Non-Hodgkin's lymphoma	Any age	Small follicular type has best prognosis, large diffuse type has worst; primary tumor may be located in GI tract
Myelodysplasia, myelofibrosis	>50 y	Anemia, teardrop cells, dry tap on bone marrow biopsy, high mean corpuscular volume and red cell distribution width index; associated with CML
Multiple myeloma	>40 y	Bence Jones protein (IgG = 50%, IgA = 25%), osteolytic lesions, high calcium level
Waldenstrom's disease	>40 y	Hyperviscosity, IgM spike, cold agglutinins (Raynaud's phenomenon with cold sensitivity)
Polycythemia vera	>40 y	High hemoglobin, pruritus (after hot bath or shower). Treat with phlebotomy
Primary thrombocythemia	>50 y	Platelet count usually >1,000,000; patients might have bleeding or thrombosis

CNS, central nervous system; GI, gastrointestinal; HTLV, human T-cell lymphotrophic virus; Ig, immunoglobulin; WBC, white blood cell

Table 9-2. CANCER STATISTICS

Rank	Overall Highest Incidence		Overall Highest Mortality Rate	
	Male	*Female*	*Male*	*Female*
First	Prostate	Breast	Lung	Lung
Second	Lung	Lung	Prostate	Breast
Third	Colon	Colon	Colon	Colon

cough in a smoker. The more pack-years of tobacco use, the more suspicious you should be. Patients also can present with hemoptysis, pneumonia, and/or weight loss. Chest x-ray might show mass (Fig. 9-4) or pleural effusion; with an effusion, perform thoracentesis and examine fluid for malignant cells. After chest x-ray, get a computed tomography (CT) scan, then a positron emission tomography (PET) scan in indeterminate cases, then a tissue biopsy to confirm the diagnosis and define the histologic type. Non–small cell

Table 9-3. GENETIC PREDISPOSITION TO CANCER

Disease or Syndrome	Inheritance	Type of Cancer (in order of most likely) and Other Information
Retinoblastoma	Autosomal dominant	Retinoblastoma, osteogenic sarcoma (later in life)
MEN type I	Autosomal dominant	Parathyroid, pituitary, pancreas (islet cell tumors)
MEN type IIA	Autosomal dominant	Thyroid (medullary cancer), parathyroid, pheochromocytoma
MEN type IIB	Autosomal dominant	Thyroid (medullary cancer), pheochromocytoma, mucosal neuromas
Familial polyposis coli	Autosomal dominant	Hundreds of colon polyps that always become colon cancer
Gardner's syndrome	Autosomal dominant	Familial polyposis plus osteomas and soft tissue tumors
Turcot's syndrome	Autosomal dominant	Familial polyposis plus CNS tumors
Peutz–Jeghers syndrome	Autosomal dominant	Look for perioral freckles and multiple noncancerous GI polyps; increased incidence of noncolon cancer (stomach, breast, ovaries)
Neurofibromatosis, type 1	Autosomal dominant	Multiple neurofibromas (Fig. 9-3), café-au-lait spots; increased number of pheochromocytomas, bone cysts, Wilms' tumor, leukemia
Neurofibromatosis, type 2	Autosomal dominant	Bilateral acoustic schwannomas
Tuberous sclerosis	Autosomal dominant	Adenoma sebaceum, seizures, mental retardation, glial nodules in brain; increased renal angiomyolipomas and cardiac rhabdomyomas
Von Hippel–Lindau disease	Autosomal dominant	Hemangiomas in cerebellum, renal cell cancer; cysts in liver and/or kidney
Xeroderma pigmentosum	Autosomal recessive	Skin cancer
Albinism	Autosomal recessive	Skin cancer
Down's syndrome	Trisomy 21	Leukemia

GI, gastrointestinal; MEN, multiple endocrine neoplasia.

cancer may be treated with surgery if the cancer remains within the lung parenchyma. Small cell cancer is treated with chemotherapy only; early metastases make surgery inappropriate.

Weird, classic and frequently tested consequences of lung cancer:

◆ **Horner's syndrome:** From invasion of cervical sympathetic chain by an apical (Pancoast) tumor. Look for *unilateral* ptosis, miosis, and anhidrosis (no sweating)

◆ **Diaphragm paralysis:** From phrenic nerve involvement

◆ **Hoarseness:** From recurrent laryngeal nerve involvement

◆ **Superior vena cava syndrome:** Look for edema and plethora (redness) of the neck and face and central nervous system symptoms (headache, visual symptoms, altered mental status). These are caused by compression of the superior vena cava with impaired venous drainage.

◆ **Cushing's syndrome:** From adrenocorticotropic hormone (ACTH) production by a small cell carcinoma

Table 9-4. AVOIDABLE RISK FACTORS FOR CANCER DEVELOPMENT

Cancer Type	Risk Factor (Greatest Impact Listed First)
All cancer overall	Smoking (second is alcohol)
Bladder	Smoking, aniline dyes (rubber and dye industry), schistosomiasis (in immigrants)
Breast*	Combined estrogen/progesterone hormone replacement therapy, nulliparity, obesity, alcohol, high-fat diet (controversial), lack of exercise
Cervical	Smoking, sex, high parity
Clear cell cancer	Mothers should avoid diethylstilbestrol (DES) during pregnancy
Colorectal	High-fat and low-fiber diet
Endometrial	Unopposed estrogen stimulation, obesity
Esophagus	Smoking, alcohol
Leukemia	Chemotherapy, radiotherapy, other immunosuppressive drugs, benzene
Liver	Alcohol, vinyl chloride (liver angiosarcomas), aflatoxins
Lung	Smoking, asbestos (also nickel, radon, coal, arsenic, chromium, uranium)
Mesothelioma	Asbestos
Oral cavity	Smoking, alcohol
Pancreas	Smoking
Pharynx, larynx	Smoking, alcohol
Skin	Ultraviolet light exposure (e.g., sun), coal tar, arsenic
Renal cell	Smoking
Stomach	Alcohol, nitrosamines, nitrites (from smoked meats and fish)
Thyroid	Childhood head, neck, or chest irradiation

*Order of importance for avoidable breast cancer risk factors is uncertain and remains controversial. This list is presented in a random order.

Table 9-5. TUMOR MARKERS

Marker	Cancer(s)
Alpha fetoprotein	Liver, testicular (yolk-sac)
Bladder tumor antigen, NMP 22	Bladder
CA 15-3, CA 27.29	Breast
CA 19-9	Pancreas, lung, breast
CA-125	Ovarian
Carcinoembryonic antigen	Colon, pancreas, other GI tumors
Chromogranin A	Carcinoid tumors, neuroblastoma
Human chorionic gonadotropin	Hydatiform moles, choriocarcinoma
β_2-Microglobulin	Multiple myeloma, chronic lymphocytic leukemia
Prostate-specific antigen	Prostate (early)
S-100	Melanoma, CNS tumors, nerve tumors
Thyroglobulin	Thyroid

CNS, central nervous system; GI, gastrointestinal.

- ◆ **Syndrome of inappropriate secretion of antidiuretic hormone (SIADH):** From antidiuretic hormone production by a small cell carcinoma
- ◆ **Hypercalcemia:** From bone metastases or production of parathyroid hormone by a squamous cell carcinoma

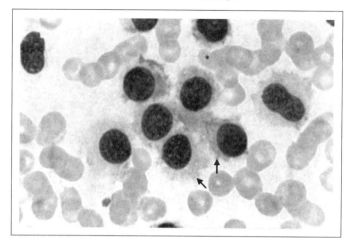

FIGURE 9-1. Peripheral blood film from a patient with hairy cell leukemia (HCL). The malignant cells show characteristic nuclear morphology and "hairy" cytoplasmic projections (*arrows*). This illustration is not typical of HCL because it is extremely unusual to find such large numbers of hairy cells circulating in the peripheral blood. (From Wood ME: Hematology/Oncology Secrets, 2nd ed. Philadelphia, Hanley & Belfus, 1999, with permission.)

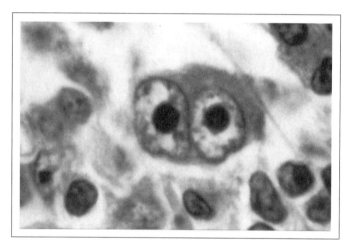

FIGURE 9-2. Lymph node from a patient with Hodgkin's disease. A Reed–Sternberg cell shows the typical "owl eye" nuclear appearance. (From Wood ME: Hematology/Oncology Secrets, 2nd ed. Philadelphia, Hanley & Belfus, 1999, with permission.)

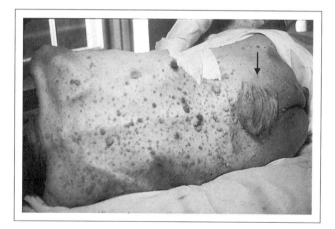

FIGURE 9-3. Neurofibromas and plexiform neurofibroma (*arrow*). (From Fitzpatrick JE, Aeling JL: Dermatology Secrets. Philadelphia, Hanley & Belfus, 1996, with permission.)

◆ **Eaton–Lambert syndrome:** Myasthenia gravis–like disease due to lung cancer that spares the ocular muscles; the muscles become stronger with repetitive stimulation (opposite of myasthenia gravis)

Solitary pulmonary nodule on chest x-ray: The first step is **comparison with previous chest x-rays.** If the nodule has remained the same size for more than 2 years, it is *not* cancer. If no old films are available and the patient is older than 35 years or has a long smoking history, get a CT scan, followed by PET scan if the nodule remains indeterminate

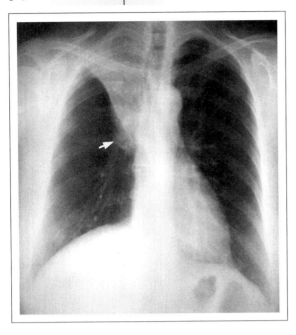

FIGURE 9-4. Convexity of the medial aspect of the minor fissure (*arrow*) is caused by a large central mass, with resulting right upper lobe atelectasis. This is known as the *reverse S sign of Golden.*

(i.e., not definitely benign). Obtain biopsy of the nodule (via bronchoscopy or transthoracic CT guided biopsy if possible) for tissue diagnosis. If the patient is younger than 35 years or has no smoking history, the cause is most likely infectious (tuberculosis or fungi), hamartoma, or collagen vascular disease. The patient may undergo *careful* observation and follow-up with repeat chest CT scans to ensure no growth.

Breast Cancer

Incidence: Roughly 1 in 10 women will develop breast cancer in their lifetime.

Risk factors for breast cancer:

◆ Personal history of breast cancer (biggest risk factor)

◆ Family history in first-degree relatives

◆ Age (breast cancer is rare before age 30; the incidence increases with age). Greatest risk in women older than 70 years.

◆ Early menarche, late menopause, and late first pregnancy or nulliparity (more menstrual cycles = more risk)

◆ Atypical hyperplasia of the breast

◆ Radiation exposure before age 30

◆ The effect of hormonal stimulation (e.g., oral contraceptive pills, estrogen therapy) on the risk of developing breast cancer is controversial, but women with active or past breast cancer are advised not to take estrogen or progesterone.

Signs and symptoms that suggest a mass indicate breast cancer until proved otherwise: fixation of breast mass to the chest wall or overlying skin, satellite nodules or ulcers on the skin, lymphedema or peau d'orange, matted or fixed axillary lymph nodes, inflammatory skin changes (red, hot skin with enlargement of the breast due to inflammatory cancer), prolonged unilateral scaling erosion of the nipple with or without discharge (may be

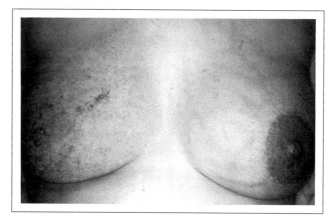

FIGURE 9-5. Paget's disease of the nipple (left side of figure, right breast).

Paget's disease of the nipple, shown in Fig. 9-5), microcalcifications on mammography, and *any new breast mass in a postmenopausal woman.*

The **conservative approach** is to biopsy every palpable breast mass in a woman older than 35 years when in doubt, especially if she has any risk factors. If the board question does not want you to biopsy the mass, it will give you clues that it is not cancer (e.g., bilateral, lumpy breasts that become symptomatic with every menses and have no dominant mass; age younger than 30 years).

IMPORTANT POINTS

1 In women younger than 30 years, breast cancer is rare. With a discrete breast mass in this age group, think of fibroadenoma and observe the patient over a few menstrual cycles before considering biopsy. Fibroadenomas are usually roundish, rubbery-feeling, and freely movable.

2 The most common histologic type of breast cancer is invasive ductal carcinoma.

3 In patients with a palpable breast mass, the decision to do a biopsy is a *clinical* one. A mammogram that looks benign (unless it is definitive) should not deter you from doing a biopsy if a lesion is clinically suspicious. On the other hand, a lesion that is detected on mammography and looks suspicious should be biopsied, even if it is not palpable (needle localization biopsy).

4 Mammograms in women younger than 30 years are rarely helpful (breast tissue is too dense to see cancer). Ultrasound is often a more important way to image the breast in younger women. MRI is increasingly being used to screen high-risk women and evaluate masses found on mammography or ultrasound.

5 Aromatase inhibitors (e.g., letrozole, anastrozole) or tamoxifen generally improve survival if the tumor is estrogen receptor–positive and even more so if the tumor is also progesterone receptor–positive. If the tumor is HER-2/neu–receptor positive, trastuzumab antibody therapy (against the receptor) is usually effective.

6 Mastectomy and breast-conserving surgery plus radiation are considered equal in efficacy. In either case, do an axillary sentinel node biopsy or full dissection to determine spread to the nodes. If nodes are positive, chemotherapy (hormone therapy and/or traditional chemo) is given.

Prostate Cancer

Risk factors:

◆ Age (not seen in men younger than 40 years; incidence increases with age; 60% of men older than 80 years have prostate cancer)

◆ Race: black > white > Asian

Patients often present late (in the absence of screening) because early prostate cancer is asymptomatic. Look for symptoms suggestive of benign prostatic hypertrophy (hesitancy, dysuria, frequency) with hematuria and/or elevated prostate-specific antigen (PSA), a test used for screening and monitoring of disease. Look for prostate irregularities (e.g., nodules) on rectal exam. Patients might present with back pain from vertebral metastases (osteoblastic).

Local prostate cancer is treated with surgery (prostatectomy). Patients with metastases have several options for hormonal therapy: orchiectomy, gonadotropin-releasing hormone agonist (leuprolide), androgen-receptor antagonist (flutamide), estrogen (diethylstilbestrol), and others (e.g., cyproterone). Chemotherapy does not work, and radiation therapy is used for local disease or pain from bony metastases.

Colorectal Cancer

Risk factors:

◆ Age (incidence begins to increase after age 40 years; peak incidence is between 60 and 75 years)

◆ Family history (especially with familial polyposis or Gardner's, Turcot's, or Lynch's syndrome)

◆ Inflammatory bowel disease (risk from ulcerative colitis is greater than risk from Crohn's disease, but both increase risk)

◆ Low-fiber, high-fat diet (weak evidence)

IMPORTANT POINTS

1 Patients might present with asymptomatic blood in stool (visible streaks of blood on stool or guaiac-positive stool), anemia with right-sided colon cancer, change in stool caliber (pencil stool) or frequency (alternating constipation and frequency) with left-sided colon cancer. As with any cancer, look for weight loss.

2 Occult blood in the stool of a patient older than 40 years should be considered colon cancer until proved otherwise. To rule out colon cancer, either do flexible sigmoidoscopy and a barium enema *or* do a total colonoscopy. If you see any lesions (Fig. 9-6) with a flexible sigmoidoscope or barium enema, you need to do a total colonoscopy with removal and histologic examination of all polyps and lesions. For this reason, most physicians now start with colonoscopy.

3 Carcinoembryonic antigen (CEA) is often elevated with colon cancer, and a preoperative level is usually measured. After surgery to remove the tumor, CEA should return to

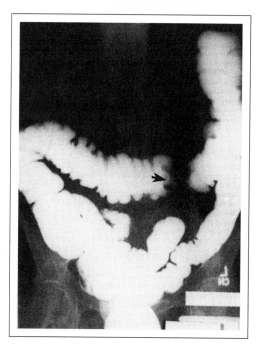

FIGURE 9-6. An apple-core lesion on barium enema (*arrow*).

normal levels. Periodic monitoring of CEA postoperatively helps to detect recurrence before it is clinically apparent. CEA is *not* used as a screening tool for colon cancer; it is used only to follow known cancer.

4 Treatment is primarily surgical, with resection of involved bowel. Adjuvant chemotherapy is sometimes done with 5-fluorouracil (5-FU) and levamisole or leucovorin.

5 Colon cancer often metastasizes to the liver; if the metastasis is solitary, surgical resection may be attempted. With metastases elsewhere, chemotherapy is the only option and prognosis is poor.

6 Colon cancer is a common cause of a large bowel obstruction in an adult.

Pancreatic Cancer

The classic presentation for adenocarcinoma (most common type and reflects 85%-90% of cases; cell of origin is ductal epithelium) is a smoker between the ages of 40 and 80 years who has lost weight and is jaundiced. May have epigastric pain, migratory thrombophlebitis (**Trousseau's syndrome,** which can also be seen with other visceral cancer), or a palpable, nontender gallbladder (**Courvoisier's sign**). Males > females, diabetics > nondiabetics, blacks > whites. Surgery is rarely curative (Whipple procedure), and the prognosis is dismal (5% 5-year survival).

Islet cell tumors (5%-10% of pancreatic cancer cases, but classic on boards):

◆ **Insulinoma (beta cell tumor):** Most common islet cell tumor. Look for two thirds of Whipple's triad: hypoglycemia (glucose <50 mg/dL) and central nervous system symptoms due to hypoglycemia (confusion, stupor, loss of consciousness). As the good doctor, you will provide the third part of Whipple's triad: give glucose to relieve symptoms. Ninety percent of insulinomas are benign and can be cured with resection. In your work-up, take history and check C peptide first to make sure that the patient is not a diabetic who accidentally took too much insulin or a patient with factitious disorder. C peptide is high with insulinoma, low with other conditions.

◆ **Gastrinoma:** Zollinger–Ellison syndrome is gastrinoma plus acid hypersecretion and peptic ulcer disease (gastrin causes acid secretion). Peptic ulcers are often multiple and resistant to therapy; they may be in an unusual location (distal duodenum or jejunum). More than half are malignant.

◆ **Glucagonoma (alpha cell tumor):** Hyperglycemia with high glucagon level and migratory necrotizing skin erythema.

Ovarian Cancer

Ovarian cancer usually manifests late, with weight loss, pelvic mass, ascites, and/or bowel obstruction in a postmenopausal woman. Any ovarian enlargement in a postmenopausal woman is cancer until proved otherwise. In women of reproductive age, most ovarian enlargements are benign. Ultrasound is a good first test to evaluate an ovarian lesion. Treatment includes debulking surgery and chemotherapy; prognosis is usually poor. Most ovarian cancer arises from ovarian epithelium. Serous cystadenocarcinoma, the most common ovarian cancer, often has psammoma bodies on histopathology.

 Oral contraceptives have been shown to reduce the incidence of ovarian cancer by 50% (also reduce endometrial cancer risk).

Germ cell tumors provide fodder for Step 2 questions:

◆ **Teratoma/dermoid cyst:** Look for a description of the tumor to include skin, hair, and/or teeth or bone; it can show up as pelvic calcifications on x-ray.

◆ **Sertoli-Leydig cell tumor:** Causes virilization (hirsutism, receding hairline, deepening voice, clitoromegaly).

◆ **Granulosa-theca cell tumor:** Causes feminization and precocious puberty.

Terms worth knowing:

◆ **Meigs' syndrome:** Ovarian fibroma, ascites, and right hydrothorax or pleural effusion

◆ **Krukenberg's tumor:** Stomach (or other gastrointestinal [GI]) cancer with metastases to the ovaries

Cervical Cancer

Papanicolaou (Pap) smears decrease the incidence and mortality of cervical cancer. Give female patients a Pap smear if they are due, even if they present with an unrelated complaint. Follow up any dysplastic Pap smear with colposcopy-directed biopsies and endocervical curettage. If the Pap smear shows microinvasive cancer, proceed to conization. Frankly invasive cancer needs surgery and/or radiation.

Risk factors for cervical cancer:

- Younger than 20 years old at first coitus, pregnancy, or marriage
- Multiple sexual partners (role of human papillomavirus and possibly herpes) or coitus with a promiscuous person
- Smoking
- Low socioeconomic status
- High parity (which protects against endometrial cancer)

IMPORTANT POINTS

1 Invasive cervical cancer begins in the transformation zone and usually manifests with vaginal bleeding or discharge (may be postcoital, intermenstrual spotting, or abnormal menstrual bleeding).

2 Maternal exposure to diethylstilbestrol causes daughters to get clear cell cancer of the cervix or vagina.

Uterine Cancer

Postmenopausal bleeding is cancer until proved otherwise; endometrial cancer is the most common cancer to manifest in this fashion (fourth most common cancer in women). Get an endometrial biopsy for any patient with postmenopausal bleeding (as well as a Pap smear, endocervical curettage, and pelvic ultrasound). Any woman with unexplained gynecologic bleeding that persists needs a Pap smear, endocervical curettage, and endometrial biopsy.

Risk factors for endometrial cancer:

- Chronic, unopposed estrogen stimulation, as in polycystic ovary syndrome, estrogen-secreting neoplasm (granulosa-theca cell tumor), and estrogen replacement (increases risk of cancer only if taken without progesterone)
- Diabetes mellitus
- Gallbladder disease
- Hypertension
- Late menopause
- Nulliparity
- Obesity

IMPORTANT POINTS

1 Oral contraceptives have been shown to reduce the incidence of endometrial as well as ovarian cancer.

> **2** Most uterine cancer is adenocarcinoma and spreads by direct extension.
>
> **3** Treat with surgery and/or radiation.

Miscellaneous Neoplasms

ADRENAL TUMORS

Adrenal tumors may be functional and cause primary hyperaldosteronism (Conn's syndrome) or hyperadrenalism (Cushing's disease). Patients also might have a pheochromocytoma; look for intermittent, severe hypertension with mental status changes, headaches, and diaphoresis. Check 24-hour urine catecholamines (vanillylmandelic acid, homovanillic acid, or metanephrines). Most adrenal tumors are benign nonfunctional adenomas and can be diagnosed by CT or MRI. Percutaneous needle biopsy can be used in uncertain cases.

BLADDER CANCER

Look for persistent, painless hematuria. Patients often are smokers or work in the rubber or dye industry (aniline dye exposure). Do CT scan with contrast first, but this is better for renal cancer than bladder cancer (both cause hematuria). Cystoscopy is usually done first to evaluate a potential bladder cancer. Local destructive therapy is done for noninvasive tumors, and cystectomy with adjuvant chemoradiotherapy is done for invasive disease.

BRAIN TUMORS

In adults, two thirds of primary tumors (metastases are more common than primary tumors) are supratentorial (i.e., cerebral hemispheres), whereas in children two thirds are infratentorial (posterior fossa; i.e., cerebellum and brainstem). In either group, look for new-onset seizures, neurologic deficits, or signs of intracranial hypertension (headache, blurred vision, papilledema, projectile nausea and vomiting). In children, also look for hydrocephalus and ataxia.

The most common types in adults are gliomas (most are intraparenchymal astrocytomas with little or no calcification) and meningiomas (usually calcified, external to the brain substance). In children, the most common types are cerebellar astrocytoma and medulloblastoma, followed by ependymoma.

Treatment is surgical removal, which may be followed by radiation and chemotherapy, depending on the tumor.

IMPORTANT POINTS

1 A young, obese woman who has headaches, papilledema, and vomiting with a negative CT or MRI has pseudotumor cerebri, *not* a malignancy.

2 The most common primary posterior fossa tumors in children are astrocytoma and medulloblastoma; in adults, it is acoustic neuroma (watch for neurofibromatosis) and hemangioblastoma (watch for von Hippel–Lindau syndrome). Metastases (Fig. 9-7) are much more likely than primary tumors in adults.

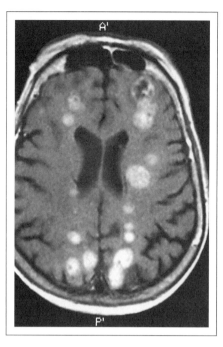

FIGURE 9-7. Axial T1-weighted magnetic resonance image of metastases from breast carcinoma following administration of contrast (gadolinium). Multiple nodular enhancing masses of varying sizes are seen. Some have low signal intensity centers signifying necrosis.

3 Children can develop craniopharyngiomas (remnant of Rathke's pouch), a classically calcified tumor in or around the sella turcica.

CARCINOID TUMORS

The most common location is the small bowel, but carcinoid is the most common appendiceal tumor (other locations are uncommon). The liver breaks down serotonin and other vasoactive secreted substances to make the tumor asymptomatic, but when carcinoid metastasizes to the liver and vasoactive products reach the systemic circulation, symptoms begin (carcinoid syndrome): episodic cutaneous flushing, abdominal cramps, diarrhea, and right-sided heart valve damage. Urinary 5-hydroxyindoleacetic acid (5-HIAA) is increased (a product of serotonin breakdown). Lung carcinoids also occur but the tumor is rarely endocrinologically active.

ESOPHAGEAL CANCER

Signs and symptoms of esophageal cancer include weight loss, possible anemia, and complaints that "my food is sticking," which progresses to dysphagia for liquid. Patients present late, because early cancer is often asymptomatic. The most common type is now adenocarcinoma, seen in obese whites and blacks with long-term history of reflux and/or heartburn. Barrett's esophagus (columnar metaplasia of esophageal squamous epithelium due to chronic acid reflux) is a precursor to adenocarcinoma and, once found, routine endoscopic surveillance for cancer is indicated. Look for chronic smoker and drinker (blacks more than whites) when the subtype is squamous cell.

HISTIOCYTOSIS

CD1+ Birbeck granules (cytoplasmic inclusion bodies that look like tennis rackets) within histiocytes.

KAPOSI'S SARCOMA

Kaposi's sarcoma is mostly seen in HIV-positive patients. It is a vascular skin tumor that starts as a papule or plaque, commonly on the upper body or in the oral cavity. The classic description is a rash that does not respond to multiple treatments.

LIVER TUMORS

Hepatocellular carcinoma is caused by alcohol, chronic hepatitis (B or C), and anything else that causes cirrhosis (hemochromatosis is especially known to cause liver cancer). Alpha fetoprotein is often elevated and can be measured postoperatively to detect recurrences. Patients have a history of alcoholism, chronic hepatitis, and/or hemochromatosis or other causes of cirrhosis and present with weight loss, right upper quadrant pain, and an enlarged liver. Surgery is the only hope for cure; prognosis is poor. Liver metastases are shown in Figure 9–8.

Other tumors of the liver:

◆ **Angiosarcoma:** Look for industrial exposure to vinyl chloride.

◆ **Cholangiosarcoma:** 50% of patients have a history of ulcerative colitis; liver flukes (*Clonorchis*) might be the cause in immigrants.

◆ **Hemangioma:** The most common primary tumor of the liver; generally left alone. Definitive diagnosis usually possible with CT, MRI, or nuclear medicine ("hemangioma scan"). Surgery is done only in the rare case of symptoms due to large size. Percutaneous needle biopsy can be done in uncertain cases.

◆ **Hepatic adenoma:** Women of reproductive age taking oral contraceptives. Stop the pills! The tumor may then regress; if not, surgical removal is generally advocated after establishing the diagnosis with percutaneous needle biopsy.

◆ **Hepatoblastoma:** The main primary liver tumor in children.

NASOPHARYNGEAL CANCER

Nasopharyngeal cancer is typically seen in Asians; remember association with Epstein–Barr virus.

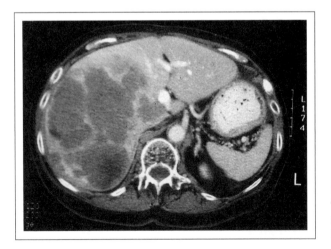

FIGURE 9-8. Large liver metastases from colon carcinoma. Contrast-enhanced computed tomography shows replacement of the right hepatic lobe and a portion of the left hepatic lobe by hypodense lesions.

ORAL CANCER

Like other head and neck malignancies, oral cancer is usually the squamous cell type and due to smoking, chewing tobacco, and/or drinking alcohol; also look for poor oral hygiene. Oral cancer often starts as leukoplakia (know the appearance), which must be differentiated from oral hairy leukoplakia, a condition associated with Epstein–Barr virus that affects HIV-positive patients.

OSTEOSARCOMA

Osteosarcoma is seen in 10- to 30-year-olds; classic x-ray finding is a "sunburst" or Codman's triangle appearance of periosteal reaction (Fig. 9-9) in the distal femur or proximal tibia.

PITUITARY TUMORS

Look for bitemporal hemianopsia (order an MRI if the patient has it) in larger, often nonfunctioning pituitary adenomas. The most common type of functioning tumor is a prolactinoma (high prolactin levels that cause galactorrhea and menstrual and sexual dysfunction). Other functional adenomas can cause Cushing's disease or hyperthyroidism.

RETINOBLASTOMA

Retinoblastoma manifests as leukocoria (red reflex is white with a penlight; Fig. 9-10) or unilateral exophthalmos in a young child; the inherited form may be bilateral.

SARCOMA BOTRYOIDES

Sarcoma botryoides is a rhabdomyosarcoma subtype that manifests in a girl with a "bunch of grapes" coming out of the vagina.

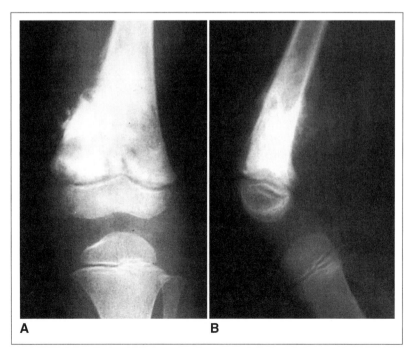

FIGURE 9-9. An aggressive osteosarcoma in the distal metaphysis of the femur. A, Anteroposterior radiograph shows bone destruction and extension into the adjacent soft tissues. **B,** Lateral radiograph shows the classic Codman's triangle–type periosteal reaction proximal to the lesion. (From Burke DL, Collins AJ: Musculoskeletal imaging. In Provenzale JM, Nelson RC (eds): Duke Radiology Case Review. Philadelphia, Lippincott, 1998, pp 229–287; with permission.)

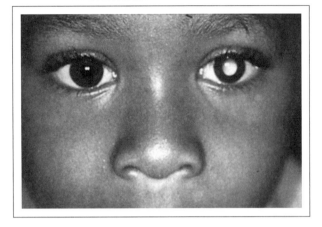

FIGURE 9-10. Leukocoria in the left eye due to a retinoblastoma. (From Klintworth GK: The eye. In Rubin E, Farber JL (eds): Pathology, 3rd ed. Philadelphia, Lippincott, 1999, pp 1537–1565; with permission.)

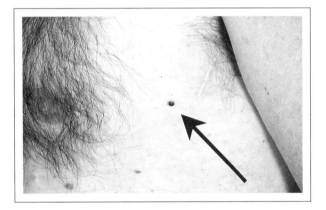

FIGURE 9-11. Skin melanoma (*arrow*) of trunk.

SKIN CANCER

Ultraviolet light increases the risk of basal, squamous, and melanoma (Fig. 9-11) skin cancer. The **ABCDs** of melanoma should make you suspicious of malignancy. Biopsy any lesion with any of these characteristics: **a**symmetry, **b**orders (irregular), **c**olor (change in color or multiple colors), or **d**iameter (the bigger the lesion, the more likely that it is malignant). Know the classic appearance of basal cell cancer (pearly, umbilicated, telangiectasias). Basal cell cancer is extremely common and almost never metastasizes. Squamous cancer rarely metastasizes, whereas melanoma commonly metastasizes. Biopsy any suspicious lesion (excisional biopsy).

STOMACH CANCER

Risk factors for stomach cancer are Japanese race, increasing age, smoking, and consumption of smoked meat. *Helicobacter pylori* also is implicated. Krukenberg's tumor is stomach cancer with bilateral ovarian metastases. Virchow's node is left supraclavicular node enlargement due to visceral cancer spread (classically stomach cancer). If a gastric ulcer is seen on upper GI barium series or endoscopy, it should be biopsied to exclude malignancy.

TESTICULAR CANCER

The most common solid malignancy in men younger than 30 years. The main risk factor is cryptorchidism. Transillumination and ultrasound help to distinguish hydrocele (fluid-filled, transilluminates) from cancer (solid). The most common type is seminoma (radiosensitive). Lymphatic drainage follows testicular veins to the retroperitoneal lymph nodes in the region of the abdominal aorta and inferior vena cava at the level of the renal veins.

THYROID CANCER

In thyroid cancer, the patient presents with a nodule in the thyroid gland. Be suspicious of cancer in any of the following scenarios: cold nodule on nuclear scan, male patient, history of childhood irradiation, nodule described as "stony hard," recent or rapid enlargement, and increased calcitonin level (medullary thyroid cancer—usually in patients with multiple endocrine neoplasia type II). To evaluate a nodule in the thyroid, get thyroid function tests and an ultrasound scan. Thyroid-stimulating hormone is the best screening test; "toxic" or functional nodules are unlikely to be cancer. On a nuclear scan, a cold nodule or area of decreased uptake is more suspicious than normal or increased uptake. Perform fine-needle aspiration for diagnosis.

UNICAMERAL BONE CYST

A unicameral bone cyst is an expansile, lytic, well-demarcated lesion in the proximal portion of the humerus in children and adolescents. It is benign but can weaken bone enough to cause a pathologic fracture.

WILMS' TUMOR AND NEUROBLASTOMA

Both Wilms' tumor and neuroblastoma manifest as flank masses in children at a peak age of around 2 years old. Neuroblastomas occur at a slightly younger age, usually arise from the adrenal gland, and classically contain calcifications, whereas Wilms' tumor arises from the kidney; thus imaging tests (e.g., CT scan or MRI) can usually tell the two apart. Rarely, neuroblastomas regress spontaneously (for unknown reasons).

 Patients with cancer, like all others, have the right to refuse treatment. However, watch for and treat depression, especially in terminal patients, before accepting a patient's refusal of treatment.

10 INFECTIOUS DISEASE

General

Table 10-1 lists empiric treatment to use while waiting for test results. Table 10-2 lists empiric treatment for various bacteria.

Staining hints:

◆ Gram-positive organisms are blue-purple; gram-negative organisms are red.

◆ Gram-positive cocci in chains = streptococci

◆ Gram-positive cocci in clusters = staphylococci

◆ Gram-positive cocci in pairs (diplococci) = *Streptococcus pneumoniae*

◆ Gram-negative coccobacilli (small rods) = *Haemophilus* spp.

◆ Gram-negative diplococci = *Neisseria* (gonorrhea, septic arthritis, meningitis) or *Moraxella* spp. (lungs, sinusitis)

◆ Gram-negative rod that is plump and has a thick capsule (mucoid appearance) = *Klebsiella* spp.

◆ Gram-positive rods that form spores = *Clostridium, Bacillus* spp.

◆ Pseudohyphae = *Candida* spp. (hyphae are a marker for the presence of fungi; Fig. 10-1)

◆ Acid-fast organisms = *Mycobacterium* tuberculosis, *Nocardia* spp.

◆ Gram-positive organism with sulfur granules = *Actinomyces* spp. (pelvic inflammatory disease in women who use intrauterine devices; rare cause of neck mass and cervical adenitis)

◆ Silver-staining = *Pneumocystis jiroveci* and cat-scratch disease

◆ Positive India ink preparation (thick capsule) = *Cryptococcus* spp.

◆ Spirochete = *Treponema, Leptospira* spp. (both seen only on dark-field microscopy), Borrelia sp. (regular light microscope)

Classic topics for infectious disease questions:

◆ Patient (perhaps a gardener) stuck with thorn: *Sporothrix schenckii* (a fungus). Treat with itraconazole, fluconazole, or oral potassium iodide.

Table 10-1. EMPIRIC THERAPY WHILE AWAITING CULTURE AND SENSITIVITY RESULTS

Condition	Main Organism(s)	Empiric Antibiotic(s)
Bronchitis	Virus, *Hemophilus influenzae, Moraxella* spp.	Amoxicillin, erythromycin
Cellulitis	Streptococci, staphylococci	Antistaphylococcal penicillin (covers both)
Endocarditis	Staphylococci, streptococci	Antistaphylococcal penicillin (or vancomycin) + aminoglycoside
Meningitis (child or adult)	*Streptococcus pneumoniae, Neisseria meningitidis**	Third-generation cephalosporin or meropenem + vancomycin
Meningitis (neonate)	Streptococci B, *Escherichia coli, Listeria* spp.	Ampicillin + aminoglycoside, third-generation cephalosporin
Osteomyelitis	*Staphylococcus aureus, Salmonella* spp.	Antistaphylococcal penicillin,† vancomycin
Pneumonia (atypical)	*Mycoplasma, Chlamydia* spp.	Macrolide antibiotic, doxycycline
Pneumonia (classic)	*S. pneumoniae, H. influenzae*	Third-generation cephalosporin, azithromycin
Septic arthritis‡	*S. aureus*	Antistaphylococcal penicillin, vancomycin
	Gonococci	Ceftriaxone, fluoroquinolone, spectinomycin
Sepsis	Gram-negative organisms, streptococci, staphylococci	Third-generation penicillin or cephalosporin + aminoglycoside, imipenem
Urinary tract infection	*E. coli*	Trimethoprim-sulfamethoxazole, nitrofurantoin, amoxicillin, quinolones

H. influenzae type b is no longer as common a cause of meningitis in children because of widespread vaccination. In a child with no history of immunization, *H. influenzae* is the most likely cause of meningitis.

†Examples: dicloxacillin, methicillin.

‡Think of staphylococci if the patient is monogamous or not sexually active. Think of gonorrhea for younger adults who are sexually active.

◆ Aplastic crisis in sickle cell disease or other hemoglobinopathy: parvovirus B19

◆ Sepsis after splenectomy (or autosplenectomy in sickle cell disease): *S. pneumoniae, H. influenzae, N. meningitidis* (encapsulated bugs)

◆ Pneumonia in the Southwest (California, Arizona): *Coccidioides immitis;* treat with itraconazole, fluconazole, or amphotericin B (for severe disease)

◆ Pneumonia after cave exploring or exposure to bird droppings in Ohio and Mississippi River valleys: *Histoplasma capsulatum*

◆ Pneumonia after exposure to a parrot or exotic bird: *Chlamydia psittaci*

◆ Fungus ball or hemoptysis after tuberculosis-induced cavitary disease: *Aspergillus* spp.

◆ Pneumonia in a patient with silicosis: tuberculosis

◆ Diarrhea after hiking or drinking from a stream: *Giardia lamblia;* cysts in stool; treat with metronidazole

◆ Pregnant women with cats: *Toxoplasma gondii*

◆ B_{12} deficiency and abdominal symptoms: *Diphyllobothrium latum*

◆ Seizures with ring-enhancing brain lesion on computed tomography (CT): *Taenia solium* (cysticercosis)

◆ Bladder cancer (squamous cell) in Middle East and Africa: *Schistosoma haematobium*

Table 10-2. EMPIRIC ANTIBIOTICS OF CHOICE FOR DIFFERENT BUGS*

Bug	Antibiotic	Other Choices
Bacteroides sp.	Metronidazole	Clindamycin
Borrelia spp.	Doxycycline, amoxicillin	Erythromycin
Chlamydia spp.	Azithromycin, doxycycline	Erythromycin, fluoroquinolone
Enterococci	Penicillin or ampicillin + aminoglycoside	Vancomycin + aminoglycoside
Escherichia coli	Third-generation cephalosporin, fluoroquinolone	Aminoglycoside
Gonococci[†]	Ceftriaxone or fluoroquinolone	Spectinomycin
Haemophilus sp.	Second- or third-generation cephalosporin	Ampicillin
Klebsiella spp.	Third-generation cephalosporin, fluoroquinolone	Third-generation penicillin + aminoglycoside
Meningococcus	Ampicillin	Cefotaxime, chloramphenicol
Mycobacterium tuberculosis	Isoniazid–rifampin	Ethambutol, pyrazinamide
Mycoplasma spp.	Azithromycin, fluoroquinolone	Doxycycline
Pseudomonas spp.	Extended spectrum pencillin + aminoglycoside	Aztreonam, imipenem
Streptococci A or B	Penicillin, cephazolin	Erythromycin
Treponema spp.	Penicillin	Doxycycline
Streptococcus pneumoniae	Third-generation cephalosporin, fluoroquinolone	Fluoroquinolone
Staphylococci	Antistaphylococcal penicillin	Vancomycin (MRSA)

*Always use culture sensitivities to guide therapy if available.
   †With genital infections, treat for presumed *Chlamydia* coinfection with azithromycin or doxycycline.
   MRSA, methicillin-resistant *S. aureus.*

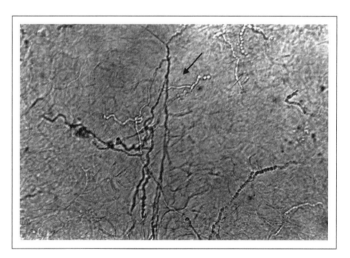

FIGURE 10-1. Hyphae in a potassium hydroxide (KOH) prep (*arrow*).

◆ Worm infection in children: *Enterobius* spp. (positive tape test, perianal itching)

◆ Fever, muscle pain, eosinophilia, and periorbital edema after eating raw meat: *Trichinella spiralis* (trichinosis)

◆ Gastroenteritis in young children: rotavirus

◆ Food poisoning after eating reheated rice: *Bacillus cereus*

◆ Food poisoning after eating raw seafood: *Vibrio parahaemolyticus*

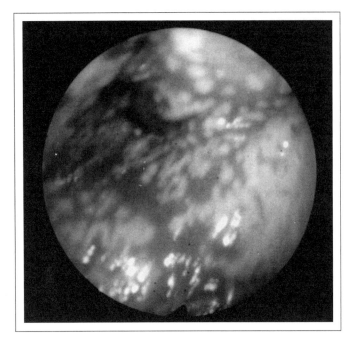

FIGURE 10-2. Colonoscopy reveals the classic "pseudo-membranes" (the light-colored, 3- to 10-mm plaques scattered about the mucosa) of *C. difficile* colitis.

◆ Diarrhea after traveling to Mexico (Montezuma's revenge): *Escherichia coli*

◆ Diarrhea after antibiotics: *Clostridium difficile* (Fig. 10-2); treat with oral metronidazole or vancomycin

◆ Infant paralyzed after eating honey: *Clostridium botulinum* (toxin blocks acetylcholine release)

◆ Genital lesions in children in the absence of sexual abuse or activity: molluscum contagiosum

◆ Cellulitis after cat or dog bites: *Pasteurella multocida* (treat cat and dog bites with prophylactic ampicillin)

◆ Slaughterhouse worker with fever: *Brucella* spp.

◆ Pneumonia after being in a hotel, near an air conditioner or water tower: *Legionella pneumophila*; treat with azithromycin or fluoroquinolone

◆ Burn wound infection with blue/green color: *Pseudomonas* spp. (*S. aureus* also common, but without blue-green color)

Pneumonia

Look for classic clues to differentiate. The gold standard for diagnosis is sputum culture; do blood cultures, too.

Common causes:

◆ ***Streptococcus pneumoniae:*** Most common cause, especially in older adults. Look for rapid onset of shaking chills after an upper respiratory infection; then fever, pleurisy, and productive cough (yellowish-green or rust-colored from blood). X-ray shows lobar consolidation (Fig. 10-3). White blood cell count is high, with large percentage of

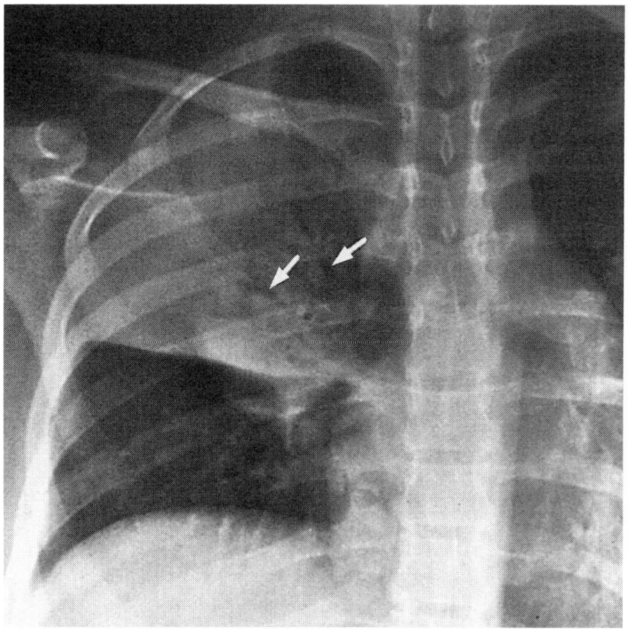

FIGURE 10-3. Alveolar lung disease—air bronchograms. Note black, air-filled airways (*arrows*) surrounded by white, fluid-filled airspaces in this patient with right upper lobe pneumococcal pneumonia. The sharply defined lower margin of the area of pneumonia is produced by the minor, or horizontal, fissure.

neutrophils. Give vaccine to all children, patients older than 65 years, splenectomized patients, patients with sickle cell disease, immunocompromised patients (HIV, malignancy, organ transplant), and all patients with chronic disease (diabetes mellitus; cardiac, pulmonary, renal, or liver disease). Good treatments include third-generation cephalosporin or fluoroquinolone.

◆ *Haemophilus influenzae:* Second only to S. *pneumoniae* as the most common cause of pneumonia; more common in young children. Resembles S. *pneumoniae* clinically. Treat with ampicillin or amoxicillin or second- or third-generation cephalosporin if gram-negative coccobacilli are seen on sputum Gram stain.

◆ *Staphylococcus aureus:* Causes hospital-acquired pneumonia and pneumonia in patients with cystic fibrosis (second to *Pseudomonas* spp.), intravenous drug abusers, and patients with chronic granulomatous disease (look for recurrent lung abscesses). Empyema and lung abscesses are relatively common. Cultures usually are positive.

◆ **Gram-negative organisms:** *Pseudomonas* spp. classically are associated with cystic fibrosis; *Klebsiella* spp. is the classic cause in skid-row alcoholics and homeless persons; enteric gram-negative organisms (e.g., *E. coli*) are common with aspiration, neutropenia, and hospital-acquired pneumonia. High mortality rate because of patients affected and severity of pneumonia (abscesses common). Treat empirically with a third-generation penicillin or cephalosporin plus aminoglycoside.

◆ *Mycoplasma* spp: Most common in adolescents and young adults (the classic case is a college student who lives in the dorm and has sick contacts). Called "atypical" pneumonia because it is different from S. *pneumoniae*, with long prodrome and gradual worsening of malaise, headaches, dry nonproductive cough, and sore throat. Chest x-ray shows a patchy, diffuse bronchopneumonia (the x-ray classically looks terrible, although the patient does not feel that bad). Look for positive cold-agglutinin antibody titers (can cause hemolysis and anemia). The classic empiric treatment of atypical pneumonia is a macrolide antibiotic (e.g., azithromycin).

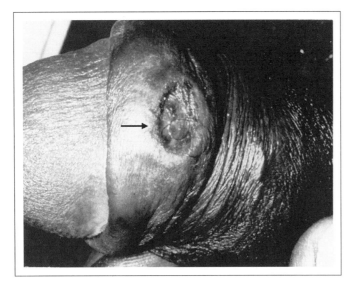

FIGURE 10-4. Primary chancre of syphilis (*arrow*).

◆ *Chlamydia pneumoniae:* Second only to *Mycoplasma* spp. as cause of pneumonia in adolescents and young adults. It manifests similarly but has negative cold-agglutinin antibody titers.

◆ **Viral pneumonia:** Viruses commonly cause respiratory infections (respiratory syncytial virus, influenza, parainfluenza, adenovirus)

◆ *Pneumocystis jiroveci* **pneumonia (PCP) and cytomegalovirus (CMV):** Always suspect in HIV-positive patients. PCP is more common; bronchoalveolar lavage often is required to obtain the diagnosis, though many treat empirically. PCP shows up with silver stains. Treat with trimethoprim–sulfamethoxazole; the alternative is pentamidine. PCP is acquired when the CD4 count is below 200, at which point you should institute PCP prophylaxis in an HIV-positive patient. CMV has intracellular inclusion bodies. Treat with ganciclovir; foscarnet is an alternative.

Syphilis

Screen with Venereal Disease Research Laboratory (VDRL) or rapid plasma reagin (RPR) test; if positive, confirm with fluorescent treponemal antibody, absorbed (FTA-ABS) or microhemagglutination *Treponema pallidum* (MHA-TP) test. *T. pallidum* also can be seen with dark-field microscopy but not with a Gram stain. Screen all pregnant women with VDRL/RPR. Treatment is penicillin; use doxycycline for penicillin allergy.

Three stages of syphilis:

1. **Primary:** Look for painless chancre (Fig. 10-4) that resolves on its own within 8 weeks.

2. **Secondary:** Roughly 6 weeks to 18 months after infection; look for condyloma lata (Fig. 10-5), maculopapular rash (especially involving palms and soles of feet), and lymphadenopathy.

3. **Tertiary:** Now quite rare, it occurs years after the initial infection. Between secondary and tertiary stages is the latent phase, when the disease is quiet and asymptomatic.

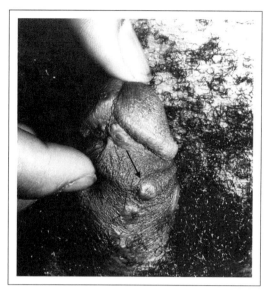

FIGURE 10-5. Condyloma lata of the penis (*arrow*).

Look for gummas (granulomas in many different organs), neurologic symptoms and signs (neurosyphilis, Argyll Robertson pupil, dementia, paresis, tabes dorsalis, Charcot joints), and/or thoracic aortic aneurysms.

 Watch for false-positive VDRL/RPR in patients with lupus erythematosus. For other sexually transmitted diseases, see Chapter 18, Gynecology.

Infectious Rashes

Infectious rashes occur most often in children. Treatment is supportive only unless otherwise specified.

CHICKENPOX (VARICELLA)

The description and progression of the rash itself should lead to the diagnosis: Discrete macules (usually on the trunk) turn into papules, which turn into vesicles that rupture and crust over. These changes occur within 1 day. The lesions appear in successive crops; therefore, the rash is in different stages of progression in different areas. The patient is infectious until the last lesion crusts over. A Tzanck smear of tissue from the base of a vesicle shows multinucleated giant cells (Fig. 10-6).

A complication is infection of the lesions (streptococci, staphylococci [erysipelas], cellulitis, sepsis). The patient should be instructed to keep clean to avoid infection. Other complications include pneumonia (especially in very young children and immunocompromised adults), encephalitis, and Reye's syndrome. Do *not* give aspirin to any child with a fever unless the diagnosis requires its use.

Varicella zoster immunoglobulin is available for prophylaxis in patients with debilitating illness (e.g., leukemia, AIDS) if you see them within 4 days of exposure or in newborns of mothers with chickenpox. Acyclovir may be used in severe cases. The

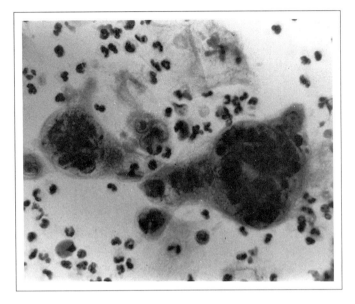

FIGURE 10-6. Positive Tzanck preparation.

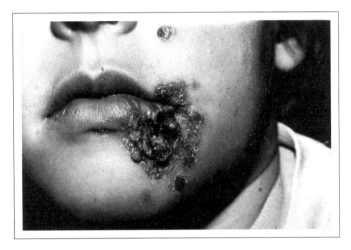

FIGURE 10-7. Impetigo.

varicella zoster virus can reactivate years later to cause shingles (zoster), which is characterized by dermatomal distribution of rash. Pain and paresthesias often precede the rash.

ERYTHEMA INFECTIOSUM (FIFTH DISEASE)

Classic "slapped-cheek" rash (confluent erythema over the cheeks) appears around the same time as mild constitutional symptoms (low fever, malaise). One day later, a maculopapular rash appears on the arms, legs, and trunk. It is caused by parvovirus B19 (the same virus that causes aplastic crisis in sickle cell disease).

IMPETIGO

Look for history of skin break (e.g., previous chickenpox, insect bite, scabies, cut). The rash starts as thin-walled vesicles that rupture and form yellowish crusts (Fig. 10-7). The skin often is described as "weeping." Classically, lesions are on the face and tend to be localized. Impetigo is infectious; look for sick contacts. Treat with oral antistaphylococcal penicillin to cover streptococci and staphylococci, the most common causative bugs.

INFECTIOUS MONONUCLEOSIS (EPSTEIN–BARR VIRUS INFECTION)

Look for fatigue, fever, pharyngitis, and lymphadenopathy (similar to streptococcal pharyngitis, but malaise tends to be more prolonged and pronounced). To differentiate from streptococcal disease, look for splenomegaly; hepatomegaly; atypical lymphocytes (bizarre forms that can resemble leukemia) with lymphocytosis, anemia, or thrombocytopenia; and positive serology (heterophile antibodies [e.g., Monospot test] or specific EBV antibodies, such as the viral capsid antigen). Patients can develop splenic rupture and should avoid contact sports and heavy lifting. Include HIV in the differential diagnosis. Remember the association of EBV with nasopharyngeal cancer and African Burkitt's lymphoma.

KAWASAKI'S SYNDROME (MUCOCUTANEOUS LYMPH NODE SYNDROME)

Kawasaki's syndrome is rare and usually occurs in patients younger than 5 years. Diagnostic criteria include fever longer than 5 days (mandatory for diagnosis); bilateral conjunctival injection; changes in the lips, tongue, or oral mucosa (strawberry tongue, fissuring, injection); changes in the extremities (desquamation, edema, erythema); polymorphous truncal rash (usually begins one day after the fever starts); and cervical lymphadenopathy. Also look for arthralgia or arthritis. The most feared complications involve the heart (coronary artery aneurysms, congestive heart failure, arrhythmias, myocarditis, myocardial infarction). Think of Kawasaki's syndrome in the differential diagnosis of any child who has a myocardial infarction. If suspicion is high, give aspirin and intravenous (IV) immunoglobulin, both of which reduce cardiac lesions. Follow up with echocardiography to detect heart involvement.

MEASLES (RUBEOLA)

Look for a reason for the patient not to be immunized. Koplik's spots (tiny white spots on buccal mucosa) are seen 3 days after high fever. Other symptoms include cough, runny nose, and conjunctivitis and photophobia. On the next day, the rash (maculopapular) begins on the head and neck and spreads downward to cover the trunk (cephalocaudal progression). Complications include pneumonia (giant-cell pneumonia, especially in very young and immunocompromised patients), otitis media, and encephalitis (which may be acute or cause subacute sclerosing panencephalitis, which usually occurs years later).

ROCKY MOUNTAIN SPOTTED FEVER (*RICKETTSIA RICKETTSII* INFECTION)

Look for history of a tick bite (especially on the East Coast) one week before the development of high fever or chills, severe headache, and prostration or severe malaise. The rash appears roughly 4 days after symptoms on the palms and wrists and the soles and ankles, rapidly spreading to the trunk and face (unique pattern of spread). Patients often look very sick (disseminated intravascular coagulation, delirium). Treat with doxycycline or chloramphenicol.

ROSEOLA INFANTUM (EXANTHEM SUBITUM)

Easy to recognize because of progression: high fever (may be >40° C) with no apparent cause for 4 days (patient may get febrile seizures), then an abrupt return to normal temperature as a diffuse macular and maculopapular rash appears on the chest and abdomen. Rare in children older than 3 years, it is caused by human herpesvirus type 6 (a DNA virus).

RUBELLA (GERMAN MEASLES)

Most important because of infection in pregnant women. Screen and immunize any woman of reproductive age *before* she becomes pregnant; the vaccine is contraindicated in pregnant women. Rubella is milder than measles, with low-grade fever, malaise, tender swelling of the suboccipital and postauricular nodes, and arthralgias. After a 2- to 3-day prodrome, the rash (maculopapular, faint) starts on the face and neck and spreads to the trunk (cephalocaudal progression). Complications include encephalitis and otitis media.

SCARLET FEVER

Look for a history of untreated streptococcal pharyngitis (caused only by *Streptococcus* species that produce erythrogenic toxin), followed by a sandpaper-like rash on the abdomen and trunk with classic circumoral pallor and strawberry tongue. The rash tends to desquamate once the fever subsides. Treat with penicillin to prevent rheumatic fever.

Endocarditis

Either acute (fulminant, most commonly caused by *S. aureus*) or subacute (insidious onset, most commonly caused by *Streptococcus viridans*). Look for general signs of infection (e.g., fever, tachycardia, malaise) plus new-onset heart murmur, embolic phenomena (stroke and other infarcts), Osler's nodes (painful nodules on tips of fingers), Roth's spots (round retinal hemorrhages with white centers), splinter hemorrhages under fingernails, and septic shock (more dramatic with acute than subacute disease). Diagnosis is made by blood cultures. Echocardiogram may be able to visualize valve vegetations.

Empiric treatment is begun with wide-spectrum antibiotics until culture and sensitivity results are known. A third-generation penicillin or cephalosporin plus aminoglycoside is a reasonable choice.

Patients more likely to be affected include IV drug abusers (who develop right-sided lesions, although left-sided lesions are much more common in the general population); patients with abnormal heart valves (prosthetic valves, rheumatic valvular disease, or congenital heart defects); and postoperative patients (especially after genitourinary, gastrointestinal, or dental surgery—hence the use of **prophylaxis** in susceptible persons).

Meningitis

The highest incidence of meningitis is seen in neonates; >75% of cases are seen in patients younger than 2 years. Thus, the decision about when to do a lumbar tap is difficult, because such patients often do not have classic physical findings (Kernig's and Brudzinski's signs). Look for lethargy, hyper- *or* hypothermia, poor tone, bulging fontanel, vomiting, photophobia, altered consciousness, and signs of generalized sepsis (hypotension, jaundice, respiratory distress). Seizures may be seen, but simple febrile seizures also are possible if the patient is between 5 months and 6 years old and has a fever >102° F in the absence of other signs of meningitis. If seizures occur in the presence of other signs of meningitis or sepsis, proceed to supportive measures, broad-spectrum antibiotics, and lumbar puncture.

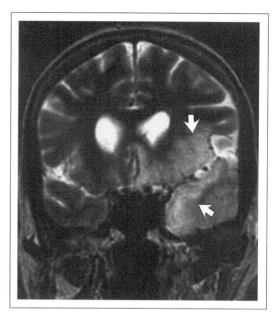

FIGURE 10-8. Magnetic resonance image of herpes encephalitis.

The most common neurologic sequela of meningitis is hearing loss. All patients need formal hearing evaluation after a bout of meningitis; vision testing also is recommended. Other sequelae include mental retardation, motor deficits or paresis, epilepsy, and learning and behavioral disorders.

IMPORTANT POINTS

1 Mumps and measles are possible causes of aseptic (nonbacterial or culture-negative) meningitis. The best prevention is immunization.

2 Watch for herpes encephalitis (Fig. 10-8) if the mother has herpes simplex lesions at the time of the infant's birth. Look for mention of temporal lobe abnormalities on a CT or MRI scan of the head. Give acyclovir.

3 If meningitis is due to *Neisseria* spp., give all contacts ciprofloxacin, ceftriaxone, or rifampin as prophylaxis.

4 For cerebrospinal fluid findings in meningitis, see Chapter 12, Neurology.

Pediatric Respiratory Infections

The big three are croup, epiglottitis, and bronchiolitis: high yield!

BRONCHIOLITIS

Look for a 0- to 18-month-old patient; usually occurs in fall or winter. More than 75% of cases are caused by the respiratory syncytial virus; other causes are parainfluenza and influenza. Patients start with symptoms of viral upper respiratory infection, followed 1 to 2 days later by rapid respirations, intercostal retractions, and expiratory wheezing. The patient also might have crackles on auscultation of the chest. Diffuse hyperinflation of the lungs is classic on chest x-ray; look for flattened diaphragms. Treat supportively (oxygen, mist tent, bronchodilators, IV fluids). Use ribavarin in patients with severe symptoms or increased risk (cyanosis, other health problems).

CROUP OR ACUTE LARYNGOTRACHEITIS

Look for patient to be 1 to 2 years old; usually occurs in fall or winter. About 50% to 75% of cases are due to parainfluenza virus; the other causative agent is influenza. Patients start with symptoms of viral upper respiratory infection (rhinorrhea, cough, and fever) and roughly 1 or 2 days later develop a barking cough, hoarseness, and inspiratory stridor. The "steeple sign" (subglottic tracheal narrowing) is classic on frontal x-ray of the neck. Treat supportively with a mist tent and racemic epinephrine.

EPIGLOTTITIS

The patient usually is 2 to 5 years old. The main cause by far used to be *Haemophilus influenzae* type b, but with widespread vaccination, *H. influenzae* and *S. aureus* are equally frequent. Pick *H. influenzae* if you have to choose. Look for little or no prodrome, with rapid progression to high fever, toxic appearance, drooling, and respiratory distress with no coughing. The "thumb sign" (enlarged, swollen epiglottis) is classic on lateral neck x-ray (Fig. 10-9). Do *not* examine the throat or irritate the patient in any way—you might precipitate airway obstruction. When a case of epiglottitis is presented, the first step is to be prepared to establish an airway. Treat with antibiotics (e.g., third-generation cephalosporin).

DIPHTHERIA AND PERTUSSIS

Diphtheria (*Corynebacterium diphtheriae*) and pertussis (*Bordetella pertussis*) should be considered if the patient is not immunized. Diphtheria is associated with grayish

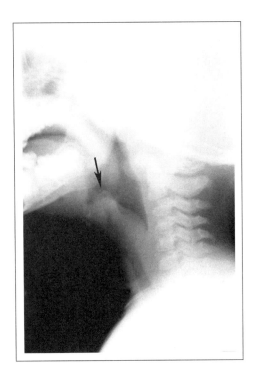

FIGURE 10-9. Classic thumb sign of enlarged, swollen epiglottis.

pseudomembranes (necrotic epithelium and inflammatory exudate) on the pharynx, tonsils, and/or uvula and myocarditis. Pertussis is associated with severe paroxysmal coughing and a high-pitched whooping inspiratory noise (classically called "whooping cough"). Treat both with antibiotics and give antitoxin for diphtheria.

Rabies

In the United States, rabies is usually due to bites from bats, skunks, raccoons, or foxes. Vaccination has eliminated dog rabies. The incubation period is usually around 1 to 2 months. Classic symptoms are hydrophobia and central nervous system signs (paralysis).

After a bite, take these steps:

1. **Local wound treatment:** Cleanse thoroughly with soap; do not cauterize or suture the wound.

2. **Observe the animal.** If possible, capture and observe a dog or cat to see if it develops rabies. If a wild animal (bat, skunk, raccoon, fox) is caught, it should be killed and the tissue examined for rabies.

3. **Prophylaxis with rabies immunoglobulin and vaccine:**
   - If a captured or killed animal has rabies, definitely give prophylaxis and vaccinate.
   - If a wild animal (bat, skunk, raccoon, fox only) bites and escapes, give prophylaxis and vaccine.
   - If a dog or cat bites and escapes, do *not* give prophylaxis or vaccine *unless* the animal acted strangely and/or bit the patient without provocation *and rabies is prevalent in the area (rare)*.
   - Do *not* give prophylaxis or vaccine for bites by rabbits or other rodents (rats, mice, squirrels, chipmunks).

Streptococcal Infection

ENTEROCOCCUS FAECALIS

Enterococcus faecalis are normal bowel flora. *E. faecalis* causes endocarditis, urinary tract infection, and sepsis.

STREPTOCOCCUS AGALACTIAE

Streptococcus agalactiae (strep B) is famous as the most common cause of neonatal meningitis and sepsis. It is acquired from the maternal birth canal, in which it is part of the normal flora. Treat with amoxicillin or ampicillin.

STREPTOCOCCUS PNEUMONIAE

Streptococcus pneumoniae is the common cause of pneumonia, otitis media, meningitis, sinusitis, and sepsis.

STREPTOCOCCUS PYOGENES

Streptococcus pyogenes (strep A) causes several important infections.

Pharyngitis. Look for sore throat with fever, tonsillar exudate, enlarged tender cervical nodes, and leukocytosis. Streptococcal throat culture confirms the diagnosis, but the rapid ''strep test'' is commonly used for convenience. Avoid treating on the boards without confirming the diagnosis. Elevated antistreptolysin O (ASO) and anti-DNase titers also are used retrospectively when needed (rheumatic fever, post-streptococcal glomerulonephritis). Treat with penicillin to avoid rheumatic fever and scarlet fever.

◆ **Rheumatic fever:** Diagnosis is made by history of streptococcal pharyngitis and Jones criteria, major (migratory polyarthritis, carditis, chorea, erythema marginatum, subcutaneous nodules) and minor (elevated erythrocyte sedimentation rate, C-reactive protein, white blood cell count, and ASO titer; prolonged PR interval on electrocardiogram [EKG]; arthralgia). Treat with aspirin; steroids are used for severe carditis (e.g., congestive heart failure).

◆ **Scarlet fever:** Some untreated cases progress to scarlet fever if the streptococcal species produces erythrogenic toxin. Symptoms include red flush in skin (which blanches with pressure, classically with circumoral pallor), truncal rash, strawberry tongue, and late skin desquamation. Kawasaki's syndrome is another cause for this set of symptoms.

◆ **Post-streptococcal glomerulonephritis:** Occurs most commonly after a skin infection, but it can occur after pharyngitis. The patient presents with a history of streptococcal infection (by a nephritogenic strain) 1 to 3 weeks earlier and abrupt onset of hematuria, proteinuria (mild, not in nephrotic range), red blood cell casts, hypertension, edema (especially periorbital), and elevated BUN and creatinine. Treat supportively: Control blood pressure, and use diuretics for severe edema. Unlike scarlet and rheumatic fever, glomerulonephritis cannot be prevented by treating streptococcal infections with antibiotics.

Skin Infections. Skin infections often occur after a break in the skin due to trauma, scabies, or insect bite. Watch for development of post-streptococcal glomerulonephritis.

◆ **Impetigo:** Maculopapules, vesicopustules or bullae, or honey-colored, crusted lesions. Staphylococci are a more common cause than streptococci. Definitely think of staphylococci if a furuncle or carbuncle is present; think of streptococci if glomerulonephritis occurs. Infection is contagious; watch for sick contacts. Treat empirically with antistaphylococcal penicillin (e.g., dicloxacillin).

◆ **Erysipelas:** A superficial cellulitis that is red, shiny, swollen, and tender; may be associated with vesicles and/or bullae, fever, and lymphadenopathy.

◆ **Cellulitis:** Involves subcutaneous tissues (deeper than erysipelas). Streptococci are the most common cause, but staphylococci also may be implicated. Treat empirically with antistaphylococcal penicillin or vancomycin to cover both. If *Pseudomonas* spp. are suspected (diabetic foot ulcers, burns, severe trauma), treat with broad-spectrum penicillin plus an aminoglycoside. If *Pasteurella multocida* is suspected (after dog or cat bites), treat with IV ampicillin. If *Vibrio vulnificus* is suspected (fishermen or other salt-water exposure), treat with tetracycline.

◆ **Necrotizing fasciitis:** Progression of cellulitis to necrosis and gangrene, crepitus, and systemic toxicity (tachycardia, fever, hypotension). Often multiple organisms (aerobes and anaerobes) are involved. Treat with IV fluids, incision and drainage or debridement, and broad-spectrum antibiotics (broad-spectrum penicillin or cephalosporin plus an aminoglycoside).

Endometritis or Puerperal Fever. Endometritis is postdelivery fever and uterine tenderness. Treat with amoxicillin or ampicillin.

STREPTOCOCCUS VIRIDANS

Streptococcus viridans causes subacute endocarditis and dental caries (*Streptococcus mutans*).

Staphylococcal Infection

Staphylococcus aureus **is a common cause of various infections:**

◆ Abscess: especially in the breast after breast-feeding or in the skin after a furuncle
◆ Cellulitis
◆ Endocarditis: especially in drug users
◆ Food poisoning: preformed toxin
◆ Furuncle or carbuncle
◆ Impetigo
◆ Osteomyelitis: most common cause except in patients with sickle cell disease
◆ Pneumonia: often forms lung abscess or empyema
◆ Scalded skin syndrome: preformed toxin that affects younger children, who often start with impetigo, then desquamate (Fig. 10-10)
◆ Septic arthritis
◆ Toxic shock syndrome: preformed toxin, classically in a woman who leaves a tampon in place too long and develops hypotension, fever, and a rash that desquamates
◆ Wound infections

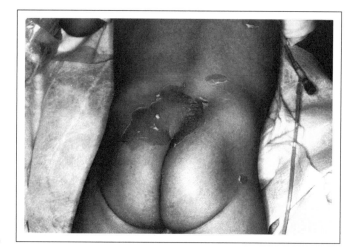

FIGURE 10-10. Staphylococcal scalded skin syndrome.

Staphylococcus epidermidis: IV catheter infections, infections of prosthetic implants (heart valves, vascular grafts), and sepsis.

Staphylococcus saprophyticus: common cause of urinary tract infection. Treat empirically with standard urinary tract infection antibiotics.

 Health care workers who are chronic *Staphylococcus* nasal carriers can cause nosocomial infections. Treat the carrier with antibiotics.

With all staph infections, treat abscesses with incision and drainage, other infections with antistaphylococcal penicillin (e.g., methicillin, dicloxacillin) or vancomycin (MRSA).

DERMATOLOGY

Table 11-1 shows common skin lesions.

ACNE

Know the description of acne: comedones (whiteheads, blackheads), papules, pustules, inflamed nodules, superficial pus-filled cysts with possible inflammatory skin changes (Fig. 11-1). *Propionibacterium acnes* is thought to be partially involved in pathogenesis as well as blockage of pilosebaceous glands. Acne has *not* been proved to be related to food (but if the patient relates it to a food, you can try discontinuing it), exercise, or sex or masturbation, but cosmetics can aggravate it.

Treatment options are numerous. Start with topical benzoyl peroxide, then try topical clindamycin, oral tetracycline, oral erythromycin (for *P. acnes* eradication), and topical tretinoin. The *last resort* is oral isotretinoin. Oral isotretinoin is highly effective, but it is teratogenic (pregnancy testing before and during therapy is mandatory), and it can cause dry skin and mucosae, muscle and joint pain, and liver function abnormalities.

ATOPIC DERMATITIS

Look for family and personal history of allergies (e.g., hay fever) and asthma. This chronic condition begins in the first year of life with red, itchy, weeping skin on the head, upper extremities, and sometimes around the diaper area (Fig. 11-2). The biggest problem is scratching, which leads to skin breaks and possible bacterial infection. Treatment involves antihistamines, topical steroids, and avoidance of drying soaps.

BALDNESS

Watch out for trichotillomania (psychiatric patients pulling out their hair) and alopecia areata (idiopathic and associated with antimicrosomal and other autoantibodies, lupus, syphilis, or chemotherapy) as exotic causes of irregular, patchy baldness. Typical male-pattern baldness is considered a genetic disorder that requires androgens to be expressed.

BASAL CELL CANCER

Basal cell cancer begins as a shiny papule and slowly enlarges and develops an umbilicated center (which later might ulcerate) with peripheral telangiectasias. Basal cell cancer rarely metastasizes. As with all skin cancer, sunlight exposure increases risk. It is more common in light-skinned people. Treat with excision. Biopsy any suspicious skin lesion in elderly patients.

Table 11-1. COMMON TERMS TO DESCRIBE SKIN FINDINGS

Primary Lesion	Definition	Morphology	Examples
Macule	Flat, circumscribed skin discoloration that lacks surface elevation or depression	Macule	Café-au-lait Vitiligo Freckle Junctional nevi Ink tattoo
Papule	Elevated, solid lesion <0.5 cm in diameter	Papule	Acrocordon (skin tag) Basal cell carcinoma Molluscum contagiosum Intradermal nevi Lichen planus
Plaque	Elevated, solid "confluence of papules" (>0.5 cm in diameter) that lacks a deep component	Plaque	Bowen's disease Mycosis fungoides Psoriasis Eczema Tinea corporis
Patch	Flat, circumscribed skin discoloration; a very large macule >1 cm in diameter	Patch	Nevus flammeus Vitiligo
Nodule	Elevated, solid lesion >0.5 cm in diameter; a larger, deeper papule	Nodule	Rheumatoid nodule Tendon xanthoma Erythema nodosum Lipoma Metastatic carcinoma
Wheal	Firm, edematous plaque that is evanescent and pruritic; a hive	Wheal	Urticaria Dermographism Urticaria pigmentosa
Vesicle	Papule that contains clear fluid; a blister	Vesicle	Herpes simplex Herpes zoster Dyshidrotic eczema Contact dermatitis
Bulla	Localized fluid collection >0.5 cm in diameter; a large vesicle	Bulla	Pemphigus vulgaris Bullous pemphigoid Bullous impetigo

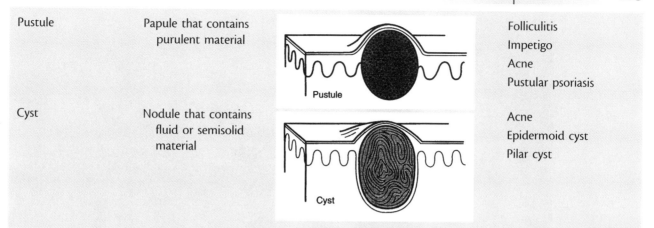

Pustule	Papule that contains purulent material		Folliculitis
			Impetigo
			Acne
			Pustular psoriasis
Cyst	Nodule that contains fluid or semisolid material		Acne
			Epidermoid cyst
			Pilar cyst

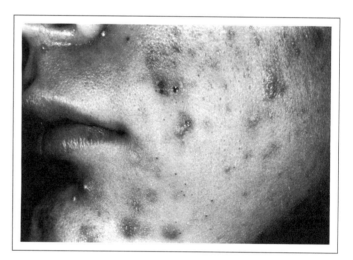

FIGURE 11-1. Acne.

CANDIDIASIS

Thrush (creamy white patches on the tongue or buccal mucosa that can be scraped off) may be seen in normal children, and candidal vulvovaginitis is seen in normal women, especially when they are pregnant or after taking antibiotics. However, at other times and in different patients, candidal infections are a classic sign of diabetes mellitus or immunodeficiency. For example, thrush in a man should make you think about the possibility of HIV/AIDS.

Treat with oral fluconazole or itraconazole or local or topical nystatin or imidazoles (e.g., miconazole, clotrimazole).

CONTACT DERMATITIS

Contact dermatitis is often due to a type IV hypersensitivity reaction; it also may be due to an irritating or toxic substance. On Step 2, look for a question that mentions new exposure to a classic offending agent (poison ivy, nickel earrings, deodorant). The rash is well circumscribed and found only in the area of exposure; skin is red and itchy and often has vesicles or bullae. Avoidance of the agent is required; patch testing can be done, if needed, to determine the antigen.

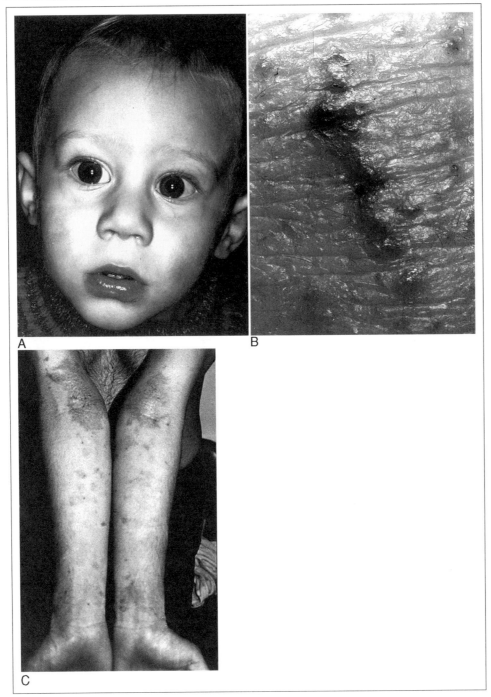

FIGURE 11-2. Phases of atopic dermatitis. A, Infantile phase. Typical erythematous, oozing, and crusted plaques seen on the cheek of an infant with atopic dermatitis. **B,** Childhood phase. Close-up view of a lichenified, excoriated, crusted, and secondarily infected plaque on the right knee of a 4-year-old girl. **C,** Adolescent or young adult phase with chronic, symmetric, pigmented and erythematous skin changes. (From Fitzpatrick JE, Aeling JL: Dermatology Secrets. Philadelphia, Hanley & Belfus, 1996, with permission.)

DERMATITIS HERPETIFORMIS

Dermatitis herpetiformis should alert you to the presence of gluten sensitivity; look for diarrhea and weight loss. Skin has IgA deposits even in unaffected areas. Patients present with intensely pruritic vesicles, papules, and wheals on the extensor aspects of the elbows and knees, possibly on the face and neck. Treat with a gluten-free diet.

DECUBITUS ULCERS

Decubitus ulcers (bedsores or pressure sores) are caused by prolonged pressure against the skin. The best treatment is prophylaxis. Periodic turning of paralyzed, bedridden, or debilitated patients prevents bedsores, as do special dynamic air mattresses. Cleanliness and dryness also help to prevent this condition, and periodic skin inspection makes sure that you catch the problem early. When missed, the lesions can ulcerate down to the bone and become infected, possibly leading to sepsis and death. Treat major skin breaks with aggressive surgical debridement and antibiotics if signs of infection are present.

DRUG REACTIONS

Penicillin, cephalosporins, and sulfa drugs commonly cause rashes; tetracycline and phenothiazines commonly cause photosensitivity.

ERYTHEMA MULTIFORME

Look for classic target (iris) lesions. These are usually caused by drugs or infections (e.g., herpes). The severe form is known as Stevens–Johnson syndrome (Fig. 11-3), which often is fatal. Treat supportively.

ERYTHEMA NODOSUM

Erythema nodosum is inflammation of the subcutaneous tissue and skin, classically over the shins (pretibial). Tender, red nodules are present. Look for "exotic" diseases such as sarcoidosis, coccidioidomycosis, and ulcerative colitis as the cause, although more commonly the cause is unknown or a streptococcal infection.

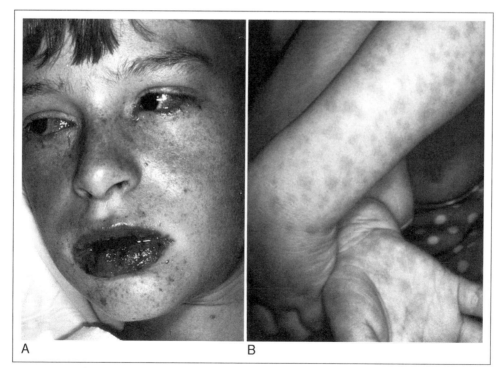

FIGURE 11-3. A, Stevens–Johnson syndrome. Typical mucosal inflammation of the mouth, lips, and conjunctiva. **B,** Erythema multiforme or Stevens–Johnson syndrome. The eruption consists of annular and papular erythema over the acral areas. (From Fitzpatrick JE, Aeling JL: Dermatology Secrets. Philadelphia, Hanley & Belfus, 1996, with permission.)

EXCESSIVE PERSPIRATION

Think of hyperthyroidism and pheochromocytoma.

FUNGAL SKIN INFECTIONS

Fungal skin infections include dermatophyte infections and ringworm. Depending on location, fungal skin infections are known as:

- **Tinea corporis (body and trunk):** Look for red ring-shaped lesions that have raised borders and tend to clear centrally while they expand peripherally.

- **Tinea pedis (athlete's foot):** Look for macerated, scaling web spaces between the toes that often itch and for thickened, distorted toenails (onychomycosis). Good foot hygiene is part of treatment.

- **Tinea unguium (onychomycosis):** Thickened, distorted nails with debris under the nail edges.

- **Tinea capitis (scalp):** Mainly affects children (highly contagious), who have scaly patches of hair loss and might have an inflamed, boggy granuloma of the scalp (known as a kerion), which usually resolves on its own.

- **Tinea cruris (jock itch):** More common in obese male patients, usually in the crural folds of the upper inner thighs.

Most fungal skin infections are due to *Trichophyton* species. Infections are diagnosed by scraping the lesion and doing a potassium hydroxide (KOH) preparation to visualize the fungus (Fig. 11-4) or a culture.

Oral agents (e.g., terbinafine, fluconazole, itraconazole, griseofulvin) should be used to treat tinea capitis and onychomycosis. The others can be treated with topical antifungals (e.g., miconazole, clotrimazole, ketoconazole) or oral agents for severe or persistent infections. In tinea capitis, if the hair fluoresces under Wood's lamp (Fig. 11-5), *Microsporum* spp. is the cause; if it does not, the probable cause is *Trichophyton* spp.

HIRSUTISM

Hirsutism is most commonly idiopathic, but classic causes include corticosteroid administration, Cushing's syndrome, polycystic ovary syndrome (Stein–Leventhal syndrome), and drugs (minoxidil and phenytoin). If other signs of virilization (deepening voice, clitoromegaly, frontal balding) are present, suspect an androgen-secreting ovarian tumor.

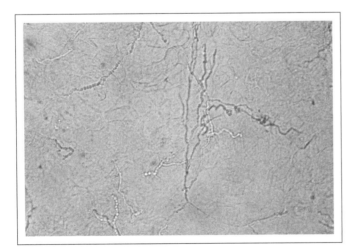

FIGURE 11-4. Potassium hydroxide (KOH) preparation revealing cylindrical, regularly shaped, branching fungal hyphae typical of tinea infections.

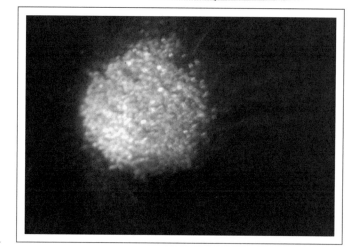

FIGURE 11-5. Wood's light–positive tinea capitis.

KERATOACANTHOMA

Keratoacanthoma is mainly important because it mimics skin cancer (especially squamous cell cancer). This flesh-colored lesion with a central crater contains keratinous material and is classically found on the face. The best way to differentiate it from cancer is that a keratoacanthoma has a *very* rapid onset, and grows to full size in 1 to 2 months. Such rapid growth almost never occurs with squamous cell cancer. The lesion involutes spontaneously in a few months and requires no treatment. If you are unsure, the best option is a biopsy, but on Step 2 choose observation/keratoacanthoma if the history is classic.

KELOID

Keloid is an overgrowth of scar tissue after an injury and is most often seen in blacks (Fig. 11-6A). Keloids are usually slightly pink and classically found on the

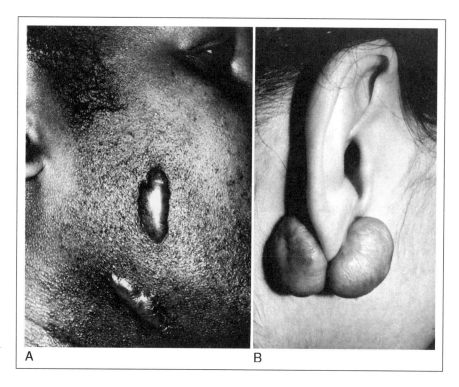

FIGURE 11-6. A, Scar tissue overgrowth after an injury. **B,** Keloid after ear piercing.

upper back, chest, and deltoid area. Also look for keloids to develop after ear piercing (Fig. 11-6B).

KAPOSI'S SARCOMA

Kaposi's sarcoma is seen in AIDS patients. Look for classic mucosal lesions or an expanding, strange rash or skin lesion that does not respond to multiple treatments (Fig. 11-7).

LICE (PEDICULOSIS)

Lice can infect the head (*Pediculus capitis*, which is common in school-aged children), body (*Pediculus corporis*, which is unusual in people with good hygiene), or pubic area (crabs—*Phthirus pubis*—transmitted sexually). Infected areas tend to itch, and diagnosis is made by seeing the lice on hair shafts. Treat with permethrin cream (preferred over lindane because of lindane's neurotoxicity), and decontaminate sources of reinfection (wash or sterilize combs, hats, bed sheets, clothing).

LICHEN PLANUS

Look for the four Ps—pruritic, purple, polygonal papules—and for oral mucosal lesions.

MALIGNANT MELANOMA

Malignant melanoma usually arises from preexisting moles. Remember your **ABCDs:** **a**symmetry, irregular **b**orders, **c**olor change, and increasing **d**iameter. Prognosis is directly related to the depth of vertical invasion. Superficial spreading melanoma tends to stay superficial and has the best prognosis. Nodular melanoma is the worst because it tends to grow downward first. Although uncommon in blacks, melanoma tends to be of the acrolentiginous type; look for black dots on the palms and soles or under the fingernails. Treat with surgery; if surgery fails, the prognosis is poor, though interferon alfa-2b might help.

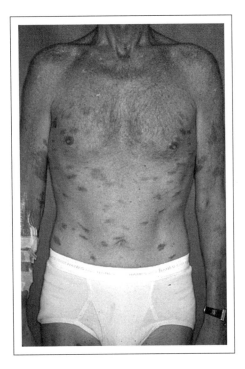

FIGURE 11-7. Kaposi's sarcoma. Multiple violaceous plaques are seen on the trunk of an HIV-positive patient. (From Fitzpatrick JE, Aeling JL: Dermatology Secrets. Philadelphia, Hanley & Belfus, 1996, with permission.)

MOLES

Moles are common and benign, but malignant transformation is possible. *Excise any mole* (or do a biopsy if the lesion is very large) if it enlarges suddenly, develops irregular borders, darkens or becomes inflamed, changes color (even if only one small area of the mole changes color), begins to bleed, begins to itch, or becomes painful. Dysplastic nevus syndrome is a genetic condition (look for family history) with multiple dysplastic-appearing nevi (usually >100). Treat with careful follow-up and excision/biopsy of any suspicious-looking lesions as well as sun avoidance and sunscreen use.

MOLLUSCUM CONTAGIOSUM

Molluscum contagiosum is a poxvirus infection that is common in children but also may be transmitted sexually. A child who has genital molluscum may or may not have contracted the infection from sexual contact; autoinoculation is possible. Do *not* automatically assume child abuse, although it must be ruled out. Diagnosis is made by the characteristic appearance of the lesions (skin-colored, smooth, waxy papules with a central depression [umbilicated] that are roughly 0.5 cm) or by looking at contents of the lesion, which include cells with characteristic inclusion bodies. Usually treated with freezing or curettage.

PAGET'S DISEASE OF THE NIPPLE

Watch for a unilateral red, oozing, and crusting nipple in a woman. An underlying breast cancer with extension to the skin must be ruled out.

PEMPHIGUS

Pemphigus is an autoimmune disease of the middle-aged and elderly that manifests with multiple bullae, starting in the oral mucosa and spreading to the skin of the rest of the body. Biopsy shows acantholysis and can be stained for antibody and shows a fish-net or lace-like immunofluorescence pattern. Treat with corticosteroids. Patients might have an underlying malignancy (often non-Hodgkin's lymphoma) as the trigger.

PITYRIASIS ROSEA

A popular topic for dermatology questions on Step 2. Pityriasis rosea is an idiopathic rash seen in adults. Look for a herald patch (slightly erythematous, ring-shaped or oval, and scaly patch classically seen on the trunk), followed 1 week later by many similar lesions that tend to itch. Look for lesions on the back with a long axis that parallels the Langerhans' skin cleavage lines, typically in a "Christmas tree" pattern. Pityriasis rosea usually remits spontaneously in 1 month. Think about syphilis and tinea-type infection in the differential diagnosis. Treat with reassurance.

PRURITUS

Pruritus may be a clue to diagnosis of serious conditions. It is seen in obstructive biliary disease, uremia, polycythemia rubra vera (classically after a warm shower or bath), contact or atopic dermatitis, scabies, and lichen planus.

PSORIASIS

Know what classic lesions look like (Fig. 11-8) and how they are described (dry, *not* pruritic, well-circumscribed, silvery, scaling papules and plaques). Family history is often

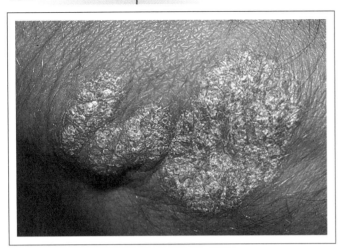

FIGURE 11-8. Psoriasis. Elbow involvement of psoriasis vulgaris, demonstrating typical well-demarcated red plaques with silvery scale. (From Fitzpatrick JE, Aeling JL: Dermatology Secrets. Philadelphia, Hanley & Belfus, 1996, with permission.)

positive. Psoriasis occurs mostly in whites with onset in early adulthood. Classic lesions are found on the scalp and extensor surfaces of the elbows and knees. Patients might have pitting of the nails and arthritis that resembles rheumatoid arthritis but is rheumatoid factor–negative. Diagnosis is made by appearance; biopsy can be used for doubtful cases. Treatment is complex, involving exposure to ultraviolet light (e.g. sunlight), lubricants, topical corticosteroids, and keratolytics (coal tar, salicylic acid, anthralin).

ROSACEA

Rosacea looks like acne, but it starts in middle age. Look for rhinophyma (bulbous red nose) and coexisting blepharitis. Treat with topical metronidazole or oral tetracycline. The pathogenesis is unknown, but it is not related to diet or caused by alcohol (which can aggravate it).

SCABIES

Scabies is caused by the mite *Sarcoptes scabei*, which tunnels into the skin and leaves visible burrows, classically in the finger web spaces and flexor surface of the wrists. Facial involvement sometimes is seen in infants. Patients have severe pruritus, and itching can lead to secondary bacterial infection. Diagnosis is made by scraping the mite out of a burrow and viewing it under a microscope (Fig. 11-9). Treat with permethrin cream applied to the whole body. Remember to treat *all* contacts (e.g., the whole family). Do *not* use

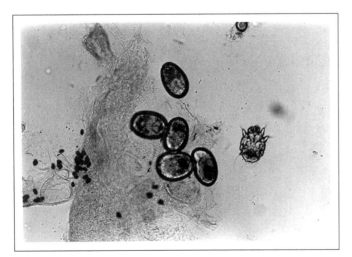

FIGURE 11-9. Scabies scraping.

lindane to treat unless permethrin is not a choice. Lindane used to be the treatment of choice but can cause neurotoxicity, especially in young children.

SEBORRHEIC DERMATITIS

Seborrheic dermatitis causes the common conditions known as cradle cap and dandruff, as well as blepharitis (eyelid inflammation). Look for scaling skin on the scalp and eyelids, and treat with dandruff shampoo.

SQUAMOUS CELL CANCER

Look for preexisting actinic keratoses (hard, sharp, red, often scaly lesions in sun-exposed areas) or burn scars that become nodular, warty, or ulcerated (Fig. 11-10). Do a biopsy if this happens! Squamous cell cancer in situ is known as *Bowen's disease.*

STOMATITIS

Watch for deficiencies of B-complex vitamins (riboflavin, niacin, pyridoxine) or vitamin C.

TINEA VERSICOLOR

Pityrosporon spp. infection that occurs most commonly in young adults. It appears as multiple patches of various size and color (brown, tan, and white) on the torso (Fig. 11-11). It often becomes noticeable in the summer because the affected areas fail to tan and look white. Diagnose from lesion scrapings (KOH preparation). Treat with oral or topical imidazoles or selenium sulfide shampoo.

VITILIGO

Vitiligo is depigmentation of unknown etiology, but it can have an autoimmune basis. It is associated with pernicious anemia, hypothyroidism, Addison's disease, and diabetes mellitus. Patients often have antibodies to melanin, parietal cells, or thyroid.

WARTS

Warts are caused by human papillomavirus (HPV); infections are most commonly seen in older children, often on the hands. Treatments include salicylic acid, liquid nitrogen, curettage, and others. Genital warts also are caused by HPV (types 16 and 18 [and others] are associated with cervical cancer).

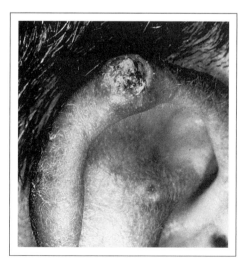

FIGURE 11-10. Squamous cell carcinoma of the ear, demonstrating a nodule with central scale and crust. (From Fitzpatrick JE, Aeling JL: Dermatology Secrets. Philadelphia, Hanley & Belfus, 1996, with permission.)

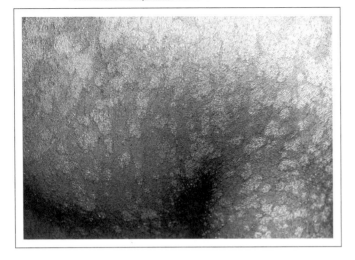

FIGURE 11-11. Tinea versicolor demonstrating hypopigmented scaly papules. (From Fitzpatrick JE, Aeling JL: Dermatology Secrets. Philadelphia, Hanley & Belfus, 1996, with permission.)

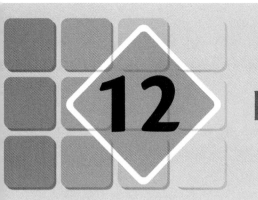

12 NEUROLOGY

Neurology Tests

Lumbar puncture is most commonly indicated for suspected meningitis or sterile inflammatory central nervous system (CNS) disorder (e.g., multiple sclerosis, Guillain-Barré syndrome). Table 12-1 shows the classic findings in various conditions. Computed tomography (CT) and magnetic resonance (MR) imaging have almost replaced lumbar puncture for routine tumor and hemorrhage evaluation (though either can occasionally exist in the setting of negative imaging studies).

IMPORTANT POINTS

1 Do *not* perform lumbar puncture in patients with acute head trauma or signs of intracranial hypertension (e.g., papilledema) until you have a negative CT or MRI. You might cause death.

Table 12-1. CLASSIC CEREBROSPINAL FLUID FINDINGS IN DIFFERENT CONDITIONS

Condition	Cells/μL*	Glucose (mg/dL)	Protein (mg/dL)	Pressure (mm Hg)
Normal cerebrospinal fluid	0–3 (L)	50–100	20–45	100–200
Bacterial meningitis	**>1000 (PMN)**	<50	Around 100	>200
Viral or aseptic meningitis	>100 (L)	Normal	Normal or slightly increased	Normal or slightly increased
Pseudotumor cerebri	**Normal**	Normal	Normal	**>200**
Guillain-Barré syndrome	0–100 (L)	Normal	**>100**	Normal
Cerebral hemorrhage†	**Bloody (RBC)**	Normal	>45	>200
Multiple sclerosis‡	Normal or slightly increased (L)	Normal	Normal or slightly increased	Normal

Note: Bold type highlights the most important considerations for each disorder.

*Main cell type is put in parenthesis after the number.

†Think of subarachnoid hemorrhage, but the same findings also can occur after an intracerebral hemorrhage.

‡On electrophoresis of cerebrospinal fluid, look for oligoclonal bands due to increased IgG production and an increased level of myelin basic protein (MBP) during active demyelination.

L, lymphocytes; PMN, polymorphonuclear neutrophils; RBC, red blood cells.

2 Tuberculosis and fungal meningitis have low glucose (<50) with high cells (>100), which are predominantly **lymphocytes**. Watch for a positive India ink preparation for *Cryptococcus* spp.

Nerve conduction velocities are slowed by demyelination (Guillain-Barré, multiple sclerosis). Repetitive stimulation can assess fatigability. Myasthenia gravis is characterized by *increasing* fatigue with stimulation; Eaton-Lambert syndrome by *decreasing* fatigue with stimulation.

Electromyography (EMG) measures the electrical (contractile) properties of muscle. Lower motor neuron lesions are associated with fasciculations and fibrillations at rest. When the disease is in the muscle itself, no electrical activity is seen at rest (which is normal), but amplitude is decreased with contraction of the muscle.

Stroke and Transient Ischemic Attack

STROKE

Cerebrovascular disease (stroke, cerebrovascular accident) is the most common cause of neurologic disability in the United States and the third leading cause of death. Ischemia from atherosclerosis is by far the most common cause; other classic causes include atrial fibrillation with resultant clot formation and emboli to the brain and septic emboli from endocarditis. Treatment for acute stroke in evolution is supportive (e.g., airway, oxygen, intravenous [IV] fluids). Heparin is controversial and should be *avoided* on Step 2, especially if the patient is hypertensive; it should not be given until a hemorrhagic stroke has been ruled out by CT (Fig. 12-1). See Chapter 25, Vascular Surgery, for a discussion of the role of carotid endarterectomy, which is *not* done emergently.

TRANSIENT ISCHEMIC ATTACK

Transient ischemic attack is a focal neurologic deficit that lasts minutes to hours, then resolves spontaneously; often a precursor to stroke. The classic presentation is ipsilateral

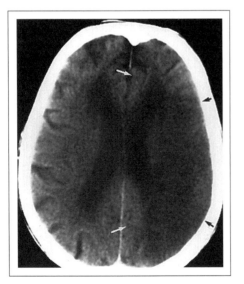

FIGURE 12-1. Large left middle cerebral artery infarct, nonhemorrhagic (*black arrows*) on computed tomograpy (CT). The sulci have been obliterated by swelling. Note sparing of the brain supplied by the left anterior and posterior cerebral arteries (*white arrows*).

Table 12-2. LOCALIZING A STROKE OR OTHER CNS LESION

Symptom or Sign	Think of this Area
Decreased or no reflexes or fasciculations	Lower motor neuron lesion (or possibly a muscle problem)
Hyperreflexia	Upper motor neuron lesion (cord or brain)
Apathy, inattention, uninhibited/labile affect	Frontal lobes
Broca's (motor) aphasia	Dominant frontal lobe*
Wernicke's (sensory) aphasia	Dominant temporal lobe*
Memory impairment, aggression, hypersexuality	Temporal lobes
Inability to read, write, name, or do math	Dominant parietal lobe*
Ignoring one side of the body, difficulty in dressing	Nondominant parietal lobe*
Visual hallucinations or illusions	Occipital lobes
Cranial nerves III and IV	Midbrain
Cranial nerves V, VI, VII, and VIII	Pons
Cranial nerves IX, X, XI, and XII	Medulla
Ataxia, dyssarthria, nystagmus, intention tremor, dysmetria, scanning speech	Cerebellum
Resting tremor, chorea	Basal ganglia
Hemiballismus	Subthalamic nucleus

*The left hemisphere is dominant in >95% of the population (99% of right-handed people and 60–70% of left-handed people).
  CNS, central nervous system.

blindness (amaurosis fugax) and/or unilateral hemiplegia, hemiparesis, weakness, or clumsiness. Get a carotid duplex ultrasound to look for stenosis. Heparin may be given acutely (if not contraindicated), but for long-term therapy use aspirin or other antiplatelet medications (e.g., clopidogrel) and/or carotid endarterectomy (if carotid stenosis is >70%).

The signs and symptoms can indicate the location of a CNS lesion (Table 12-2).

Cranial Nerve Lesions

The **olfactory nerve (cranial nerve [CN] I)** is rarely important clinically. Kallmann's syndrome is anosmia plus hypogonadism due to deficiency of gonadotropin-releasing hormone.

Optic (CN II), oculomotor (CN III), trochlear (CN IV), and abducens (CN VI) lesions are discussed in Chapter 21, Ophthalmology.

The **trigeminal nerve (CN V)** innervates muscles of mastication and facial sensation (including the afferent limb of the corneal reflex). Patients may have trigeminal neuralgia (tic douloureux), which is characterized by unilateral shooting pains in the face in older adults and is often triggered by activity (e.g., brushing teeth). Treat with carbamazepine, gabapentin, or other antiepilepsy medication. If the patient is young and/or female and/or the disease is bilateral, consider multiple sclerosis. Make sure to think about other possible causes, such as tumor or stroke.

The **facial nerve (CN VII)** innervates muscles of facial expression, taste in the anterior two thirds of the tongue, the skin of the external ear, the lacrimal and salivary glands (except parotid gland), and the stapedius muscle. Differentiate between *upper* motor neuron lesions (the forehead is spared on the affected side, and the cause is usually stroke or tumor) and *lower* motor neuron lesions (the forehead is involved on the affected side, and the cause is usually Bell's palsy or tumor) of the facial nerve. Patients may be unable to close the eye; give artificial tears to prevent corneal ulceration. Some physicians treat with acyclovir (underlying herpes virus reactivation is a common underlying cause) and/or prednisone, which are variably effective. Patients with Bell's palsy can get hyperacusis (things sound much louder than they are) due to stapedial muscle paralysis. If CNs VII and VIII are affected, think of possible cerebellopontine angle tumor (e.g., acoustic neuroma or schwannoma, especially in neurofibromatosis).

The **vestibulocochlear nerve (CN VIII)** is for hearing and balance. Lesions cause deafness, tinnitus, and vertigo. In children, think of meningitis as a cause. In adults, think of toxins and medications (aspirin, aminoglycosides, loop diuretics, cisplatin), tumors (with CN VII coinvolvement, think of acoustic neuroma, Fig. 12-2), or stroke.

The **glossopharyngeal nerve (CN IX)** innervates pharyngeal muscles and mucous membranes (afferent limb of gag reflex), parotid gland, taste in the posterior third of the tongue, skin of the external ear, and carotid body and sinus. Look for loss of gag reflex and loss of taste in the posterior third of the tongue.

The **vagus nerve (CN X)** innervates the muscles of the palate, pharynx, larynx (efferent limb of gag reflex), taste buds in the base of the tongue, abdominal viscera, and skin of the external ear. Look for hoarseness, dysphagia, and loss of gag or cough reflex. If the cause is not a stroke or brainstem tumor, think of peripheral tumors, especially Pancoast left lung tumors, or thoracic aortic aneurysms, which affect the peripheral left recurrent laryngeal nerve *only*.

The **spinal accessory nerve (CN XI)** innervates the sternocleidomastoid and trapezius muscles. With a CN XI lesion, the patient has trouble turning the head to the opposite side of the lesion and the ipsilateral shoulder droops.

The **hypoglossal nerve (CN XII)** innervates muscles of the tongue. With a CN XII lesion, a protruded tongue deviates to the side of the lesion.

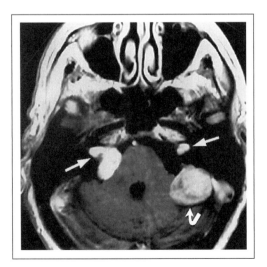

FIGURE 12-2. Contrast-enhanced axial MR image of bilateral acoustic neuromas (*straight arrows*) in a patient with neurofibromatosis type 2. A posterior fossa meningioma (*curved arrow*) is also present.

Table 12-3. DIFFERENTIAL DIAGNOSIS OF DELIRIUM AND DEMENTIA

Feature	Delirium	Dementia
Onset	Acute and dramatic	Chronic and insidious
Common causes	Illness, toxin, withdrawal	Alzheimer's, multiinfarct dementia, HIV/AIDS
Reversible	Usually	Usually not
Attention	Poor	Usually unaffected
Arousal level	Fluctuates	Normal

AIDS, acquired immunodeficiency syndrome; HIV, human immunodeficiency virus.

Delirium and Dementia

Table 12-3 shows the differential diagnosis for delirium and dementia.

IMPORTANT POINTS

1 Both delirium and dementia can feature hallucinations, illusions, delusions, memory impairment (usually global in delirium, whereas remote memory is spared in early dementia), orientation difficulties (time, place, person), and sundowning (worsened symptoms at night).

2 In the elderly watch for pseudodementia, which is caused by depression and is reversible with treatment.

3 Treatable causes of dementia include vitamin B_{12} deficiency, endocrine disorders (especially thyroid and parathyroid), uremia, syphilis, brain tumors, and normal-pressure hydrocephalus. Treatment of Parkinson's syndrome also can reverse dementia.

4 Watch for thiamine deficiency in alcoholics as the cause of delirium (Wernicke's encephalopathy, which classically manifests with ataxia, ophthalmoplegia, nystagmus, and confusion). If untreated, it can progress to Korsakoff's syndrome (memory loss with confabulation; usually irreversible).

For **delirious or unconscious patients in the emergency department** with no history of trauma, think first of hypoglycemia (give glucose), opioid overdose (give naloxone), and thiamine deficiency (give thiamine before giving glucose in a suspected alcoholic). Other common causes are alcohol, illicit drugs, prescription medications, diabetic ketoacidosis, stroke, and epilepsy or postictal state.

Headache

Causes of headache:

◆ **Tension headaches:** Most common cause. Look for long history of headaches and stress plus a feeling of tightness or stiffness, usually frontal or occipital and bilateral. Treat with stress reduction and acetaminophen or nonsteroidal antiinflammatory drugs (NSAIDs).

◆ **Cluster headaches:** Unilateral, severe, tender; occur in clusters. Oxygen might abort an attack acutely.

◆ **Migraine headache:** Look for aura, photophobia, nausea and vomiting, and positive family history. Patients might have neurologic symptoms during attacks; attacks usually begin between ages 10 and 30 years. Treat and prevent with antimigraine medication (e.g., sumatriptan).

◆ **Tumor or mass:** Look for progressive neurologic symptoms, papilledema, intracranial hypertension (classically with nausea and vomiting, which may be projectile), mental status changes, and headache every day (classically worse in the morning). Order CT or MRI.

◆ **Pseudotumor cerebri:** Can mimic tumor or mass; both cause intracranial hypertension, papilledema, and daily headaches that classically are worse in the morning and may be accompanied by nausea and vomiting. Found in young obese women, who are unlikely to have a brain tumor; CT and MRI are negative. Pseudotumor cerebri can cause permanent vision loss. Treatment is usually supportive, including cerebrospinal fluid removal periodically or with a permanent shunt; weight loss usually helps. Large doses of **vitamin A,** tetracyclines, and withdrawal from corticosteroids are possible causes.

◆ **Meningitis:** Look for fever, Brudzinski's or Kernig's sign, cerebrospinal fluid findings (see Table 12-1).

◆ **Subarachnoid hemorrhage:** "Worst headache" of patient's life; usually due to aneurysm rupture or trauma. Shows up on CT scan and can cause grossly bloody cerebrospinal fluid. Treat supportively, and order a CT, MR, or traditional angiogram for aneurysm detection once the patient is stable, unless you're given a significant trauma history.

◆ **Extracranial causes:** Eye pain (optic neuritis, eyestrain from refractive errors, iritis, glaucoma), middle ear pain (otitis media, mastoiditis), sinus pain (sinusitis), oral cavity pain (toothache), herpes zoster with cranial nerve involvement, and nonspecific (malaise from any illness).

Myasthenia Gravis

Myasthenia gravis is an autoimmune disease that destroys acetylcholine receptors. It usually manifests in women aged 20 to 40 years. Look for ptosis, diplopia, and general muscle fatigability, especially toward the end of the day.

Diagnosis is made with the Tensilon test. Injection of edrophonium (Tensilon), a short-acting anticholinesterase, improves muscle weakness. Watch for associated thymomas; most patients improve after removal of the thymus, which can be part of standard treatment. Antibodies to acetylcholine receptors are usually present in the serum. Electromyography reveals jitter in muscle fibers, and repetitive nerve stimulation reveals declining amplitude of response over time.

Treat with long-acting anticholinesterase (pyridostigmine, neostigmine); plasmapheresis is used for an acute severe crisis.

Eaton–Lambert Syndrome

Eaton–Lambert is a paraneoplastic syndrome (classically seen with small cell lung cancer) characterized by muscle weakness, with sparing of the extraocular muscles (myasthenia gravis almost always has prominent involvement of extraocular muscles). Eaton–Lambert syndrome has a different mechanism of disease (impaired release of acetylcholine from nerves) and a differential response to repetitive nerve stimulation (myasthenia gravis worsens, Eaton–Lambert improves).

IMPORTANT POINTS

1 Do not forget organophosphate poisoning as a cause for myasthenia-like muscle weakness. Usually it occurs with agricultural exposure. Symptoms of parasympathetic excess also are present (e.g., miosis, excessive bronchial secretions, urinary urgency, diarrhea). Edrophonium causes worsening of the muscle weakness. Treatment is atropine and pralidoxime.

2 Aminoglycosides in high doses can cause myasthenia-like muscle weakness and prolong the effects of muscle blockade in anesthesia.

Neuromuscular and Movement Disorders

AMYOTROPHIC LATERAL SCLEROSIS

Amyotrophic lateral sclerosis (Lou Gehrig's disease) is an idiopathic degeneration of both upper and lower motor neurons that is more common in men. The mean age at onset is 55 years. The key is to notice a combination of upper motor neuron lesion signs (spasticity, hyperreflexia, positive Babinski's sign) and lower motor neuron lesion signs (fasciculations, atrophy, flaccidity) in the same patient. Treatment is supportive, but 50% of patients die within 3 years of onset.

CEREBELLAR DISORDERS

In children, think of brain tumor (cerebellar astrocytoma, medulloblastomas), hydrocephalus (enlarging head in infants younger than 6 months, possibly due to Arnold–Chiari or Dandy–Walker syndrome), Friedreich's ataxia (autosomal recessive), or ataxia–telangiectasia (the diagnosis is in the name). Friedreich's ataxia starts between 5 and 15 years of age and manifests with areflexia, loss of vibration or position sense, and cardiomyopathy. In adults, think of alcoholism, tumor, ischemia or hemorrhage, or multiple sclerosis.

FLOPPY BABY SYNDROME

Infants have hypotonia or flaccidity. It can be caused by two disorders:

◆ **Werdnig-Hoffmann disease:** Autosomal recessive degeneration of anterior horn cells in the spinal cord and brainstem (lower motor neurons). Most infants are hypotonic at birth, and all are affected by 6 months. Look for a positive family history and a long and slowly progressive course of disease. Treatment is supportive.

◆ **Infant botulism:** Look for sudden onset and a history of honey ingestion (or other home-canned foods). Diagnosis is made by finding *Clostridium botulinum* toxin or organisms in the feces. Treat on an inpatient basis with close monitoring of respiratory status. Patients might need intubation for respiratory muscle paralysis. Spontaneous recovery usually occurs within 1 week.

GUILLAIN-BARRÉ SYNDROME

Look for history of mild infection or immunization roughly 1 week before onset of symmetric, distal weakness, paralysis, or mild paresthesias with loss of deep tendon reflexes in affected areas. As the ascending paralysis and weakness progress, respiratory paralysis can occur. Patients must be watched carefully; usually spirometry is used to follow inspiratory ability. Intubation may be required. Diagnosis depends on clinical signs and symptoms, analysis of cerebrospinal fluid (usually normal except for *markedly increased protein*), and nerve conduction velocities (slowed). Disease usually stops spontaneously. Plasmapheresis reduces the severity and length of disease. Do *not* use corticosteroids; you might make the patient worse.

HUNTINGTON'S DISEASE

Huntington's disease is an autosomal dominant condition that usually begins at 35 to 50 years of age. Look for choreiform movements (irregular, spasmodic, involuntary movements of the limbs or facial muscles) and progressive intellectual deterioration, dementia, and psychiatric disturbances. Atrophy of the caudate nucleus may be seen on CT or MRI. Treatment is supportive; antipsychotics might help.

MUSCULAR DYSTROPHY

Muscular dystrophy is most commonly due to **Duchenne's muscular dystrophy**, an X-linked recessive disorder of dystrophin that usually manifests in boys aged 3 to 7 years. Look for muscle weakness, markedly elevated creatine kinase, and pseudohypertrophy of the calves (due to fatty and fibrous infiltration of the degenerating muscle). IQ often is less than normal. Gowers' sign is classic (in trying to rise from a prone position, the patient walks the hands and feet toward each other). Muscle biopsy establishes the diagnosis. Treatment is supportive. Most patients die by age 20 years.

Other muscular dystrophies:

◆ **Becker's muscular dystrophy:** This is also an X-linked recessive dystrophin disorder, but milder.

◆ **Myotonic dystrophy:** An autosomal dominant disorder that manifests between 20 and 30 years of age. Myotonia (inability to relax muscles) classically manifests as *inability to relax the grip* (inability to release a handshake). Look for coexisting mental retardation, baldness, and testicular or ovarian atrophy. Treatment is supportive and includes genetic counseling. Diagnosis is clinical.

◆ **Mitochondrial myopathies (e.g., Lever's hereditary optic atrophy):** These are interesting because they are inherited mitochondrial defects (passed only from mother to offspring; male carriers cannot transmit). The key phrase is "ragged red fibers" on biopsy specimen. Ophthalmoplegia usually is present.

Do not forget the rare glycogen storage diseases (autosomal recessive) as a cause for muscle weakness (especially McArdle's disease, a deficiency in glycogen phosphorylase that is relatively mild and manifests with weakness and cramping after exercise).

PARKINSON'S DISEASE

Signs are the classic tetrad of slowness or poverty of movement, muscle rigidity (lead pipe and cogwheel), resting pill-rolling tremor (which disappears with movement and sleep), and postural instability (shuffling gait and festination). Patients also might have dementia and depression. The mean age of onset is around 60 years. The cause is loss of dopaminergic neurons, especially in the substantia nigra, which projects to the basal ganglia; the result is decreased dopamine in the basal ganglia. Drug therapy aims to increase dopamine. Options include levodopa or carbidopa, bromocriptine or pergolide, monoamine oxidase type B inhibitors (selegiline), amantidine, anticholinergics (trihexyphenidyl, benztropine), and antihistamines (diphenhydramine).

 Antipsychotics can cause Parkinson-like symptoms in schizophrenics. Treat with anticholinergics (benztropine, trihexyphenidyl) or antihistamines (diphenhydramine).

TREMOR AND CHOREA

Resting tremor is generally due to basal ganglia disease (chorea), intention tremor is due to cerebellar disease, and hemiballismus (random, violent, unilateral flailing of the limbs) is due to a lesion in the subthalamic nucleus. Besides Parkinson's disease, a resting tremor may be due to hyperthyroidism, anxiety, drug withdrawal or intoxication, or a benign (essential) hereditary tremor (usually autosomal dominant; look for a positive family history, and use β-blockers to reduce the tremor). Also watch for Wilson's disease (hepatolenticular degeneration) and asterixis (outstretched hands flap slowly and involuntarily) in patients with liver or kidney failure.

Seizures

Five main types of seizures are tested on the boards (although there are others):

- **Simple partial (local, focal) seizures:** These may be motor (e.g., Jacksonian march), sensory (e.g., hallucinations), or psychic (cognitive or affective symptoms). The key point is that consciousness is *not* impaired. Treat with phenytoin, valproate, or carbamazepine.

- **Complex partial (psychomotor) seizures:** Any simple partial seizure followed by impairment of consciousness. Patients perform purposeless movements and can become aggressive if restraint is attempted (people who get in fights or kill people are *not* having a seizure!). The first-line agents are phenytoin, valproate, and carbamazepine.

- **Absence (petit mal) seizures:** These *never* begin after the age of 20. They are brief (10 to 30 seconds' duration), generalized seizures in which the main manifestation is loss of consciousness, often with eye or muscle flutterings. The classic description is a child in a classroom who stares off into space in the middle of a sentence (the child is not daydreaming but having a seizure), then 20 seconds later resumes the sentence. There is no postictal state (an important differential point). The first-line agents are ethosuximide and valproate.

- **Tonic–clonic (grand mal) seizures:** The classic seizures that can have an aura; tonic muscle contraction is followed by clonic contractions, usually lasting 2 to 5 minutes. Patients often have incontinence and a postictal state (drowsiness, confusion, headache, muscle soreness). Treat with phenytoin, valproate or carbamazepine.

- **Febrile seizures:** Between the ages of 6 months and 5 years old, children might have a seizure due to fever. The seizure is usually short in duration (less than 1 or 2 minutes) and of the tonic–clonic, generalized type. Often, no specific seizure treatment is required. Treat the underlying cause of the fever, if possible, and give acetaminophen. Such children do *not* have epilepsy, and the chances of their getting it are just barely higher than in the general population's. Make sure that affected children do not have meningitis, tumor, or other serious cause of seizure. The board question will give clues in the case description if you are expected to pursue work-up for a serious condition.

Secondary seizure disorder may be caused by:

- Mass (tumor, hemorrhage)
- Metabolic disorder (hypoglycemia, hypoxia, phenylketonuria, hyponatremia)
- Toxins (lead, cocaine, carbon monoxide)
- Drug withdrawal (alcohol, barbiturates, benzodiazepines, too-rapid anticonvulsant withdrawal)
- Cerebral edema (severe or malignant hypertension; also watch for pheochromocytoma)
- Eclampsia
- Central nervous system infections (meningitis, encephalitis, toxoplasmosis, cysticercosis)
- Trauma
- Stroke

Treatment: For all seizures, secure the airway and, if possible, roll the patient onto his or her side to prevent aspiration. In secondary seizures of *any* etiology, treat the underlying disorder and use diazepam acutely or phenytoin acutely to control seizure.

Status epilepticus: Seizures of any type following one after the other with no intervening periods of consciousness. These can occur spontaneously or result from too-rapid withdrawal of anticonvulsants. Treat with IV diazepam, lorazepam, or phenytoin. Remember to protect the airway and intubate if necessary.

IMPORTANT POINTS

1 Hypertension can cause seizures or convulsions, headache, confusion, or mental status changes.

2 All anticonvulsants are teratogenic, and women need counseling about the risks of pregnancy. Do a pregnancy test before starting an anticonvulsant.

3 **Cysticercosis** is due to infection with the larval form of *Taenia solium*, the pork tapeworm, and most often is seen in AIDS patients and in immigrants. On CT scan with contrast, the lesion is classically described as "ring-enhancing" or may be calcified. Treat with niclosamide or praziquantel.

Other Neurologic Disorders

MULTIPLE SCLEROSIS

Look for insidious onset of neurologic symptoms in women aged 20 to 40 years with exacerbations and remissions. Common presentations include paresthesias and numbness, weakness and clumsiness, visual disturbances (decreased vision and pain due to *optic neuritis*, diplopia due to cranial nerve involvement), gait disturbances, incontinence or urgency, and vertigo. Also look for emotional lability or other mental status changes. Internuclear ophthalmoplegia and scanning speech are classic; Babinski's sign may be positive.

MRI, the most sensitive diagnostic tool, shows demyelination plaques (Fig. 12-3). Look for increased IgG or oligoclonal bands and possibly myelin basic protein in the cerebrospinal fluid.

Disease course is variable, but long-term prognosis poor. Treatment is variably effective and includes corticosteroids, interferon-β, and glatiramer.

PERIPHERAL NEUROPATHIES

Nerve conduction velocity is slowed with a peripheral neuropathy, which can be motor (lower motor neuron signs), sensory, and/or autonomic.

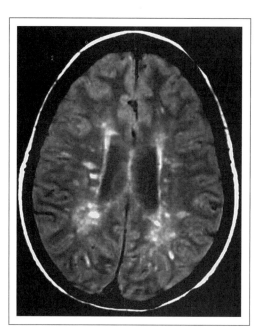

FIGURE 12-3. Multiple sclerosis on MR. The periventricular distribution and oval shape are typical of demyelination.

Multiple causes include:

◆ **Metabolic:** Diabetes mellitus (autonomic and sensory neuropathy), uremia, hypothyroidism

◆ **Nutritional:** Deficiencies of vitamin B_{12}, B_6 (look for history of isoniazid), thiamine (dry beriberi), or vitamin E

◆ **Toxins and medications:** Lead (classic symptom is wristdrop or footdrop; look for coexisting central nervous system or abdominal symptoms) or other heavy metals, isoniazid, vincristine, ethambutol (especially optic neuritis), aminoglycosides (especially CN VIII)

◆ **Postinfection, postimmunization, and autoimmune:** Guillain-Barré syndrome, systemic lupus erythematosus, polyarteritis nodosa, scleroderma, sarcoidosis, amyloidosis

◆ **Trauma:** Carpal tunnel syndrome (median nerve entrapment at the wrist), pressure paralysis (radial nerve palsy in alcoholics), or fractures. Carpal tunnel syndrome usually is due to repetitive physical activity but may be a manifestation of acromegaly or hypothyroidism. Look for positive Tinel's and Phalen's signs.

◆ **Infectious:** Lyme disease, diphtheria, HIV, tick bite, leprosy

SYNCOPE

The most common cause is vasovagal (e.g., from stress, fear, or other emotional states). Other causes include cardiac events (especially arrhythmias; get an electrocardiogram [EKG]), TIAs (consider carotid artery ultrasound), and neurologic disorders (especially seizures; consider CT or MRI of brain if other neurologic symptoms are present).

VITAMIN DEFICIENCIES

Vitamin deficiencies can present with neurologic signs and symptoms:

◆ **Vitamin A:** Vision loss

◆ **Thiamine (vitamin B_1):** Peripheral neuropathy, confusion, ophthalmoplegia, nystagmus, ataxia, confusion, delirium, dementia

◆ **Vitamin B_6:** Peripheral sensory neuropathy (watch for isoniazid as a cause, and give prophylactic B_6 to patients taking isoniazid if given the choice on Step 2)

◆ **Vitamin B_{12}:** Dementia, peripheral neuropathy, loss of vibration sense in lower extremities, loss of position sense, ataxia, spasticity, hyperactive reflexes, and positive Babinski's sign

◆ **Vitamin E:** Loss of proprioception or vibratory sensation, areflexia, ataxia, and gaze palsy

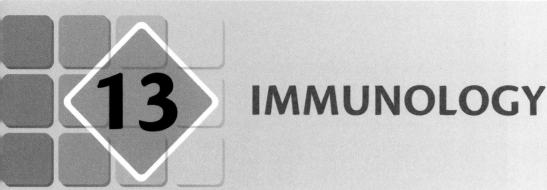

IMMUNOLOGY

Hypersensitivity

There are four types of hypersensitivity reactions: type I (anaphylactic), type II (cytotoxic), type III (immune complex–mediated), and type IV (cell-mediated [delayed]).

TYPE I (ANAPHYLACTIC)

Type I reaction is due to preformed immunoglobulin E (IgE) antibodies, which cause release of vasoactive amines (e.g., histamine, leukotrienes) from mast cells and basophils. Examples are anaphylaxis (bee stings, food allergy [especially peanuts and shellfish], medications [especially penicillin and sulfa drugs], rubber glove allergy), atopy, hay fever, urticaria, allergic rhinitis, and some forms of asthma.

With chronic type I hypersensitivity (atopy, some asthma, allergic rhinitis), look for eosinophilia, elevated IgE levels, family history, and seasonal exacerbations. Patients also might have allergic shiners (bilateral infraorbital edema) and a transverse nasal crease (from frequent nose rubbing). Pale, bluish, edematous nasal turbinates with many eosinophils in clear, watery nasal secretions also are classic.

If patients have nasal polyps, do *not* give aspirin; you might precipitate a severe asthmatic attack.

True systemic anaphylaxis causes a dramatic and rapid change in status (e.g., severe respiratory distress, hypotension, or shock) that classically occurs within seconds (intravenous [IV] drug) to minutes (oral) of exposure to medication or iodinated contrast. Patients can die within minutes. Treat immediately by securing the airway. Laryngeal edema can prevent intubation, in which case do a cricothyrotomy, if needed. Give subcutaneous (second choice is IV) epinephrine. Steroids are sometimes given for severe reactions, but they take hours to have an effect and are a secondary consideration, not primary therapy in this setting.

C1 esterase inhibitor (complement) deficiency is a cause of hereditary angioedema. Patients have diffuse swelling of lips, eyelids, and possibly the airway or bowel, unrelated to any allergen exposure. The deficiency is autosomal dominant; look for a positive family history. C4 complement is low. Treat acutely as anaphylaxis; androgens are used for long-term treatment to increase liver production of C1 esterase inhibitor.

Skin testing might identify an allergen if it is not obvious.

TYPE II (CYTOTOXIC)

Type II reaction is due to preformed IgG and IgM, which react with antigen and cause secondary inflammation. Examples are autoimmune hemolytic anemia (classic causes are methyldopa or penicillin or sulfa drugs) and other cytopenias caused by antibodies, such as idiopathic thrombocytopenic purpura, transfusion reactions, erythroblastosis fetalis (Rh incompatibility), Goodpasture's syndrome (watch for linear immunofluorescence on kidney biopsy), myasthenia gravis, Graves' disease, pernicious anemia, pemphigus, and hyperacute transplant rejection (as soon as the anastomosis is made at transplant surgery, the transplanted organ deteriorates in front of your eyes).

 With anemia, watch for a positive Coombs' test; in pregnancy, watch for a positive indirect Coombs' test.

TYPE III (IMMUNE COMPLEX–MEDIATED) REACTION

Type III (immune complex–mediated) reaction is due to deposits of antigen–antibody complexes (usually in vessels) that cause an inflammatory response. Examples are serum sickness, lupus, rheumatoid arthritis, polyarteritis nodosa, chronic hepatitis, cryoglobulinemia, and glomerulonephritis.

TYPE IV (CELL-MEDIATED) REACTION

Type IV (cell-mediated [delayed]) reaction is due to sensitized T lymphocytes, which release inflammatory mediators. Examples include tuberculosis skin test, contact dermatitis (especially poison ivy, nickel earrings, cosmetics, medications), chronic transplant rejection, and granulomas.

Human Immunodeficiency Virus and Acquired Immunodeficiency Syndrome

Initial seroconversion can manifest as a mononucleosis-type syndrome (fever, malaise, pharyngitis, rash, lymphadenopathy). Keep HIV seroconversion in the back of your mind as a differential diagnosis for any sore throat or Epstein–Barr virus–type presentation. Diagnosis is made with the enzyme-linked immunosorbent assay (ELISA), which, if positive, should be confirmed with a Western blot test. Do all tests before you tell the patient anything! It takes 1 to 6 months for antibodies to develop; therefore, if a patient comes to you for testing because of recent risk-taking behavior, you should retest the patient in 6 months if the initial test is negative.

IMPORTANT POINTS

1 Once the diagnosis of HIV infection is made, the patient should get a CD4 count every 6 months.

2 Antiretroviral therapy should be started when the CD4 count falls below 350/mm^3 (or sooner).

3 Once the CD4 count is less than 200/mm³, start prophylaxis for *Pneumocystis jiroveci* pneumonia (PCP). Use trimethoprim–sulfamethoxazole (TMP-SMX) or pentamidine (if the patient is allergic to or intolerant of TMP-SMX).

4 Once the CD4 count is less than 100/mm³, start prophylaxis for *Mycobacterium avium intracellulare* with azithromycin, clarithromycin, or rifabutin; consider cryptococcal and candidal prophylaxis with fluconazole.

5 Once the CD4 count is less than 200/mm³, the patient is automatically considered to have AIDS (even without opportunistic infections).

6 Give measles, mumps, and rubella (MMR) vaccine to HIV-positive patients, the only live vaccine given to HIV patients.

7 Give pneumococcal, hepatitis B, inactivated polio vaccine, and annual influenza vaccines to all HIV-positive patients.

8 Do an annual purified protein derivative (PPD) test for tuberculosis in HIV patients; get an annual chest x-ray if the patient is anergic.

9 Do *not* give oral polio vaccine to HIV-positive patients *or* their contacts.

10 Classic AIDS-associated malignancies: Kaposi's sarcoma and non-Hodgkin's lymphoma (especially primary B-cell lymphomas of the central nervous system).

11 A positive India ink preparation of the cerebrospinal fluid means *Cryptococcus neoformans* meningitis.

12 Ring-enhancing lesions in the brain usually mean toxoplasmosis (Fig. 13-1) or lymphoma. Also consider cysticercosis (*Taenia solium*) in Latin American patients.

13 Other commonly seen HIV sequelae include wasting syndrome (progressive weight loss), dementia, peripheral neuropathies, thrombocytopenia, and loss of delayed hypersensitivity (type IV) on skin testing (anergy).

14 Give pregnant HIV-positive patients zidovudine (AZT), and give the infant AZT (or other antiretrovirals) for 6 weeks after birth. This protocol reduces mother-to-child transmission from roughly 25% to 8%. The infant can have a falsely positive HIV antibody test for 6 to 12 months because of maternal antibodies. Check DNA or RNA polymerase

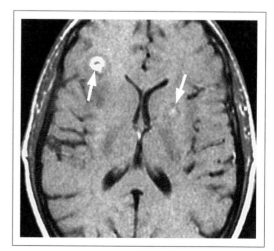

FIGURE 13-1. Toxoplasmosis in an immunosuppressed patient.
Lesions on contrast-enhanced magnetic resonance image may be either ring-enhancing (*left arrow*) or nodular (*right arrow*).

chain reaction test (or perform culture) to detect the virus directly. Cesarean section also can reduce transmission.

15 HIV-positive mothers should *not* breast-feed, because they can transmit the disease to their infants through breast milk.

16 Use ganciclovir or valganciclovir for cytomegalovirus retinitis; foscarnet or cidofovir are second-choice agents.

17 In any patient with HIV and pneumonia, think of PCP first (though plain community-acquired pneumonia is probably more common). Look for severe hypoxia with normal x-ray or diffuse, bilateral interstitial and air-space infiltrates. Usually the patient has a dry, nonproductive cough. PCP may be detectable with silver stains (Wright–Giemsa, Giemsa, methenamine silver) of induced sputum; if not, bronchoscopy with bronchoalveolar lavage and brush biopsy can make the diagnosis if needed, but patients are generally treated empirically initially and, if response occurs, invasive testing not needed.

18 Any adult patient with thrush should make you think of HIV, leukemia, or diabetes.

19 Any young adult who presents with herpes zoster should make you consider HIV.

20 *Cryptosporidium* and *Isospora* spp. are diarrheal infections uniquely seen in HIV-positive patients.

Primary Immunodeficiencies

Because primary immunodeficiencies are rare, your job is simply to recognize the classic case presentation.

- **IgA deficiency:** The most common primary immunodeficiency. Look for recurrent respiratory and gastrointestinal (GI) infections. IgA is low, and IgG subclass 2 may be low. Do *not* give immunoglobulins; you might cause anaphylaxis due to development of anti-IgA antibodies. Alternatively, in any patient who develops anaphylaxis after immunoglobulin exposure, you should think of IgA deficiency.

- **X-linked agammaglobulinemia (Bruton's agammaglobulinemia):** X-linked recessive disorder (i.e., affects male patients). B cells are low or absent; infections begin after 6 months when maternal antibodies disappear. Look for recurrent lung and sinus infections with *Streptococcus* and *Haemophilus* spp.

- **DiGeorge syndrome:** Caused by hypoplasia of the third and fourth pharyngeal pouches. Look for **hypocalcemia** and **tetany** (from absent parathyroids) in the first 24 to 48 hours of life. Also look for absent or hypoplastic thymus and congenital heart defects.

- **Severe combined immunodeficiency (SCID):** May be autosomal recessive or X-linked. Many cases are due to adenosine deaminase deficiency (autosomal recessive). Patients have B- and T-cell defects and severe infections in the first few months of life, and cutaneous anergy usually is present. Other signs include an absent or dysplastic thymus and lymph nodes.

- **Wiskott–Aldrich syndrome:** X-linked recessive disorder that affects male patients. Look for classic triad: **eczema, thrombocytopenia** (look for bleeding), and **recurrent infections** (usually respiratory).

- **Chronic granulomatous disease:** Usually an X-linked recessive disorder (i.e., male patients). Patients have a defect in reduced nicotinamide adenine dinucleotide phosphate (NADPH) oxidase activity and thus get recurrent infections with catalase-positive organisms (e.g., *Staphylococcus aureus, Pseudomonas* spp.). The diagnosis is clinched if the question mentions deficient nitroblue tetrazolium dye reduction by granulocytes (measures respiratory burst, which patients lack) or positive superoxide production testing.

- **Chediak–Higashi syndrome:** Usually autosomal recessive. Look for giant granules in neutrophils and associated oculocutaneous albinism. The cause is a defect in microtubule polymerization.

- **Complement deficiencies:** C5 through C9 deficiencies cause recurrent *Neisseria* infections; specific complement component is low.

- **Chronic mucocutaneous candidiasis:** A cellular immunodeficiency specific for *Candida* spp. Patients have candidal thrush, scalp, skin, and nail infections and anergy to *Candida* spp. with skin testing. Hypothyroidism is often an associated finding. The rest of immune function is intact.

- **Hyper IgE syndrome (Job–Buckley syndrome):** Patients get recurrent staphylococcal infections (especially of the skin) and have extremely high IgA levels. They also commonly have fair skin, red hair, and eczema.

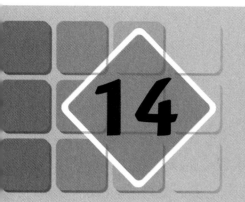

14 GENETICS

Step 2 questions often ask you to give genetic counseling to a parent or to predict the likelihood of having a second affected child after the first is born with a given disease. Because it is assumed that you know the inheritance pattern of the disease, the following information should come in handy.

Autosomal Dominant

Look for affected mother or father who passes the disease to 50% of offspring:

- von Willebrand's disease
- Neurofibromatosis: café-au-lait spots (Fig. 14-1), profuse peripheral nerve tumors, acoustic neuroma
- Multiple endocrine neoplasia (MEN) type I and II syndromes
- Achondroplasia: diagnosis by picture of a patient

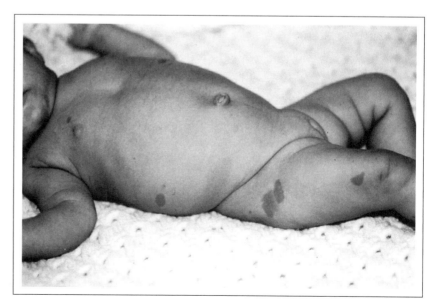

FIGURE 14-1. Café-au-lait spots.

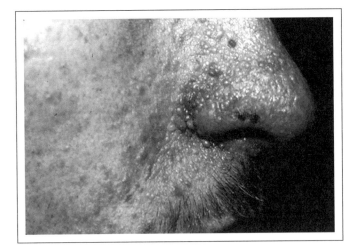

FIGURE 14-2. Facial angiofibromas.

- Marfan's syndrome: tall patient with arachnodactyly, mitral valve prolapse, aortic dissection, lens dislocation
- Huntington's disease
- Familial hypercholesterolemia: look for xanthomas, early coronary artery disease, markedly elevated cholesterol
- Familial polyposis coli
- Adult polycystic kidney disease
- Hereditary spherocytosis
- Tuberous sclerosis: hypopigmented skin macules, facial angiofibromas (i.e., adenoma sebaceum; Fig. 14-2), seizures, mental retardation, central nervous system hamartomas, rhabdomyomas, renal tumors
- Myotonic dystrophy: muscle weakness with inability to release grip, balding, cataracts, mental retardation, cardiac arrhythmias

Autosomal Recessive

Look for family history and unaffected parents who pass the disease to 25% of children:
- Sphingolipidoses (e.g., Tay-Sachs disease, Gaucher's disease; exception is Fabry's disease, which is X-linked)
- Mucopolysaccharidoses (e.g., Hurler's disease; exception is Hunter's disease, which is X-linked)
- Glycogen storage diseases (e.g., Pompe's and McArdle's disease)
- Cystic fibrosis
- Galactosemia: look for congenital cataracts, neonatal sepsis; avoid galactose- and lactose-containing foods
- Amino acid disorders (e.g., phenylketonuria, alkaptonuria)
- Sickle cell disease
- Children's polycystic kidney disease

◆ Wilson's disease

◆ Hemochromatosis (usually)

◆ Adrenogenital syndrome (e.g., 21-hydroxylase deficiency)

X-Linked Recessive

Look for affected fathers to pass the gene *only* to their daughters, who become carriers but do not get the disease. Carrier mothers (family history in male relatives) pass the gene to their sons, who get the disease:

◆ Hemophilia

◆ Glucose-6-phosphatase deficiency

◆ Fabry's disease

◆ Hunter's disease

◆ Lesch–Nyhan syndrome: hypoxanthine-guanine phosphoribosyltransferase enzyme deficiency. Look for mental retardation and self-mutilation (patients may bite off their own fingers).

◆ Duchenne's (and Becker's) muscular dystrophy

◆ Wiscott–Aldrich syndrome

◆ Bruton's agammaglobulinemia

◆ Fragile X syndrome: second most common cause of mental retardation in males (after Down's syndrome). Patients have large testes.

Polygenic Disorders

Relatives are more likely to have disease, but there is no obvious heritable pattern (yet...):

◆ Pyloric stenosis

◆ Cleft lip and/or palate

◆ Type 2 diabetes

◆ Obesity

◆ Neural tube defects

◆ Schizophrenia

◆ Bipolar disorder

◆ Ischemic heart disease

◆ Alcoholism

Chromosomal Disorders

Down's syndrome (trisomy 21; Fig. 14-3) is the most common known cause of mental retardation. The major risk factor is age of the mother (1 in 1500 offspring of 16-year-old

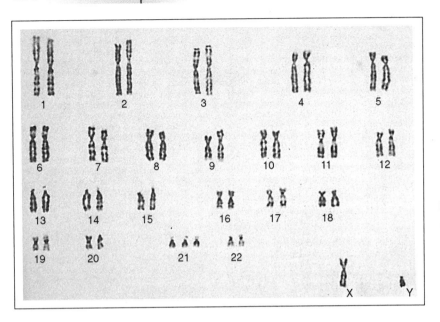

FIGURE 14-3. This karyotype in Down's syndrome reveals three copies of chromosome 21. (From Rubin E, Farber JL: Developmental and genetic diseases. In Rubin E, Farber JL (eds): Pathology, 2nd ed. Philadelphia, Lippincott, 1994, pp 200–261; with permission.)

mothers, 1 in 25 for 45-year-old mothers). At birth look for hypotonia, transverse palmar crease, and characteristic facies. Congenital cardiac defects (especially ventral septal defect) are common, and patients are at increased risk for **leukemia, duodenal atresia** (and other bowel atresias), **Hirschsprung's disease**, celiac disease, hypothyroidism, obstructive sleep apnea, gastroesophageal reflux, upper respiratory tract infections, infertility, visual problems, and **early Alzheimer's disease**.

Edwards' syndrome (trisomy 18) is more common in females than males. Patients are small for their age and have mental retardation, small head, hypoplastic mandible, low-set ears, and clenched fist with index finger overlapping third and fourth fingers (almost pathognomonic). Early pediatric death is typical.

Patau's syndrome (trisomy 13) includes mental retardation, apnea, deafness, holoprosencephaly (fusion of cerebral hemispheres), myelomeningocele, cardiovascular abnormalities, rocker-bottom feet. Early pediatric death is typical.

Patients with **Turner's syndrome** (XO instead of XX) have lymphedema of the neck at birth, short stature, webbed neck, widely spaced nipples, amenorrhea, and lack of breast development (due to primary ovarian failure). Coarctation of the aorta is common, and patients may have horse-shoe kidneys or cystic hygroma (benign neck mass or lymphangioma).

In **Klinefelter's syndrome** (XXY) the patient is tall and has microtestes (<2 cm in length), gynecomastia, sterility (the classic presentation is for infertility), and mildly decreased IQ.

Cri-du-chat is due to a deletion on the short arm of chromosome 5; look for **high-pitched cry like a cat** along with severe mental retardation.

15 GERIATRICS

IMPORTANT POINTS

1 The most rapid increase in population in the United States (percentage-wise) is in people older than 65 years (now roughly 15% of the population). Within this group, the over-85 subgroup is increasing most rapidly.

2 At age 80, patients have half the lean body mass of a 30-year-old. Because basal metabolic rate depends on lean body mass, elderly patients need fewer calories.

3 Normal changes in the elderly include slightly impaired immune response, visual (presbyopia) and hearing (presbycusis) impairment, decreased muscle mass, increased fat deposits, osteoporosis, brain changes (decreased weight, enlarged ventricles and sulci), and slightly decreased ability to learn new material.

4 Normal sexual function changes in men: Elderly men take longer to get an erection and have an increased refractory period (after ejaculation it takes longer before the patient can have another erection). Delayed ejaculation is common, and the patient might ejaculate only one of every three times that he has sex. Impotence and lack of sexual desire are *not* normal and should be investigated. Look for psychological (depression) as well as physical causes. Medications, especially antihypertensives, are notorious culprits.

5 Normal sexual function changes in women: For decreased lubrication, advise water-soluble lubricants. Atrophy of clitoris, labia, and vaginal tissues can cause dyspareunia; treat with estrogen cream (or hormone replacement therapy if desired by the patient). Delayed orgasm is common, but lack of sexual desire is *not* normal and should be investigated (psychological or physical causes).

6 The best prophylaxis for pressure ulcers in an immobilized patient is frequent turning.

7 Sleep changes: Elderly people sleep less deeply, wake up more frequently during the night, and awaken earlier in the morning. They take longer to fall asleep (longer sleep latency) and have less stage 3 and 4 and rapid-eye-movement (REM) sleep.

8 Depression in the elderly can manifest as dementia (i.e., pseudodementia). Look for a history that would trigger depression (e.g., loss of a spouse, terminal or debilitating disease).

9 After age 65 years, 15% of people suffer from dementia. The most common causes of dementia, in decreasing order, are Alzheimer's disease (gradually progressive, neurofibrillary tangles) and multi-infarct (step-wise, risk factors for cerebrovascular accident). Other causes include hypothyroidism, HIV, and Pick's disease.

10 Only 5% of people older than 65 years live in nursing homes.

11 More than 90% of hip fractures are associated with falls. Most occur in patients older than 70 years. Decrease the risk of falls in the elderly with mobility problems by fall-proofing the home (e.g., repair broken hand rails or steps and slippery floors, remove items that can be tripped over) and watching for medications that decrease the patient's sense of balance (the classic offenders are sedatives and anticholinergic drugs).

PREVENTIVE MEDICINE, EPIDEMIOLOGY, AND BIOSTATISTICS

16

Preventive Medicine

Guidelines for cancer screening are given in Table 16-1. Table 16-2 gives vaccination guidelines for adults.

In general, urinalysis (screening for urinary tract cancer that results in hematuria), alpha fetoprotein (liver and testicular cancer), and other serum markers are not appropriate for screening asymptomatic patients with no physical findings, but look for these abnormal lab values to show up in Step 2 questions as a clue to diagnosis. Prostate-specific antigen (PSA) is becoming popular as a prostate cancer screening test, but it does *not* replace a rectal exam.

Epidemiology

- **Incidence:** The number of new cases of disease in a unit of time (generally 1 year, but any time frame can be used). Incidence rate also equals the absolute risk (to be differentiated from relative or attributable risk).
- **Prevalence:** The total number of cases of disease that exist (new or old).

IMPORTANT POINTS

1 The classic question about incidence and prevalence: When a disease can be treated and people can be kept alive longer but the disease cannot be cured, what happens to the incidence and prevalence? Answer: Nothing happens to incidence, but prevalence will increase as people live longer. In short-term diseases, such as the flu, incidence may be higher than prevalence, whereas in chronic diseases, such as diabetes mellitus, prevalence is greater than incidence.

2 An epidemic occurs when the observed incidence greatly exceeds the expected incidence.

Table 16-1. AMERICAN CANCER SOCIETY GUIDELINES FOR CANCER SCREENING IN ASYMPTOMATIC PATIENTS*

Cancer	Procedure	Age (y)	Frequency
Colorectal	Sigmoidoscopy or double contrast barium enema[†]	>50	Every 5 years
	Stool occult blood test	>50	Annually
Colon, prostate	Digital rectal exam	>40	Annually
Prostate	Prostate specific antigen test	>50	Offer to patients annually (still controversial)
Cervical	Pap smear	18–65[‡]	After 2 normal exams 1 year apart, every 3 years
Gynecologic	Pelvic examination	20–40	Every 3 years
		>40	Annually
Endometrial	Endometrial biopsy	Menopause	Once at menopause
Breast	Breast self-examination	>20	Monthly
	Physician exam	20–40	Every 3 years
		>40	Annually
	Mammography	>40	Annually
Cancer checkup[§]	Health counseling/exam	20–39	Every 3 years
		≥40	Annually

*This table is for screening of asymptomatic, healthy patients. Other guidelines exist, but you'll be fine if you follow this table for boards (controversial areas are not generally tested).

[†]Colonoscopy every 10 years is an alternative option.

[‡]Start Pap smears at <18 years if the patient is sexually active.

[§]Includes examination for cancers of the thyroid, testis, ovary, lymph nodes, oral region, and skin.

Table 16-2. IMMUNIZATIONS IN ADULTS

Vaccine	Which Adults Should Receive the Vaccination
Hepatitis B	Give to any adult who wants it and anyone at risk of hepatitis B (including health care workers).
Influenza	Advised for all adults older than 50 years and any high-risk patients (e.g., those with chronic respiratory, cardiovascular, renal, or metabolic disease). Also give to women who will be pregnant during the influenza season (winter), household contacts of high-risk patients (to protect the high-risk patient), and health care workers (to protect your patients, not you!).
Pneumococcus	All adults older than 65 years and anyone with higher risks of morbidity or mortality from infection (e.g., patients with heart, lung, liver, or kidney disease; diabetes; immunocompromised including prior splenectomy).
Rubella	All women of child-bearing age who lack immunity or history of immunization. Do not give to pregnant women. Women should avoid pregnancy for 3 months after the vaccine. Also give to health care workers (to protect pregnant women's unborn children). Do not give to immunocompromised patients (except HIV-positive patients).
Tetanus (Td)	All people every 10 years. Give for any wound if vaccination history is unknown or patient has received <3 total doses. Give booster in people with full vaccination history if more than 5 years have passed since last dose for all wounds other than clean, minor wounds (including burns). Give tetanus immunoglobulin with vaccine for patients with unknown or incomplete vaccination and nonclean or major wounds.

Per-year rates commonly used to compare groups:

◆ **Birth rate:** Live births per 1000 population

◆ **Fertility rate:** Live births per 1000 population of females age 15–45 years

◆ **Death rate:** Deaths per 1000 population

◆ **Neonatal mortality rate:** Neonatal deaths (in the first 28 days) per 1000 live births; the rate in the United States is roughly 6/1000 (higher in blacks)

◆ **Perinatal mortality rate:** Neonatal deaths plus stillbirths and deaths in the first 7 days of life per 1000 total births. A stillbirth (fetal death) is defined as a prenatal or natal death after 20 weeks' gestation. In the United States, the major cause is prematurity and the rate is higher in nonwhites.

◆ **Infant mortality rate:** Deaths (from 0 to 1 year old) per 1000 live births. The top three causes in the United States, in descending order, are congenital abnormalities, low birth weight, and sudden infant death syndrome.

◆ **Maternal mortality rate:** Maternal pregnancy-related deaths (deaths during pregnancy or in the first 42 days after delivery) per 100,000 live births. The top three causes in the United States are pulmonary embolism, pregnancy-induced hypertension, and hemorrhage. The risk increases with age and is higher in blacks.

Insurance and the government:

◆ Medicare is health insurance for people who are eligible for Social Security (primarily people older than 65 years as well as the permanently and totally disabled and patients with end-stage renal disease).

◆ Medicaid covers the indigent who are deemed eligible by the individual states.

Biostatistics

THE 2 × 2 TABLE AND ITS DERIVATIVES

Review this section of Step 1 material for some easy (hopefully) points.

When faced with these types of questions, get in the habit of drawing a **2 × 2 table** to make calculations easier:

		Disease (+)	Disease (−)	
Test	(+)	A	B	Sensitivity = A/(A + C)
or				Specificity = D/(B + D)
Exposure	(−)	C	D	PPV = A/(A + B)

Sensitivity = A/(A + C)
Specificity = D/(B + D)
PPV = A/(A + B)
NPV = D/(C + D)
Odds ratio = (A × D)/(B × C)
Relative risk = [A/(A + B)] / [C/(C + D)]
Attributable risk = [A/(A + B)] − [C/(C + D)]

SENSITIVITY AND SPECIFICITY

Sensitivity is the ability to detect disease. Mathematically, sensitivity is calculated by dividing the number of true positives by the number of people with the disease. Tests with high sensitivity are used for screening. They might have false positives but do not miss many people with the disease (low false-negative rate).

Specificity is the ability to detect health (or nondisease). Mathematically, specificity is calculated by dividing the number of true negatives by the number of people without the disease. Tests with high specificity are used for disease confirmation. They might have false negatives but do not call anyone sick who is actually healthy (low false-positive rate). The ideal confirmatory test must have high sensitivity *and* high specificity; otherwise, people with the disease may be called healthy.

The **trade-off between sensitivity and specificity** is a classic statistics question. Understand how changing the cut-off glucose value in screening for diabetes (or changing the value of any of several screening tests) will change the number of true and false negatives and true and false positives. For example, if the cut-off value of glucose is raised, fewer people will be called diabetic (more false negatives, fewer false positives), whereas if the cut-off value is lowered, more people will be called diabetic (fewer false negatives, more false positives).

PREDICTIVE VALUES

When a test comes back positive for disease, the **positive predictive value (PPV)** measures how likely it is that the patient has the disease (probability of having a condition, given a positive test). Mathematically, PPV is calculated by dividing the number of true positives by the number of people with a positive test. PPV depends on the prevalence of a disease (the higher the prevalence, the greater the PPV) and the sensitivity and specificity of the test (e.g., an overly sensitive test that gives more false positives has a lower PPV).

When a test comes back negative for disease, the **negative predictive value (NPV)** measures how likely it is that the patient is healthy and does not have the disease (probability of not having a condition, given a negative test). Mathematically, NPV is calculated by dividing the number of true negatives by the number of people with a negative test. NPV depends on prevalence and the sensitivity and specificity, just like PPV. The higher the prevalence, the lower the NPV. In addition, an overly sensitive test with lots of false positives will make the NPV higher.

RISK

Odds ratio (OR) is used only for retrospective studies (e.g., case-control). OR compares disease in exposed and nondisease in unexposed populations with disease in unexposed and nondisease in exposed populations to determine whether there is a difference between the two. Of course, there should be more disease in exposed than unexposed populations and more nondisease in unexposed than exposed populations. OR is a less than perfect way to estimate relative risk.

Relative risk (RR) compares the disease risk in the exposed population to the disease risk in the unexposed population. RR can be calculated only after prospective or experimental studies; it *cannot* be calculated from retrospective data. RR greater than 1 is clinically significant.

Attributable risk is the number of cases attributable to one risk factor; in other words, the amount by which you can expect the incidence to decrease if a risk factor is removed. For example, if the incidence rate of lung cancer in the general population is 1/100 and in smokers it is 10/100, the attributable risk of smoking in causing lung cancer is 9/100 (assuming a properly matched control).

ACCURACY AND PRECISION

Reliability of a test (synonymous with precision) measures the reproducibility and consistency of a test (e.g., the concept of interrater reliability: If two different people administer the same test, they will get the same score if the test is reliable). Random error reduces reliability/precision (e.g., limitation in significant figures).

Validity of a test (synonymous with accuracy) measures the trueness of measurement—whether the test measures what it claims to measure. For example, if you give a valid IQ test to a genius, the test should not indicate that he or she is retarded. Systematic error reduces validity/accuracy (e.g., miscalibrated equipment).

THE BELL CURVE AND ITS VARIATIONS

Standard deviation: With a normal or bell-shaped distribution, one standard deviation (1 SD) holds 68% of values, 2 SD holds 95% of values, and 3 SD holds 99.7% of values. The classic question gives you the mean and standard deviation and asks you what percentage of values will be above a given value; variations on this question are also common. In a normal distribution, the mean = median = mode. The mean is the average, the median is the middle value, and the mode is the most common value. Questions might give you several numbers and ask for their mean, median, and mode.

Skewed distribution: A positive skew is asymmetry with an excess of high values (tail on right, mean > median > mode); a negative skew is asymmetry with an excess of low values (tail on left, mean < median < mode). These are *not* normal distributions; thus, standard deviation and mean are less meaningful values.

Hypothesis Testing, Data Comparisons and Confidence Interval

CORRELATION COEFFICIENT

The correlation coefficient measures the degree of relationship between two values. The range of the coefficient is −1 to +1. Zero equals no association whatsoever; positive one (+1) equals a perfect positive correlation (when one variable increases, so does the other); and negative one (−1) equals a perfect negative correlation (when one variable increases, the other decreases). Use the absolute value to give you the strength of the correlation (e.g., −0.3 is a stronger correlation than +0.2).

COMPARISON OF DATA

- **Chi-square test:** Used to compare percentages or proportions (nonnumeric data, also called nominal data)
- **T-test:** Used to compare two means
- **Analysis of variance (ANOVA):** Used to compare three or more means

CONFIDENCE INTERVAL

When you take a set of data and calculate a mean, you want to say that it is equivalent to the mean of the whole population, but usually they are not exactly equal. The confidence interval (CI; usually set at 95%) says that you are 95% confident that the population mean is within a certain range (usually within two standard deviations of the experimental or derived mean). For example, if you sample the heart rate of 100 people and calculate a mean of 80 bpm and a standard deviation of 2 bpm, your confidence interval (confidence limits) would be written as $76 < X < 84 = 0.95$. This means that you are 95% certain that the mean heart rate of the whole population (X) is between 76 and 84.

P-VALUE

The board exam always contains one or more questions about the significance of the p-value. If someone tells you $p < 0.05$ for a given set of data, there is less than a 5% chance (because $0.05 = 5\%$) that these data were obtained by random error or chance. If $p < 0.01$, the chance that the data were obtained by random error or chance is less than 1%. For example, if I tell you that the blood pressure in my controls is 180/100 mm Hg but decreases to 120/70 mmHg after administration of drug X and that $p < 0.10$, there is less than a 10% chance that the difference in blood pressure was due to random error or chance. However, there is up to a 9.99% chance that the result *is* due to random error or chance. Somewhat arbitrarily chosen, $p < 0.05$ is commonly used as the cutoff number for statistical significance in medicine.

Three points to remember:

◆ The study might still have serious flaws.

◆ A low p-value does not imply causation.

◆ A study that has statistical significance does *not* necessarily have clinical significance.

For example, if I tell you that drug X can lower the blood pressure from 130/80 to 128/80, p < 0.00001, you still would not use drug X (due to cost and potential side effects relative to the minimal clinical benefit).

The p-value also ties into the **null hypothesis** (the hypothesis of no difference). For example, in a drug study about hypertension, the null hypothesis is that the drug does not work; any difference in blood pressure is due to random error or chance. When the drug works beautifully and lowers the blood pressure by 60 points, we don't accept (i.e., we reject) the null hypothesis, because clearly the drug works. If that lowering of blood pressure is accompanied by a calculated p-value < 0.05, we can confidently reject the null hypothesis, because the p-value tells us that there is less than a 5% chance that the null hypothesis is correct. If the null hypothesis is incorrect, the difference in blood pressure is *not* due to chance and must be due to the new drug. In other words, the p-value represents the chance of making a **type I error** (claiming an effect or difference when none exists, rejecting the null hypothesis when it is true). If $p < 0.07$, there is less than a 7% chance that you are making a type I error. A **type II error** is to accept the null hypothesis when it is false (e.g., the hypertension drug works, but you say that it does not).

POWER

Power is the probability of rejecting the null hypothesis when it is false (a good thing). The best way to increase power (and thus reduce the risk of making a type II error) is to **increase sample size**.

STUDY TYPES AND ERRORS

Different types of studies (listed in decreasing order of quality and desirability):

- **Experimental:** The gold standard, which compares two equal groups in which one variable is manipulated and its effect is measured. Remember to use double-blinding (or at least single-blinding) and well-matched controls.

- **Prospective (aka longitudinal, cohort, incidence, or follow-up):** Choose a sample and divide it into two groups based on presence or absence of a risk factor and follow the group over time to see what diseases they develop (e.g., follow people with and without asymptomatic hypercholesterolemia to see whether people with hypercholesterolemia have a higher incidence of myocardial infarction later in life). This approach is sometimes called an observational study because all you do is observe. Relative risk and incidence can be calculated. Prospective studies are time-consuming, expensive, and good for common diseases, whereas retrospective studies are less expensive, less time-consuming, and good for rare diseases.

- **Retrospective or case-control:** Samples are chosen after the fact based on presence (cases) or absence (controls) of disease. Information can then be collected about risk factors; for example, look at people with lung cancer versus people without lung cancer and see if the people with lung cancer smoke more. An odds ratio can be calculated, but you *cannot* calculate a true relative risk or measure incidence from a retrospective study.

- **Case series:** Good for extremely rare diseases (as are retrospective studies). Case series simply describe the clinical presentation of people with a certain disease and might suggest the need for a retrospective study.

- **Prevalence survey or cross-sectional survey:** Looks at prevalence of a disease and prevalence of risk factors. When comparing two different cultures, you might get an idea about the cause of a disease, which can be tested with a prospective study (e.g., more colon cancer and higher-fat diet in the United States vs. less colon cancer and low-fat diet in Japan).

EXPERIMENTAL CONCLUSIONS AND ERRORS

The exam might give you data and the experimenter's conclusion and ask you to explain why the conclusion should not be drawn or to point out flaws in the experimental design.

- **Confounding variables:** An unmeasured variable affects both the independent (manipulated, experimental variable) and dependent (outcome) variables. For example, an experimenter measures the number of ashtrays owned and the incidence of lung cancer and finds that people with lung cancer have more ashtrays. He or she concludes that ashtrays cause lung cancer. Smoking tobacco is the confounding variable, because it causes the increase in both ashtrays and lung cancer.

- **Nonrandom or nonstratified sampling:** City A and city B can be compared but might not be equivalent. For example, if city A is a retirement community and city B is a college town, of course city A will have higher rates of mortality and heart disease if the groups are not stratified into appropriate age-specific comparisons.

◆ **Nonresponse bias:** People fail to return surveys or answer the phone for a phone survey. If nonresponse is a significant percentage of the results, the experiment will suffer. The first strategy is to visit or call the nonresponders repeatedly in an attempt to reach them and get their response. If this strategy is unsuccessful, list the nonresponders as unknown in the data analysis and see if any results can be salvaged. *Never make up or assume responses!*

◆ **Lead time bias:** Due to time differentials. The classic example is a cancer screening test that claims to have prolonged survival compared with old survival data, when in fact the measured difference in survival (i.e., elapsed time from diagnosis until death) is due only to earlier detection, *not* to improved treatment or prolonged survival.

◆ **Admission rate bias:** In comparing hospital A with hospital B for mortality due to myocardial infarction, you find that hospital A has a higher mortality rate. But this finding may be due to tougher hospital admission criteria at hospital A, which admits only the sickest patients with myocardial infarction and thus has higher mortality rates, although their care may be superior. The same bias can be found in a surgeon's mortality and morbidity rates if the surgeon takes only tough cases.

◆ **Recall bias:** Risk for retrospective studies. When patients cannot remember, they might inadvertently over- or underestimate risk factors. For example, John died of lung cancer, and his angry wife remembers him as smoking "like a chimney," whereas Mike died of a non–smoking-related cause and his loving wife denies that he smoked "much." In fact, both men smoked 1 pack per day.

◆ **Interviewer bias:** Due to lack of blinding. A scientist gets big money to do a study and wants to find a difference between cases and controls. Thus, he or she inadvertently labels the same patient comment or outcome as "no significance" in controls and "serious difference" in treated cases.

◆ **Unacceptability bias:** Patients in experiments want to be "acceptable" to the person conducting the study; thus, they might not admit to embarrassing behavior or might claim to take experimental medications when in fact they spit them out.

PSYCHIATRY

Antipsychotic Medications

Features of antipsychotic medications are listed in Table 17-1.

Extrapyramidal side effects:

◆ **Acute dystonia:** First few hours or days of treatment. The patient has muscle spasms or stiffness (e.g., torticollis, trismus), tongue protrusions and twisting, opisthotonos, and oculogyric crisis (forced sustained deviation of the head and eyes). Most common in young men. Treat by giving antihistamines (diphenhydramine) or anticholinergics (benztropine, trihexyphenidyl).

◆ **Akathisia:** First few days of treatment. The patient has a subjective feeling of restlessness. Look for constant pacing, alternate sitting and standing, and inability to sit still. β-Blockers can be tried for treatment.

◆ **Parkinsonism:** First few months of treatment. The patient has stiffness, cogwheel rigidity, shuffling gait, mask-like facies, and drooling. Parkinsonism is most common in older women. Treat by giving antihistamines (diphenhydramine) or anticholinergics (benztropine, trihexyphenidyl).

Table 17-1. FEATURES OF ANTIPSYCHOTIC MEDICATIONS

Feature	Antipsychotic Medication		
	High Potency	*Low Potency*	*Atypical**
Example(s)	Haloperidol	Chlorpromazine	Risperidone, olanzapine
Extrapyramidal side effects	High incidence	Low incidence	Low incidence
Autonomic side effects†	Low incidence	High incidence	Medium incidence
Positive symptoms	Works well	Works well	Works well
Negative symptoms	Works poorly	Works poorly	Works somewhat

*Atypical, newer agents are the drugs of choice for maintenance therapy because of reduced extrapyramidal side effects and potential effect on negative symptoms. Choose them over older agents.

†Autonomic side effects include anticholinergic (dry mouth, urinary retention, blurry vision, mydriasis), α-1 blockade (orthostatic hypotension), and antihistamine (sedation) effects.

◆ **Tardive dyskinesia:** Occurs after years of treatment. Most commonly, the patient has perioral movements (darting, protruding movements of the tongue, chewing, grimacing, puckering). The patient also can have involuntary, choreoathetoid movements of head, limbs, and trunk. There is no known treatment for tardive dyskinesia. If you have to make a choice when the patient develops tardive dyskinesia, discontinue the antipsychotic and consider switching to newer antipsychotic (e.g., olanzapine, clozapine).

◆ **Neuroleptic malignant syndrome:** Life-threatening condition that can develop at any time during treatment. The patient has rigidity, mutism, obtundation, agitation, **high fever** (up to 107° F), **high creatine phosphokinase** (often > 5000 U/L), sweating, and myoglobinuria. Treatment: **First** discontinue the antipsychotic; then provide supportive care for fever and renal shutdown due to myoglobinuria; finally, consider giving **dantrolene** (as in malignant hyperthermia).

Other antipsychotic medication pearls:

◆ **Dopamine blockade** causes increases in prolactin (dopamine is a prolactin-inhibiting factor in the tuberoinfundibular tract), which can cause galactorrhea, impotence, menstrual dysfunction, and decreased libido.

◆ **Individual antipsychotic side effects:** Thioridazine causes retinal pigment deposits; clozapine causes agranulocytosis (white blood cells counts must be monitored); chlorpromazine causes jaundice and photosensitivity.

Schizophrenia

The **diagnostic criteria** (Box 17-1) provide clues: delusions, hallucinations, disorganized speech, grossly disorganized or catatonic behavior, and negative symptoms (flat affect, refusal to talk, avolition, apathy). Factors indicating prognosis are listed in Table 17-2.

Time period is important: less than 1 month = acute psychotic disorder, 1 to 6 months = schizophreniform disorder, longer than 6 months = schizophrenia

Typical **age of onset** is 15 to 25 years for men (look for someone going to college and deteriorating) and 25 to 35 years for women.

Suicide: Up to 10% of schizophrenics eventually commit suicide (past attempt is best predictor of eventual success).

Box 17-1. SYMPTOMS OF SCHIZOPHRENIA

Positive symptoms	Negative symptoms
Delusions	Flat affect
Hallucinations	Alogia (no speech)
Bizarre behavior	Avolition (apathy)
Thought disorder	Anhedonia
Poor attention	

Table 17-2. PROGNOSIS FOR SCHIZOPHRENIA

Good Prognostic Factors	Poor Prognostic Factors
Good premorbid functioning	Poor premorbid functioning
Late onset	Early onset
Obvious precipitating factors	No precipitating factors
Married	Single, divorced, widowed
Family history of mood disorders	Family history of schizophrenia
Positive symptoms	Negative symptoms
Good support system	Poor support system

Antipsychotic medications are the mainstay of therapy, but psychosocial treatment has been shown to improve outcome. Medications are used first, but the best treatment (as in most of psychiatry) is medications plus therapy.

 Roughly 1% of people have schizophrenia (in all cultures).

In the United States, most schizophrenic patients are born in the winter (not known why).

Psychiatric patients can be hospitalized against their will if they are a danger to themselves (suicidal or unable to take care of themselves) or others (homicidal).

Bipolar Disorder

◆ Mania is the only symptom required for a diagnosis of bipolar disorder, but a history of mania alternating with depression is classic.

◆ Mania symptoms: decreased need for sleep, pressured speech, sexual promiscuity, shopping sprees, and exaggerated self-importance or delusions of grandeur.

◆ Look for initial onset between 16 and 30 years of age.

◆ Lithium and valproic acid are first-line treatments. Carbamazepine, olanzapine and gabapentin are second-line agents. Lithium can cause renal dysfunction (e.g., diabetes insipidus), thyroid dysfunction, tremor, and central nervous system (CNS) effects at toxic levels. Valproic acid can cause liver dysfunction and carbamazepine can cause bone marrow depression. Antipsychotics may be needed if the patient becomes psychotic; use at the same time as mood stabilizer.

◆ *Bipolar II disorder* is **hypomania** (mild mania without psychosis that does not cause occupational dysfunction) plus major depression. *Cyclothymia* is at least 2 years of **hypomania** alternating with depressed mood (*no* full-blown mania or depression).

Depression

Patients might not directly say: "I'm depressed." You have to watch for clues, such as change in sleep habits (classically, insomnia), vague somatic complaints, anxiety, low energy or fatigue, change in appetite (classically, decreased appetite), poor concentration, psychomotor retardation, and/or anhedonia (loss of pleasure).

Patients might or *might not* have obvious precipitating factors in history, such as loss of loved one, divorce or separation, unemployment or retirement, or chronic or debilitating disease. Depression is more common in women.

ADJUSTMENT DISORDER WITH DEPRESSED MOOD

When a bad situation occurs, the patient does not handle it well and feels "bummed out" for less than 6 months but does not meet criteria for full-blown depression. For example, the patient gets a divorce, seems to cry a lot for the next few weeks, and leaves work early on most days.

DYSTHYMIA

Depressed mood on most days for more than 2 years, but no episodes of major depression, mania, hypomania, or psychosis.

 Antidepressants can trigger mania or hypomania, especially in bipolar patients.

TREATMENT

Treat with both antidepressants and psychotherapy (combination works better than medications alone).

Antidepressants:

◆ **Tricyclic antidepressants** (TCAs; e.g., nortriptyline, amitriptyline) prevent reuptake of norepinephrine and serotonin. They also block α-adrenergic receptors (watch for orthostatic hypotension, dizziness, and falls) and muscarinic receptors, cause sedation, and lower the seizure threshold (especially bupropion, which technically is not a tricyclic). TCAs are dangerous in overdose primarily because of **cardiac arrhythmias,** which might respond to bicarbonate.

◆ **Selective serotonin reuptake inhibitors** (SSRIs; e.g., fluoxetine, paroxetine) prevent reuptake of serotonin only and have less serious side effects (e.g., insomnia, anorexia, **sexual dysfunction**).

◆ **Monoamine oxidase inhibitors** (MAOIs; e.g., phenelzine, tranylcypromine) are older medications and rarely used. They may be good for atypical depression (look for hypersomnia and hyperphagia, the opposite of classic depression). When patients eat tyramine-containing foods (especially wine and cheese), they may get a hypertensive crisis. Do *not* give MAOIs at the same time as SSRIs or meperidine; severe reactions can occur, possibly death.

◆ **Trazodone** is a notorious cause of priapism (persistent, painful erection without sexual arousal or desire).

Grief

Normal versus pathologic grief, mourning, bereavement:

◆ **Initial grief after a loss** (e.g., death of a loved one) can include a state of shock, feeling of numbness or bewilderment, distress, crying, sleep disturbances, decreased appetite, difficulty with concentrating, weight loss, and guilt (survivor guilt) **for up to 1 year**—in other words, the same symptoms as depression.

- It is **normal** to have an illusion or hallucination about the deceased, but a normal grieving person *knows* that it is an illusion or hallucination, whereas a depressed person believes that the illusion or hallucination is real.
- **Intense yearning** (even years after the death) and even searching for the deceased are normal.
- Feelings of worthlessness, psychomotor retardation, and suicidal ideation are *not* normal expressions of grief; they are signs of depression.

Personality Disorders

Personality disorders are lifelong disorders with no real treatment, although psychotherapy may be tried.

- **Antisocial:** Most frequently tested personality disorder. Patients have a long criminal record (con artists) and torture animals or set fires as children (a history of conduct disorder is required for this diagnosis). They are aggressive, do not pay bills or support children, often lie, and have no remorse or conscience. Strong association with alcoholism and drug abuse as well as somatization disorder. Most patients are male.
- **Avoidant:** Patients have no friends but want them; they are afraid of criticism or rejection and avoid others (inferiority complex).
- **Borderline:** Unstable mood, behavior, relationships (many bisexual), and self-image. Look for splitting (people are all good or all bad and may frequently change categories), suicide attempts, micropsychotic episodes (2 minutes of psychosis), impulsiveness and constant crisis (see Glenn Close in the movie *Fatal Attraction*).
- **Dependent:** Patients cannot be (or do anything) alone; highly dependent on others; e.g., a wife who stays with a severely abusive husband.
- **Histrionic:** Overly dramatic, attention seeking, and inappropriately seductive; the patient must be the center of attention.
- **Narcissistic:** Egocentric and lacking empathy; patients use others for their own gain or have a sense of entitlement.
- **Obsessive-compulsive:** Anal-retentive, stubborn; rules more important than objectives; restricted affect, cheap.
- **Paranoid:** Patients think that everyone is out to get them (friends, too) and often start law-suits.
- **Schizoid:** The classic loner; no friends and no interest in having friends.
- **Schizotypal:** Bizarre beliefs (extrasensory perception, cults, superstition, illusions) and manner of speaking, but no psychosis.

Suicide

The major **risk factors** are age older than 45 years, alcohol or substance abuse, history of rage or violence, prior suicide attempts, male sex (men commit suicide three times more often than women, but women attempt it four times more often than men), prior psychiatric history, depression, recent loss or separation, loss of health, unemployment or retirement, and single, widowed, or divorced status.

Always ask patients about suicide (it does *not* make them more likely to commit the act). If you need to do so, acutely hospitalize suicidal patients against their will.

When patients come out of a deep depression, they are at increased risk for suicide. The antidepressant begins to work, and the patient gets more energy—just enough to carry out suicide plans.

> **Note**
>
> If you have to choose on Step 2, the best predictor of future suicide is a past attempt.
>
> Suicide rates are rising the fastest in 15- to 24-year-olds, but the greatest risk is in people older than 65 years.

Other Psychiatric Disorders

- **Adjustment disorder:** Normal life experience (e.g., relationship break-up, failing grade, loss of job) is not handled well. Patients often are depressed (adjustment disorder with depressed mood) but do *not* meet the criteria for full-blown depression. For example, a high-school girl who breaks up with her boyfriend may mope around the house, crying and not wanting to attend school or go out with her friends for a few weeks.

- **Dissociative fugue/psychogenic fugue:** The patient has amnesia and travels, assuming a new identity.

- **Dissociative identity disorder** (old name: **multiple personality disorder**): The disorder most likely to be associated with childhood sexual abuse.

- **Generalized anxiety disorder:** Patients worry about everything (e.g., career, family, future, relationships, money) at the same time. Symptoms are not as dramatic as in panic disorder; patients are just severe worriers. Treat with buspirone or SSRI (both nonaddictive, nonsedating). Second-line treatment is benzodiazepines (addictive, sedating).

- **Homosexuality and homosexual experimentation:** Considered normal variants (not pathologic) at any age. Kinky fantasies or occasional kinky activities (a man wearing women's underwear, mild foot fetish) are normal.

- **Narcolepsy:** Daytime sleepiness; decreased rapid-eye-movement (REM) latency (patients go into REM as soon as they fall asleep); cataplexy (loss of muscle tone, falls); hypnopompic (as patient wakes up) and hypnagogic (as patient falls asleep) hallucinations. Treat with modafinil (a nonamphetamine stimulant) or amphetamines.

- **Obsessive-compulsive disorder:** Patients have recurrent thoughts or impulses (obsessions) and/or recurrent behavior or acts (compulsions) that cause marked dysfunction in occupational and/or interpersonal lives. Look for **washing** (e.g., wash hands 30 times a day) and/or **checking rituals** (check to see if door is locked 30 times a day). Onset usually is in adolescence or early adulthood. Treat with SSRIs (especially fluvoxamine) or clomipramine. Behavioral therapy also may be effective (e.g., flooding).

- **Panic disorder:** Look for 20- to 40-year-old patient who thinks that he or she is dying or having a heart attack, but is healthy and has a negative work-up for organic disease. Patients often hyperventilate and are extremely anxious. A common association is agoraphobia (fear of leaving the house). Treat with SSRIs (e.g., fluoxetine) over benzodiazepines (which are addicting and sedating).

- **Posttraumatic stress disorder:** Look for someone who has been through a life-threatening event (Vietnam or Iraq war veteran, victim of severe accident or rape) who recurrently experiences the event in nightmares or flashbacks, tries to avoid thinking about it, and has depression or poor concentration as a result. Treat with group therapy and/or SSRI.

- **Simple phobias:** For example, to needles, blood products, animals, or heights. Treat with behavioral therapy (flooding, systematic desensitization, biofeedback, mental imagery—know what these terms mean) if patient desires treatment.

- **Social anxiety disorder** (social phobia): A specific simple phobia that is best treated with behavioral therapy. β-Blockers may be used to reduce symptoms before a public appearance that cannot be avoided, and SSRIs might help.

- **Somatoform disorders:** Patients do *not* behave inappropriately on purpose. Treat with frequent return clinic visits and/or psychotherapy.

  - **Somatization disorder:** Multiple *different* complaints in multiple *different* organ systems over many years with extensive work-ups in the past.

  - **Conversion disorder:** Obvious precipitating factor (fight with boyfriend) followed by unexplainable neurologic symptoms (blindness, stocking-and-glove numbness).

  - **Hypochondriasis:** Patients keep believing that they have the *same* specific disease despite extensive negative work-up.

  - **Body dysmorphic disorder:** Preoccupation with imagined physical defect (e.g., a teenager who thinks that his or her nose is too big when it is of normal size).

Somatoform disorders versus factitious disorder versus malingering:

- **Somatoform disorders:** Patients do *not* intentionally create symptoms.

- **Factitious disorders:** Patients *intentionally* create their illness or symptoms (e.g., inject themselves with insulin to provoke hypoglycemia) and subject themselves to procedures to assume the role of a patient (no financial or other secondary gain).

- **Malingering:** Patients intentionally create their illness for *secondary gain* (e.g., money, to get out of work or jail).

Psychological Tests

Many different psychological tests are available to aid in a difficult diagnosis; they are *not* used for a straightforward case. There are two types of tests: **objective**—multiple choice, scored by a computer; and **subjective**—no right answers, scored by the test giver.

- **Beck Depression Inventory:** Objective test to screen for depression.

- **Halstead–Reitan Battery:** Used to determine the location and effects of specific brain lesions.
- **Luria–Nebraska Neuropsychological Battery:** Assesses a wide range of cognitive functions and tells you the patient's cerebral dominance (left or right).
- **Minnesota Multiphasic Personality Inventory:** Objective test designed to measure personality type.
- **Rorschach test:** Subjective test in which patients describe what they see in an inkblot.
- **Stanford-Binet:** Objective IQ test for adults.
- **Thematic Apperception Test:** Subjective test in which the patient describes what is going on in a cartoon drawing of people.
- **Wechsler Intelligence Scale for Children:** Objective IQ test for children (4–17 years old).

Child Psychiatry

ANOREXIA

Look for a female adolescent who is a good athlete and/or student with a perfectionistic personality. Patients have body weight at least 15% below normal, intense fear of gaining weight (or "feel fat" even though emaciated), and amenorrhea (all three are required for diagnosis). Death occurs in roughly 10% to 15% of patients as a result of complications of starvation and/or bulimia (electrolyte imbalances, cardiac arrhythmias, infections). Some patients are hospitalized against their will for intravenous (IV) nutrition. Roughly half of anorexics also have bulimia.

ATTENTION-DEFICIT/HYPERACTIVITY DISORDER

In attention-deficit/hyperactivity disorder (ADHD), as the name implies, affected children are hyperactive and have short attention spans. Boys are affected more often than girls. Look for a fidgety child who is impulsive and cannot pay attention but is not cruel. Treat with stimulants (paradoxical calming effect) such as modafinil, methylphenidate (Ritalin), or dextroamphetamine, which can all cause insomnia, abdominal pain, anorexia, and weight loss or growth suppression. Hot topic due to concerns about overdiagnosis and treatment. Use drug holidays (temporarily stop drug) to combat side effects.

AUTISM

Autism usually starts at a very young age. Look for impaired social interaction (isolative, unaware of surroundings), impaired verbal and nonverbal communication (strange words, babbling, repetition), and restricted activities and interests (head banging, strange movements). Autism is usually idiopathic, but look for congenital rubella as a potential cause. See Dustin Hoffman in the movie *Rain Man*.

BULIMIA

Look for a female adolescent who is of normal weight or overweight (unless anorexia coexists). Patients have binge-eating episodes during which they feel a lack of control and then engage in purging behavior (vomiting, laxatives, exercise, fasting). Patients might require hospitalization for electrolyte disturbances. In the classic patient, the tooth enamel has been eroded because of frequent vomiting; the skin over the knuckles may also be eroded from putting fingers into the throat.

CONDUCT DISORDER

Conduct disorder is the pediatric form of antisocial disorder. Look for fire setting, cruelty to animals, lying, stealing, and/or fighting. As adults, patients often have antisocial disorder. *Note:* Conduct disorder in childhood is required to make a diagnosis of antisocial personality disorder in an adult.

ENCOPRESIS AND ENURESIS

Encopresis and enuresis are not disorders until after age 4 years (encopresis) or 5 years (enuresis). This is obviously an important diagnostic point to remember when the mother complains (normal finding if the child is 3 years old). Rule out physical problems (e.g., Hirschsprung's disease, urinary tract infection), then treat with behavioral therapy ("gold star for being good" charts, alarms, biofeedback). Imipramine is used only for refractory cases of enuresis; it is *not* a first-line agent.

LEARNING DISORDER

This disorder can include impairment in math, reading, writing, speech, language, or coordination, but everything else is normal and no mental retardation is present ("Chris just can't do math").

MENTAL RETARDATION

Most cases are idiopathic, and 85% of cases are mild (IQ range: 55–70). Patients often have a reasonable level of independence but need assistance or guidance during periods of stress. **Fetal alcohol syndrome** is the number-one *preventable* cause, whereas **Down's syndrome** is the number-one *overall* cause. Fragile X syndrome (in boys) is another common cause of mental retardation.

OPPOSITIONAL DEFIANT DISORDER

This includes negative, hostile, and defiant behavior toward authority figures (parents, teachers). The child misbehaves around adults, but behaves normally around peers and is not a cruel, lying criminal (as in conduct disorder).

SEPARATION ANXIETY DISORDER

Look for a child who refuses to go to school. Basically, affected children think that something will happen to them or their parents if they separate; thus, they will do anything to avoid separation (stomachache, headache, temper tantrums).

TOURETTE'S DISORDER

Only 10% to 30% of patients utter obscenities. Look for boys with motor tics (eye-blinking, grunting, throat-clearing, grimacing, barking, or shoulder shrugging) that are exacerbated by stress and remit during activity or sleep. Tourette's disorder can be caused or unmasked by use of stimulants (e.g., for presumed ADHD). Antipsychotics (e.g., haloperidol) are used if the symptoms are severe. Tourette's disorder tends to be a lifelong problem.

IMPORTANT POINTS

1 Depression in children often manifests as irritable mood instead of depressed mood.

2 The top three causes of adolescent deaths in order are **accidents, homicide,** and **suicide.** Together they account for about 75% of teenage deaths.

Drugs of Abuse

AMPHETAMINES

Amphetamines are classically associated with psychotic symptoms (patients may appear to be full-blown schizophrenics), but effects are similar to cocaine's.

BENZODIAZEPINES AND BARBITURATES

Benzodiazepines and barbiturates cause sedation and drowsiness as well as reduced anxiety and disinhibition. Overdose may be fatal (respiratory depression); treat with **flumazenil** if needed. Withdrawal also may be fatal (just as with alcohol) because of seizures and/or cardiovascular collapse. Treat withdrawal on an inpatient basis with a long-acting benzodiazepine; gradually taper the dose over several days. Benzodiazepines and barbiturates are especially dangerous when mixed with alcohol (all three are CNS depressants).

COCAINE

Look for sympathetic stimulation (insomnia, tachycardia, mydriasis, hypertension, sweating) with hyperalertness and possible paranoia, aggression, delirium, psychosis, or formications ("cocaine bugs"—patients think that bugs are crawling on them). Overdose can be fatal (arrhythmia, myocardial infarction, seizure, or stroke). On withdrawal, patients become sleepy, hungry (versus anorexic with intoxication), and irritable, possibly with severe depression. Withdrawal is not dangerous, but psychological cravings usually are severe. Cocaine is teratogenic (vascular disruptions in fetus).

INHALANTS

Inhalant (e.g., gasoline, glue, varnish remover) intoxication causes euphoria, dizziness, slurred speech, a feeling of floating, ataxia, and/or a sense of heightened power. Intoxication usually is seen in younger teenagers (11–15 years). Can be fatal in overdose (respiratory depression, cardiac arrhythmias, asphyxiation) or cause severe permanent sequelae (CNS, liver, and kidney toxicity; peripheral neuropathy). There is no known withdrawal syndrome.

LSD AND MUSHROOMS

Symptoms of intoxication with lysergic acid diethylamide (LSD) and mushrooms include hallucinations, mydriasis, tachycardia, diaphoresis, and perception and mood disturbances. Hallucinations usually are visual rather than auditory (opposite of schizophrenia). Overdose is not dangerous (unless the patient thinks that he or she can fly and jumps out a window). No withdrawal symptoms are noted. Patients can have flashbacks months to years later (brief feeling of being on drug again, although none was taken) or a bad trip (acute panic reaction or dysphoria). Treat bad trips with reassurance or benzodiazepine or antipsychotic medication (if needed).

MARIJUANA

Marijuana is the most commonly abused illegal drug. Look for a teenager who listens to rebellious music, has red eyes, and acts "weird." Other symptoms include "amotivational syndrome" (chronic use can cause laziness and lack of motivation), time distortion, and munchies (eating binge when intoxicated). No physical withdrawal symptoms are noted, although patients can have psychological cravings. Overdose is not dangerous, but patients can have temporary dysphoria. Marijuana is not a proven teratogen.

OPIOIDS

Heroin and other opioids cause euphoria, analgesia, drowsiness, miosis, constipation, and CNS depression. Overdose can be fatal (respiratory depression); treat with naloxone. Because the drug is usually taken intravenously, there are associated morbidities and mortalities (endocarditis, HIV, cellulitis, talc damage). Withdrawal is not life-threatening, but patients act as though they are going to die. Symptoms include gooseflesh, diarrhea, insomnia, and cramping or pain. Methadone treatment sometimes is given for addicts. Methadone is a longer-acting opioid that allows patients to function by keeping them on a chronic, free, lower dose. Its use is controversial.

PHENCYCLIDINE

Phenyclidine (PCP) causes LSD or mushroom symptoms in intoxication plus confusion, agitation, and aggressive behavior. Also look for **vertical and/or horizontal nystagmus,** plus possible schizophrenic-like symptoms (paranoia, auditory hallucinations, disorganized behavior and speech). Overdose can be fatal (convulsions, coma, respiratory arrest). Treat with supportive care and urine acidification to hasten elimination. No withdrawal symptoms are noted.

 Caffeine withdrawal can cause headaches, irritability, and fatigue.

18 GYNECOLOGY

Adenomyosis

In adenomyosis, endometrial glands are found within the uterine musculature (i.e., part of the spectrum of endometriosis, but confined to the uterus). Patients usually are older than 40 years and have dysmenorrhea and menorrhagia. Physical exam reveals a large, boggy uterus. Ultrasound might suggest and magnetic resonance image (MRI) can confirm this diagnosis, which is usually clinical.

Do dilation and curettage (D&C) to rule out endometrial cancer, and consider total abdominal hysterectomy to relieve severe symptoms. Gonadotropin-releasing hormone agonists also can relieve symptoms.

Amenorrhea

PRIMARY AMENORRHEA

Any girl who has not menstruated by age 16 has primary amenorrhea. In the absence of secondary sexual characteristics by age 14 or absence of menstruation within 2 years of developing secondary sex characteristics, patients also should be evaluated.

IMPORTANT POINTS

1 The first step is to rule out pregnancy! (Yes, pregnancy can manifest as primary amenorrhea.)

2 If the patient is older than 14 years and has no secondary sexual characteristics, she most likely has a congenital problem.

3 In a phenotypically normal female patient (normal breast development) with an absence of both axillary and pubic hair, think of androgen insensitivity syndrome. The uterus is absent.

4 In the presence of normal breast development and a uterus, the first step is to get a prolactin level to rule out pituitary adenoma. If prolactin is high, get an MRI. If it is normal, administer progesterone and follow the same procedures as for evaluation of secondary amenorrhea.

SECONDARY AMENORRHEA

In a previously menstruating, sexually active woman of reproductive age, the diagnosis is pregnancy until proved otherwise (with a negative human chorionic gonadotropin [hCG] assay). Amenorrhea is not uncommon in hard-training athletes (due to exercise-induced depression of gonadotropin-releasing hormone [GRH]). Watch for amenorrhea as a presenting symptom for anorexia (amenorrhea is required for a diagnosis of anorexia), especially in a ballet dancer or model. Another common cause is polycystic ovarian syndrome (PCOS; see later). Secondary amenorrhea also may be due to endocrine disorders (headaches, galactorrhea, and visual field defects can indicate a pituitary tumor), antipsychotics (due to increased prolactin), or previous chemotherapy (which causes premature ovarian failure and menopause).

The first step after a negative pregnancy test and no obvious abnormality in the history or physical exam is to **administer progesterone**, which tells you the patient's estrogen status:

◆ If the patient has vaginal bleeding within 2 weeks, she has sufficient estrogen. Next, check luteinizing hormone (LH). If the level is high, think of PCOS. If it is low or normal, check the prolactin level to rule out pituitary adenoma and the thyroid-stimulating hormone (TSH) level to rule out hypothyroidism (high TSH level causes high prolactin level). If prolactin is high with normal TSH, get an MRI of the brain. If prolactin is normal, look for drug-, stress-, or exercise-induced depression of GRH. Any of these patients may try clomiphene to become pregnant.

◆ If the patient does not have vaginal bleeding, she has insufficient estrogen. Check follicle-stimulating hormone (FSH) next. If the level is elevated, the patient has premature ovarian failure (i.e., menopause); check for autoimmune disorder, karyotype abnormalities, and history of chemotherapy. If FSH is low or normal, the patient might have a craniopharyngioma or other central nervous system (CNS) tumor; get an MRI of the brain.

When in doubt, follow these steps _in order_ to evaluate any amenorrhea:

1. Do a pregnancy test.
2. Administer progesterone.
3. Further testing depends on results of progesterone challenge (bleeding or no bleeding).

Any sexually active woman of reproductive age who has amenorrhea should have a pregnancy test as the first step in evaluation.

Birth Control

◆ The best choice is oral contraceptives if the patient is a candidate and does not desire sterilization. Oral contraceptives do _not_ reduce transmission of sexually transmitted diseases.

◆ An intrauterine device should be used only in older women, preferably those who are monogamous, because it increases the risk of ectopic pregnancy and pelvic inflammatory disease (PID) (look for _Actinomyces_ spp.).

◆ Condoms are good because they prevent transmission of sexually transmitted diseases.

Breast Disorders

BREAST DISCHARGE

First get the patient's history of oral contraceptives, hormone therapies, antipsychotic medications, or hypothyroidism symptoms, all of which can cause discharge. When bilateral and nonbloody, the discharge is *not* due to breast cancer; the cause may be a prolactinoma (check prolactin) or endocrine disorder. A discharge that is unilateral, bloody, and/or associated with a mass should raise concern about breast cancer. Biopsy any mass.

BREAST MASS IN A WOMAN YOUNGER THAN 35 YEARS

- **Fibrocystic disease:** *Bilateral*, multiple, tender (especially premenstrually) *cystic lesions*. Most common of all breast diseases. Generally, no further work-up is needed—just routine follow-up. Progesterone for 1 week at the end of each month or danazol might help to relieve symptoms.

- **Fibroadenoma:** Painless, discrete, sharply circumscribed, rubbery, mobile mass. Most common benign tumor of the female breast. Observe the patient for one or more menstrual cycles in the absence of symptoms. Pregnancy or oral contraceptives can stimulate growth; menopause causes regression (estrogen-dependent growths). Excision is curative but not required (unless patient desires it or there is clinical concern for cancer).

- **Mastitis or abscess:** Lactating women typically in the first few months postpartum develop painful, swollen erythematous breast(s). The nipple may be cracked or fissured. The patient should be treated with analgesics (e.g., acetaminophen, ibuprofen) and instructed to continue breast-feeding with the affected breast(s) even though it is painful (use breast pump to empty breast if needed) to prevent further milk duct blockage and abscess formation. Antistaphylococcal antibiotic (e.g., cephalexin, dicloxacillin) is given for more than mild symptoms. If a fluctuant mass develops or there is no response to antibiotics within a few days, an abscess is likely present and must be drained.

- **Fat necrosis:** History of trauma.

 Avoid mammography in women younger than 30 years (breast tissue is too dense to give interpretable films). If suspicious of cancer (exceedingly rare in this age group), use ultrasound for evaluation.

BREAST MASS IN A WOMAN 35 YEARS OR OLDER

- **Fibrocystic disease:** As above, but aspiration of cyst fluid and baseline mammography are recommended. If the cyst fluid is nonbloody and the mass resolves after aspiration, the patient needs only reassurance, follow-up, and a baseline mammogram. If the fluid is bloody or the cyst recurs quickly, do a biopsy to rule out cancer.

- **Fibroadenoma:** Get baseline mammogram. Observe briefly if the mass is small *and* seems benign clinically *and* the woman is premenopausal *and* she has no risk factors for breast cancer. Otherwise, do a biopsy. Watch for cystosarcoma phylloides that masquerades as fibroadenoma.

- **Fat necrosis:** As for younger women.

- **Mastitis or abscess:** As for younger women.
- **Breast cancer:** You might not get a classic presentation of nipple retraction and/or peau d'orange in a nulliparous woman with a strong family history. In a woman 35 years or older, you will rarely be faulted for doing a biopsy of any new mass. In the absence of a classic benign presentation (such as trauma to the breast with fat necrosis or bilaterality with premenstrual mastalgia), always consider biopsy. Also get a diagnostic mammogram (first imaging study) and potentially ultrasound and/or breast MRI. (See Chapter 9, Oncology.)

IMPORTANT POINTS

1 If the patient is postmenopausal (or older than 50 years) and develops a new lesion, you should be highly suspicious of malignancy on the boards.

2 In patients with a clinically evident breast mass, the decision to perform a biopsy is a clinical one. Mammography (and ultrasound and increasingly MRI) is often done to help evaluate the mass, and in a woman older than 35 years can serve as a baseline for future comparison. If a mass is detected on imaging and not clearly or probably benign, biopsy is generally recommended.

3 Conversely, any suspicious lesion found on mammogram (or other imaging) should be biopsied, even if it is inapparent or seems benign on physical exam.

Dysfunctional Uterine Bleeding

Dysfunctional uterine bleeding (DUB) is defined as abnormal uterine bleeding not associated with tumor, inflammation, or pregnancy. DUB is the most common cause of abnormal uterine bleeding and is a diagnosis of exclusion. More than 70% of cases are associated with anovulatory cycles (unopposed estrogen, as occurs in the polycystic ovarian syndrome). The age of the patient is important. After menarche and just before menopause, DUB is extremely common and, in fact, physiologic. Most other patients have polycystic ovaries.

Always do a D&C to rule out **endometrial cancer** in women older than 35 years. Also get hemoglobin and hematocrit to make sure that the patient is not anemic from excessive blood loss.

Uncommon causes of DUB are infections, endocrine disorders (thyroid, adrenal, pituitary/prolactin), coagulation defects, and estrogen-producing neoplasm.

IMPORTANT POINTS

1 In the absence of pathology, treat first with nonsteroidal antiinflammatory drugs (NSAIDs) (first-line agents for DUB and dysmenorrhea).

2 Oral contraceptives are also a first-line agent for menorrhagia and DUB if the patient does not desire pregnancy and cycles are irregular.

3 Progesterone can be used to help stop severe bleeding.

Endometriosis

Endometriosis is endometrial glands outside the uterus (ectopic). Patients usually are nulliparous and older than 30 years with the following symptoms: **dysmenorrhea, dyspareunia** (painful intercourse), **dyschezia** (painful defecation), and/or perimenstrual spotting. The most common site is the ovaries (look for tender adnexae in an afebrile patient), followed by the broad or uterosacral ligament (classic signs are nodularities on physical exam and sequela of retroverted uterus), and peritoneal surface. The gold standard of diagnosis is laparoscopy with visualization of endometriosis. Ultrasound or MRI can sometimes make the diagnosis noninvasively.

IMPORTANT POINTS

1 Endometriosis is the most likely cause of infertility in a menstruating woman older than 30 years (in the absence of a PID history).

2 Treat first with oral contraceptives (danazol and GRH agonists are second-line agents).

3 Surgery and cautery may be used to destroy endometrioma in an attempt to restore fertility. In an older patient, consider total abdominal hysterectomy and bilateral salpingo-oophorectomy for severe symptoms.

Infertility

In two thirds of couples, infertility is a female problem; in one third, it is a male problem. If nothing is apparent after history and physical exam, the first step is **semen analysis** (cheap, easy, noninvasive). Normal semen has the following properties:

- Ejaculate volume >1 mL
- Sperm concentration >20 million/mL
- Initial forward motility >50% of sperm
- Normal morphology >60% of sperm

The next step is **documentation of ovulation**. History might suggest an ovulatory problem (irregular cycle length, duration, or amount of flow; lack of premenstrual symptoms). Basal body temperature, luteal phase progesterone levels, and/or endometrial biopsy can be done to check for ovulation.

Tubal and uterine evaluation is done by a **hysterosalpingogram** (Figs. 18-1 and 18-2). History might suggest a tubal problem (PID, previous ectopic pregnancy) or a uterine problem (previous D&C can cause intrauterine synechiae, adhesions, scarring [Asherman's syndrome], history of fibroids or endometriosis symptoms).

Cervical factor may be a cause of infertility and is suggested by a history of cervicitis, birth trauma, or previous cone biopsy. Evaluate cervical mucus, and do a postcoital test.

Laparoscopy is a last resort or is done in patients with a history suggestive of endometriosis. Lysis of adhesions and destruction of endometriosis lesions can restore fertility.

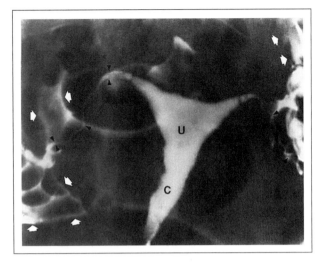

FIGURE 18-1. Normal hysterosalpingogram. Contrast is seen filling the endocervical canal (*C*) and the uterine cavity (*U*). The fallopian tubes (*black arrowheads*) and bilateral free spillage of contrast (*white arrows*) are demonstrated.

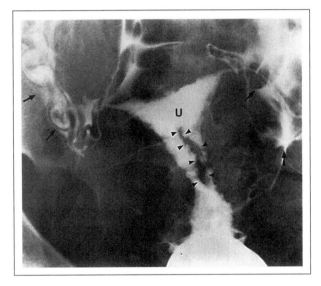

FIGURE 18-2. Uterine synechiae (Asherman's syndrome) shown as an irregular filling defect (*arrowheads*) in the lower uterine cavity (*U*) on this abnormal hysterosalpingogram. Bilateral free spillage of contrast (*arrows*) confirms patency of the fallopian tubes.

Medical therapy for infertility is usually clomiphene citrate to induce ovulation, but this approach requires that the woman is producing adequate estrogen. If the woman is hypoestrogenic, use human menopausal gonadotropin (hMG), which is a combination of FSH and LH. If these methods fail, use in vitro fertilization.

Leiomyoma

Leiomyomas are also called fibroids and are benign tumors (Fig. 18-3). However, they are the most common indication for hysterectomy (when they grow too large or cause symptoms). Look for rapid growth during pregnancy or use of oral contraceptives with regression after menopause (tumors are estrogen dependent). Fibroids can cause infertility; myomectomy might restore fertility. Other symptoms include pain and menorrhagia or metrorrhagia. Anemia due to leiomyoma is an indication for hysterectomy. D&C rules out endometrial cancer and malignant transformation in women older than 40 years. Patients might present with a polyp protruding through the cervix. Malignant transformation is rare (<1%).

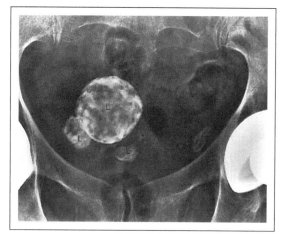

FIGURE 18-3. Plain film of the pelvis shows typical calcifications within three separate uterine leiomyomas (*L*).

 Any sexually active woman of reproductive age with abnormal uterine bleeding should have a pregnancy test as the first diagnostic step.

Menopause

The average age at menopause is 51. Patients have irregular cycles or amenorrhea, hot flushes, mood swings, and an elevated FSH level. Patients also might complain of dysuria, dyspareunia, incontinence, and/or vaginal itching, burning, or soreness—symptoms that often are due to atrophic vaginitis in this age group. Look for vaginal mucosa to be thin, dry, and atrophic, with increased parabasal cells on cytology. Estrogen, either topical or systemic, improves symptoms but is now rather controversial as a systemic therapy due to side effects.

Pelvic Inflammatory Disease

Look for a female patient aged 13 to 35 years with abdominal pain, adnexal tenderness, *and* cervical motion tenderness (all three must be present). PID also requires one or more of the following: elevated erythrocyte sedimentation rate (or C-reactive protein), leukocytosis, fever, purulent cervical discharge, or purulent fluid from culdocentesis. Treat with more than one antibiotic (e.g., cefoxitin or ceftriaxone and doxycycline on outpatient basis; clindamycin and gentamicin on an inpatient basis) to cover multiple organisms (e.g., *Neisseria gonorrhoeae*, *Chlamydia* spp., *Escherichia coli*). With a history of intrauterine device use, think *Actinomyces israelii*.

IMPORTANT POINTS

1 PID is the most common cause of preventable infertility (causes scarring of tubes) and the most likely cause of infertility in a *normally* menstruating woman under age 30.

2 Watch for progression to tuboovarian abscess (palpable on exam) and its rupture. Treat with antibiotics on an inpatient basis initially; perform laparotomy with excision of affected tube (unilateral disease) or total abdominal hysterectomy and bilateral salpingo-oophorectomy (bilateral disease) if there is no response or worsening symptoms over the first 24 to 48 hours.

Pelvic Relaxation and Vaginal Prolapse

Pelvic relaxation and vaginal prolapse are caused by weakening of pelvic supporting ligaments. Look for history of several vaginal deliveries, feeling of heaviness or fullness in the pelvis, backache, worsening of symptoms with standing, and resolution with lying down.

- **Cystocele:** Bladder bulges into the *upper anterior* vaginal wall. Symptoms: urinary urgency, frequency, incontinence.
- **Rectocele:** Rectum bulges into the *lower posterior* vaginal wall. Major symptom: difficulty with defecating.
- **Enterocele:** Loops of bowel bulge into the *upper posterior* vaginal wall.
- **Urethrocele:** Urethra bulges into the *lower anterior* vaginal wall. Symptoms: urinary urgency, frequency, incontinence.

 Conservative treatment involves pelvic strengthening exercises and/or a pessary (artificial device inserted into the vagina to provide support). Surgery is used for refractory or severe cases.

Polycystic Ovarian Syndrome

Classic presentation is an overweight woman with hirsutism, amenorrhea, and infertility. PCOS is the most likely cause of infertility in a woman younger than 30 years with *abnormal* menstruation. Multiple ovarian cysts may be seen on ultrasound (though not needed for diagnosis). A high LH level and androgen excess (e.g., testosterone, androstenedione) are present and the ratio of LH to FSH is greater than 2:1. Unopposed estrogen increases the risk for **endometrial hyperplasia and cancer.**

Treat with oral contraceptives or cyclic progesterone. If the patient desires pregnancy, use clomiphene. Patients have an increased risk of insulin resistance and diabetes.

Vaginal Infections

Vaginal infections are described in Table 18-1. Figure 18-4 shows gram-negative diplococci that probably indicate gonorrhea.

IMPORTANT POINTS

1 Chlamydia is treated with erythromycin or amoxicillin if the patient is pregnant. If compliance is an issue (alcoholic, drug-abusing, homeless, or unreliable patient), you can give azithromycin, 1 g orally all at once, and watch the patient take it.

Table 18-1. VAGINAL INFECTIONS 101

Bug	Findings	Treatment
Candida albicans	"Cottage cheese" discharge, pseudohyphae on KOH preparation, history of diabetes mellitus, antibiotic treatment, pregnancy	Topical or oral antifungal
Chlamydia trachomatis	Most common sexually transmitted disease; dysuria, positive culture or antibody test	Doxycycline, azithromycin
Gardnerella vaginalis	Malodorous discharge; fishy smell on KOH preparation, clue cells	Metronidazole
Herpes	Multiple shallow, painful ulcers; recurrence and resolution	Acyclovir, valacyclovir
Human papillomavirus	Venereal warts, koilocytosis on Pap smear	Many (acid, cryotherapy, laser, podophyllin)
Molluscum contagiosum	Characteristic appearance of lesions, intracellular inclusions	Many (curettage, cryotherapy, coagulation)
Neisseria gonorrhoeae	Mucopurulent cervicitis; gram-negative bugs on Gram stain	Ceftriaxone, ciprofloxacin
Pediculosis	"Crabs"; itching, lice on pubic hairs	Permethrin cream
Primary syphilis	Painless chancre, spirochete on dark-field microscopy	Penicillin
Secondary syphilis	Condyloma lata, maculopapular rash on palms, serology	Penicillin
Trichomonas vaginalis	See bugs swimming under microscope; pale green, frothy, watery discharge, "strawberry" cervix	Metronidazole

KOH, potassium hydroxide.

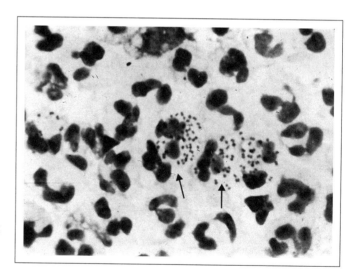

FIGURE 18-4. Gram stain of an endocervical or urethral exudate or discharge revealing leukocytes containing gram-negative diplococci (*arrows*). This is virtually diagnostic for gonorrhea.

2 Any patient with gonorrhea is generally treated for presumed chlamydial coinfection (e.g., give ceftriaxone *and* doxycycline). The reverse, however, is not true.

3 With all infections but *Candida* and *Gardnerella* spp., treat the patient's sexual partners and give counseling (e.g., condoms).

4 All of the above information is similar for men (except candidal infection), but any lesions and discharges are on, or come from, the penis.

Pediatric Gynecology

In a child with **ambiguous genitalia,** look for congenital adrenal hyperplasia (also called adrenogenital syndrome), which usually is due to 21-hydroxylase deficiency (90% of cases). Patients are female; boys with this disease show precocious sexual development. Patients with 21-hydroxylase deficiency have salt-wasting (low sodium levels), hyperkalemia, hypotension, and elevated 17-hydroxyprogesterone. Treat with corticosteroids and intravenous (IV) fluids immediately to prevent death. No patient with ambiguous genitalia should be assigned a gender until the work-up is complete. A karyotype must be done.

IMPORTANT POINTS

1 Any child with a "bunch of grapes" protruding from her vagina probably has sarcoma botryoides, a malignant tumor (rhabdomyosarcoma subtype).

2 Premature or precocious puberty is usually idiopathic but may be caused by a hormone-secreting tumor or CNS disorder, which must be ruled out. By definition, the patient must be younger than 8 years (9 years for boys). Treat the underlying cause or, if idiopathic, treat with **gonadotropin-releasing hormone analogue** (e.g., leuprolide) to prevent premature epiphyseal closure and to arrest or reverse puberty until the appropriate age.

3 Most cases of pediatric vaginitis or vaginal discharge are nonspecific or physiologic. But look for foreign body, sexual abuse (especially with sexually transmitted disease), or candidal infection (as a presentation of diabetes; measure serum glucose and/or check for glycosuria).

4 Imperforate hymen is seen in a patient of menarche age with hematocolpos (blood in vagina) that cannot escape (hymen bulges outward). Treatment is surgical opening of the hymen.

5 Vaginal bleeding in the neonate is usually physiologic as a result of maternal estrogen withdrawal and resolves by itself.

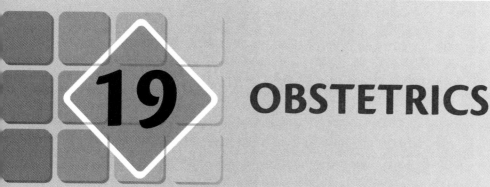

19 OBSTETRICS

General Pregnancy

IMPORTANT POINTS

1 The most common cause of secondary amenorrhea is pregnancy. *Always* do a pregnancy test first when a patient presents with amenorrhea. Pregnancy also must be ruled out as a cause of primary amenorrhea.

2 A woman may be (or say that she is) taking oral contraceptives and still be pregnant. No contraception is 100% effective, especially when you factor in compliance.

3 **Signs of pregnancy:** Amenorrhea, morning sickness, Hegar's sign (softening and compressibility of the lower uterine segment), Chadwick's sign (dark discoloration of the vulva and vaginal walls), linea nigra, chloasma, auscultation of fetal heart tones, visibility of gestational sac and/or fetus on ultrasound, uterine contractions, weight gain, and palpation or ballottement of fetus.

4 Give all pregnant patients folate to prevent neural tube defects. Ideally, all women of reproductive age should take folate, because it is most effective in the first trimester when most women do not know that they are pregnant. Iron is often given routinely during pregnancy to prevent anemia.

5 Macrosomia (or positive history in previous children) is caused by maternal diabetes mellitus until proved otherwise.

Routine laboratory tests in a pregnant patient:

- **Blood type, Rh type, and antibody screen:** At first visit (for identification of possible isoimmunization or Rh incompatibility).
- **Complete blood count:** At first visit to see if the patient is anemic (pregnancy can aggravate anemia).
- **Glucose screen:** At first visit if the patient has risk factors for diabetes mellitus (obesity, family history, age >30 years); otherwise, do at 24 to 28 weeks. Screen with fasting serum glucose *and* serum glucose 1 or 2 hours after an oral glucose load.

- **Pap smear:** Give to every patient at first visit, unless she had a normal Pap smear in the past 6 months.
- **Rubella antibody screen:** In the absence of a good vaccination history, obtain at first visit (otherwise not needed).
- **Serum alpha fetoprotein (AFP) or triple or quadruple screen:** Between 16 and 20 weeks for older or other high-risk patients. Positive triple screen (low AFP, low estriol, and high human chorionic gonadotropin [hCG]) means likely Down's syndrome. The fourth value in a quad screen is inhibin A, which is high with Down's syndrome.
- **Syphilis test:** At first visit (mandated in most states) and subsequent visits if the patient is at high risk.
- **Urinalysis:** At first visit and every visit (screen for preeclampsia and bacteriuria; not a good screen for diabetes mellitus).

Hepatitis B serology, tuberculous skin test, HIV test, *Chlamydia* sp. and gonorrhea cultures, and ultrasound are used only when the patient has a suggestive history or risk factors. If asked, you should do *Chlamydia trachomatis* and gonorrhea cultures for any pregnant teenager.

Common pregnancy changes, signs, and complaints include nausea and vomiting (morning sickness), amenorrhea, heavy (possibly even painful) feeling of the breasts, increased pigmentation of the nipples and areolae (and Montgomery tubercles), backache, linea nigra, chloasma, striae gravidarum, *mild* ankle edema, heartburn, and increased frequency of urination.

Normal physiologic changes in pregnancy:

- **Laboratory tests:** Erythrocyte sedimentation rate is markedly elevated (*worthless* test in pregnancy). Thyroxine and thyroxine-binding globulin increase, but free thyroxine is *normal*. Hemoglobin increases, but plasma volume increases more, so net result is a decreased hematocrit and hemoglobin; BUN and creatinine decrease because glomerular filtration rate (GFR) increases (high end of normal range for BUN and creatinine indicate renal disease in pregnancy); alkaline phosphatase increases markedly. Mild proteinuria and glycosuria are *normal* in pregnancy. Electrolytes and liver function tests remain normal.
- **Cardiovascular changes:** Blood pressure decreases slightly, heart rate increases by 10 to 20 bpm, stroke volume increases, and cardiac output increases (up to 50%).
- **Pulmonary changes:** Minute ventilation increases because of increased tidal volume with the same or only slightly increased respiratory rate. Residual volume and carbon dioxide decrease (together, these changes result in physiologic hyperventilation and respiratory alkalosis of pregnancy).
- **The average weight gain** in pregnancy is 28 lb (12.5 kg). With a greater weight gain, think of diabetes mellitus. With a smaller weight gain, think of hyperemesis gravidarum or psychological or major systemic disease.

Prenatal Care

At every prenatal visit, listen for fetal heart tones and evaluate uterine size for any **size/date discrepancy.** Uterine size is evaluated by measuring the distance from the symphysis pubis to the top of the fundus in centimeters. Between roughly 20 and 35 weeks, the measurement in centimeters should equal the number of weeks of gestation. A discrepancy greater than 2 to 3 cm is called a size/date discrepancy, and ultrasound should be done to evaluate further. Possible explanations include inaccurate dates, intrauterine growth retardation, and multiple gestation.

IMPORTANT POINTS

1 At 12 weeks' gestation, the uterus enters the abdomen; at roughly 20 weeks, it reaches the umbilicus.

2 Fetal heart tones and cardiac activity can be detected with transvaginal ultrasound at 5.5 to 7 weeks, heard with Doppler at 10 to 12 weeks, and heard with a stethoscope at 16 to 20 weeks.

3 Between 16 and 20 weeks, ultrasound is most accurate at estimating fetal age (using the biparietal diameter).

4 Quickening (when the mother first detects fetal movements) usually occurs at 18 to 20 weeks in a primigravida and 16 to 18 weeks in a multigravida.

Treat asymptomatic bacteriuria in pregnancy (but not in other patients), because 20% of patients develop cystitis and/or pyelonephritis if untreated. Thought to be due to progesterone decreasing the tone of the ureters, and the uterus compressing the ureters. Give penicillin, cephalosporin, or nitrofurantoin.

hCG roughly doubles every two days in the first trimester of pregnancy. An hCG that stays the same or increases only slowly with serial testing indicates a fetus in trouble or fetal demise. A rapidly increasing hCG or one that does not decrease after delivery can indicate a hydatiform mole or choriocarcinoma. The standard hCG home pregnancy test becomes positive roughly 2 weeks after conception.

Prepartum Pregnancy Issues

ABORTION

Abortion is defined as termination of a pregnancy at less than 20 weeks (fetus <500 g). The following specific terms also imply that the event occurs at earlier than 20 weeks' gestation:

◆ **Threatened abortion:** Uterine bleeding without cervical dilation and no expulsion of tissue. Treat with IV fluids (or blood, if needed), bedrest, pelvic rest, and RhoGAM (Rh immune globulin) if the patient is Rh-negative. Do dilation and curettage (D&C) if the fetus dies and is not promptly expelled.

◆ **Inevitable abortion:** Uterine bleeding with cervical dilation and crampy abdominal pain and no tissue expulsion. Treat with IV fluids, RhoGAM if the patient is Rh-negative, and D&C.

◆ **Incomplete abortion:** Passage of some products of conception through the cervix. Treat with IV fluids, RhoGAM if the patient is Rh-negative, and D&C.

- **Complete abortion:** Expulsion of all products of conception from the uterus. Treat with serial hCG testing to make sure that hCG drops to zero, consider D&C, and give RhoGAM if the patient is Rh-negative.

- **Missed abortion:** Fetal death with no expulsion of tissue (often for several weeks). Treat with D&C if less than 14 weeks, attempted delivery if greater than 14 weeks. Give RhoGAM if the patient is Rh-negative.

- **Induced abortion:** Intentional termination of pregnancy <20 weeks; may be elective (requested by patient) or therapeutic (to maintain the health of the mother).

- **Recurrent abortion:** Two or three successive unplanned abortions. History and physical exam may show:

  - Infectious etiology (*Listeria, Mycoplasma,* or *Toxoplasma* spp., syphilis)
  - Environmental influences (alcohol, tobacco, drugs)
  - Diabetes mellitus
  - Hypothyroidism
  - Systemic lupus erythematosus (especially with positive antiphospholipid/lupus anticoagulant antibodies)
  - Cervical incompetence (watch for history of patient's mother taking diethylstilbestrol (DES) during pregnancy and patient with recurrent second-trimester abortions; treat future pregnancies with a cervical cerclage at 14–16 weeks)
  - Congenital female tract abnormalities (correct if possible to restore fertility)
  - Fibroids (remove them)
  - Chromosomal abnormalities (e.g., maternal or paternal translocations)

 In women with antiphospholipid antibodies and previous problem pregnancies, low-dose aspirin may help in subsequent pregnancies. Normally, aspirin and other nonsteroidal antiinflammatory drugs (NSAIDs) should be *avoided* in pregnancy; use acetaminophen instead.

TESTING

Alpha fetoprotein levels:

- Low AFP: Down syndrome, fetal demise, or inaccurate dates
- High AFP: neural tube defects (e.g., anencephaly, spina bifida), ventral wall defects (e.g., omphalocele, gastroschisis), multiple gestation, or inaccurate dates
- If AFP or triple screen is positive (at 16–20 weeks), the patient should undergo amniocentesis (also done at 16–20 weeks) for a definitive diagnosis of chromosomal disorders (cell culture) or neural tube defects (amniotic fluid AFP).

Chorionic villus sampling (CVS) can be done at 9 to 12 weeks (earlier than amniocentesis) and generally is reserved for women with previously affected offspring or known genetic disease. CVS gives women the advantage of first-trimester abortion if a fetus is affected. It is associated with a slightly higher miscarriage rate than amniocentesis and *cannot* detect neural tube defects.

DIABETES MELLITUS

◆ **Problems in pregnant diabetic mothers:** polyhydramnios, preeclampsia, and complications of diabetes

◆ **Problems in infants born to diabetic mothers:** macrosomia or intrauterine growth retardation (IUGR); respiratory distress syndrome; cardiovascular, colon (e.g., left colon hypoplasia), craniofacial (e.g., cleft lip or palate), and neural tube defects; caudal regression syndrome (lower half of body incompletely formed), and **postdelivery hypoglycemia** in the fetus (from fetal islet-cell hypertrophy due to maternal and thus fetal hyperglycemia). After birth, the infant is cut off from the mother's glucose and the hyperglycemia goes away, but islet cells still overproduce insulin and cause hypoglycemia. Treat with IV glucose.

◆ **Treat diabetes mellitus** with diet, exercise, and/or insulin (*no* oral hypoglycemics). Tighter control results in better outcomes for mother and infant. Check hemoglobin A1c (Hb_{A1c}) to determine compliance and glucose fluctuations.

◆ **In evaluating amniotic fluid** to determine fetal lung maturity, phosphatidylglycerol concentration is better than the lecithin-to-sphingomyelin ratio when the mother is diabetic.

ECTOPIC PREGNANCY

Major risk factor is a history of pelvic inflammatory disease (10-fold increase in ectopic pregnancies). Other risk factors include previous ectopic pregnancy, history of tubal sterilization or tuboplasty, pregnancy that occurs with an intrauterine device in place, and DES exposure (which can cause tubal abnormalities in women exposed in utero).

Classic symptoms of ectopic pregnancy are amenorrhea, vaginal bleeding, and abdominal pain. Patients also have positive hCG test. If you palpate an adnexal mass, you may be palpating an ectopic pregnancy or a corpus luteum cyst, which can coexist with a tubal pregnancy or a threatened abortion (both can have similar symptoms). When in doubt and the patient is doing poorly (hypovolemia, shock, severe abdominal pain, or rebound tenderness), do urgent ultrasound while stabilizing the patient and prepare for laparoscopy for definitive diagnosis and treatment, if necessary. Ultrasound can often make or exclude the diagnosis.

Tubal Pregnancy. If the patient is stable and the conceptus is <3 cm in greatest diameter, tubal pregnancy can be treated with salpingostomy and removal, leaving the tube open to heal on its own. In reliable patients who desire to avoid surgery, methotrexate can be given to cause medical abortion. If the patient is unstable or the ectopic pregnancy has ruptured or is >3 cm, salpingectomy is required. Give RhoGAM after treatment for Rh-negative patients.

HYPEREMESIS GRAVIDARUM

Hyperemesis gravidarum is intractable nausea and vomiting leading to dehydration and possible electrolyte disturbances. The condition occurs in the **first trimester,** usually in younger patients with their first pregnancy and underlying social stressors or psychological problems. Treat with supportive care, including small, frequent meals and antiemetics (fairly safe in pregnancy). Outpatient treatment sometimes is acceptable unless the patient has severe dehydration and/or electrolyte disturbances, in which case admit for treatment.

PHARMACOLOGY

Drugs that are not safe in pregnancy are shown in Table 19-1.

Drugs that are generally **safe in pregnancy**: acetaminophen (*not* NSAIDs or aspirin), penicillin, cephalosporins, erythromycin, nitrofurantoin, H_2 blockers, antacids, heparin, hydralazine, methyldopa, labetalol, insulin, docusate.

TRANSVAGINAL ULTRASOUND

Transvaginal ultrasound detects an intrauterine gestational sac at roughly 5 weeks and a fetus at 5.5 to 7 weeks. Use this information in trying to determine the possibility of an ectopic pregnancy. If the patient's last menstrual period (LMP) was 4 weeks ago and the pregnancy test is positive, you cannot rule out an ectopic pregnancy with ultrasound. If, however, the patient's LMP was 10 weeks ago, there is a positive pregnancy test, and an ultrasound of the uterus shows no gestational sac, think of ectopic pregnancy. If hCG is >2000 mIU, you should be able to visualize a gestational sac with transvaginal ultrasound.

Table 19-1. TERATOGENIC AGENTS

Agent	Defect(s) Caused
Alcohol	Fetal alcohol syndrome
Aminoglycosides	Deafness
Aminopterin	Intrauterine growth retardation, CNS defects, cleft lip, cleft palate
Antineoplastics	Many
Birth control pills	VACTERL syndrome (**v**ertebral, **a**nal, **c**ardiac, **t**racheoesophageal, **r**enal, and **l**imb malformations)
Carbamazepine	Fingernail hypoplasia, craniofacial defects
Cigarettes	Intrauterine growth retardation, low birth weight, prematurity
Cocaine	Cerebral infarcts, mental retardation
Diazepam	Cleft lip, cleft palate
Diethylstilbestrol	Clear cell vaginal cancer, adenosis, cervical incompetence
Iodine	Goiter, cretinism
Isotretinoin[*]	CNS, craniofacial, ear, and cardiovascular defects
Lithium	Cardiac (Ebstein's) anomalies
Phenytoin[†]	Craniofacial and limb defects, mental retardation, cardiovascular defects
Progesterone	Masculinization of female fetus
Radiation	Intrauterine growth retardation, CNS and face defects, leukemia
Tetracycline	Yellow or brown teeth
Thalidomide	Phocomelia
Trimethadione	Craniofacial and cardiovascular defects, mental retardation
Valproic acid	Spina bifida, hypospadias
Warfarin	Craniofacial and central nervous system defects, intrauterine growth retardation, stillbirth

Note: Marijuana and LSD (lysergic acid diethylamide) have not been confirmed as teratogens.
   [*]Vitamin A in general is considered teratogenic when recommended intake levels are exceeded.
   [†]Diphenylhydantoin.
   CNS, central nervous system.

Maternal-to-Fetal Infections

TORCH INFECTIONS

Most intrauterine fetal infections can cause mental retardation, microcephaly, hydrocephalus, hepatosplenomegaly, jaundice, anemia, low birth weight, and/or IUGR.

- *Toxoplasma gondii:* Look for exposure to cats; specific defects include intracranial calcifications, chorioretinitis.

- **Other:** Varicella zoster (limb hypoplasia and scarring of the skin) and syphilis (rhinitis, saber shins, Hutchinson's teeth, interstitial keratitis, skin lesions).

- *Rubella:* Worst in first trimester (some authorities recommend abortion if the mother contracts rubella in the first trimester). Always check antibody status on first visit if the patient has a poor immunization history. Look for cardiovascular defects (patent ductus arteriosus, ventral septal defect), deafness, cataracts, and microphthalmia.

- **Cytomegalovirus: Most common;** look for deafness, cerebral calcifications, microphthalmia.

- *Herpes:* Look for vesicular skin lesions (with positive Tzanck smears), history of maternal herpes lesions.

With all in utero infections that can cause problems with the fetus, the mother may be asymptomatic (subclinical infection) and the infant may even be asymptomatic at birth, only to develop symptoms later (e.g., learning disability, mental retardation).

HUMAN IMMUNODEFICIENCY VIRUS

In untreated HIV-positive patients, transmission to the fetus occurs in roughly 25% of cases. With prenatal zidovudine (AZT) treatment for the mother and administration of AZT (or other antiretroviral) to the infant for 6 weeks after birth, HIV transmission is reduced to less than 10%. A noninfected infant might still be HIV-positive on ELISA testing because maternal antibodies can cross the placenta. Within 6 months, the test reverts to negative. Children are thus tested with a DNA polymerase chain reaction (PCR) test after birth to directly detect the HIV virus. HIV-positive mothers should *not* breast-feed because milk can transmit HIV to the infant.

HERPES

When the mother has genital herpes simplex virus (HSV) infection, delay the decision of whether to do a cesarean section until the mother goes into labor. If at the time of true labor she has lesions of HSV, do a cesarean section. If at the time of true labor the mother has no HSV lesions, deliver vaginally.

HEPATITIS B

If the mother has hepatitis B, give the infant the first hepatitis B vaccine shot and hepatitis B immunoglobulin at birth.

VARICELLA

If the mother gets chickenpox in the last 5 days of pregnancy or first 2 days after delivery, give the infant varicella zoster immunoglobulin.

CHLAMYDIA

In pregnancy, treat chlamydial infection with erythromycin or amoxicillin (not doxycycline). Remember association with neonatal conjunctivitis and pneumonia.

GROUP B STREPTOCOCCUS (GBS)

Treat maternal carriers (can be a normal member of vaginal flora) during labor and delivery. For example, if the patient is GBS-positive at 26 to 28 weeks, wait until labor and give ampicillin. The goal of treatment is to prevent neonatal sepsis and endometritis.

IMPORTANT POINTS

1 Immunoglobulin G (IgG) is the only maternal antibody that crosses the placenta. An elevated neonatal IgM concentration is *never* normal, whereas an elevated neonatal IgG often represents maternal antibodies.

2 **If a woman has tuberculosis in pregnancy** (positive purified protein derivative [PPD] test and suspicious chest x-ray, plus a positive sputum culture), treat as you would any other patient. If the patient is a known recent PPD converter or has additional risk factors (such as HIV positivity or household contact with an active case of tuberculosis), treat with isoniazid as in a nonpregnant patient. Make sure to give the mother vitamin B_6 with isoniazid to prevent nutritional defect in her and the fetus. Avoid streptomycin, which can cause deafness and nephrotoxicity in fetus.

Other Conditions in Pregnancy

CHOLESTASIS OF PREGNANCY

Cholestasis of pregnancy presents with itching, abnormal liver function tests, and/or jaundice during pregnancy. The only treatment is delivery, but cholestyramine can help with symptoms.

Acute fatty liver of pregnancy is a more serious disorder that occurs in the third trimester or after delivery and usually progresses to hepatic coma. Treatment includes IV fluids, IV glucose, and fresh frozen plasma. Vitamin K does not work, because the liver is in temporary failure.

HYDATIDIFORM MOLE

In a sense, the products of conception become a tumor. Look for preeclampsia before the third trimester; an hCG that does not return to zero after delivery or abortion or that rapidly rises during pregnancy; first- or second-trimester bleeding with possible expulsion of "grapes"; uterine size/date discrepancy; and/or a *"snow-storm"* pattern on ultrasound. Complete moles are 46 XX (all chromosomes from the father) and have no fetal tissue; incomplete moles are usually 69 XXY and contain fetal tissue. Gross appearance suggests a *bunch of grapes.*

Treat with uterine D&C, then follow hCG until it falls to zero. If hCG does not fall to zero or rises, the patient has either an invasive mole or choriocarcinoma; in either case, the patient needs chemotherapy (usually *methotrexate* or actinomycin D).

INTRAUTERINE GROWTH RETARDATION

Intrauterine growth retardation (IUGR) is defined as size below the tenth percentile for age. The causes are many and are best understood in broad terms as caused by one of three factors: maternal (e.g., smoking, alcohol or drugs, lupus erythematosus), fetal (e.g., TORCH infections, congenital anomalies), or placental (e.g,. hypertension, preeclampsia). Do ultrasound on all patients who have a size/date discrepancy greater than 2 to 3 cm or risk factors for pregnancy problems (e.g., hypertension; diabetes mellitus; renal disease; lupus erythematosus; cigarette, alcohol, or drug use; history of previous problems). Ultrasound parameters measured for IUGR determination include biparietal diameter, head circumference, abdominal circumference, and femur length.

MULTIPLE GESTATIONS

If sex or blood type is different, twins are dizygotic. If the placentas are monochorionic, the twins are monozygotic. These three simple factors differentiate monozygotic from dizygotic twins in 80% of cases. The remaining 20% require HLA-typing studies. Complications of multiple gestations (the higher the number of fetuses, the higher the risk of most of these conditions) include the following:

◆ **Maternal:** Anemia, hypertension, premature labor, postpartum uterine atony, postpartum hemorrhage, preeclampsia

◆ **Fetal:** Polyhydramnios, malpresentation, placenta previa, abruptio placentae, velamentous cord insertion or vasa previa, premature rupture of membranes (PROM), prematurity, umbilical cord prolapse, IUGR, congenital anomalies, increased perinatal morbidity and mortality

With vertex–vertex presentations, you can try vaginal delivery for both infants; with any other combination of presentations, do a cesarean section.

OLIGOHYDRAMNIOS

Oligohydramnios is defined as amniotic fluid (AF) <500 mL, AF index <5. Causes include IUGR, PROM, postmaturity, and renal agenesis (Potter's disease). Oligohydramnios can cause fetal problems such as pulmonary hypoplasia, cutaneous and skeletal abnormalities due to compression, and hypoxia due to cord compression.

POLYHYDRAMNIOS

Polyhydramnios is defined as AF >2000 to 2500 mL, AF index >25. Causes include maternal diabetes mellitus, multiple gestation, neural tube defects (anencephaly, spina bifida), GI anomalies (omphalocele, esophageal atresia), and hydrops fetalis. Polyhydramnios can cause maternal dyspnea (overdistended uterus compromising pulmonary function) and postpartum uterine atony with resultant postpartum hemorrhage.

POSTTERM PREGNANCY

Postterm pregnancy is defined as pregnancy after 42 weeks of gestation. Generally, if gestational age is known to be accurate, labor is induced (e.g., by oxytocin) if the cervix is favorable. If the cervix is not favorable or the dates are uncertain, do twice-weekly nonstress test (NST) and biophysical profile (BPP) (see later). At 43 weeks, most authorities advise induction of labor or cesarean section. Both prematurity and postmaturity increase perinatal morbidity and mortality. Prolonged gestation is common in association with anencephaly and placental sulfatase deficiency.

PREECLAMPSIA

Look for hypertension (in patients with preexisting hypertension, blood pressure should increase by >30/15 mm Hg over baseline); urinalysis with 2+ or more proteinuria; oliguria; swelling or edema of hands and/or face; headache; visual disturbances; and/or **HELLP** syndrome (hemolysis, elevated liver enzymes, low platelets). Preeclampsia often involves right upper quadrant and epigastric pain and **develops in the third trimester**.

The main **risk factors** for preeclampsia (in order of importance) are chronic renal disease, chronic hypertension, family history, multiple gestation, primiparity, age older than 40 years (although the classic case is a young woman with her first child), diabetes mellitus, and black race. **Treatment** is delivery if the patient is at term. If the patient is premature and has mild disease, treat hypertension with labetalol or hydralazine and bedrest. Observe the patient carefully. If the patient has severe disease (oliguria, mental status changes, headache, blurred vision, pulmonary edema, cyanosis, HELLP syndrome, blood pressure >160/110 mm Hg, or progression to eclampsia [seizures]), deliver regardless of gestational age, because both mother and infant might die.

IMPORTANT POINTS

1 Mild ankle edema is normal in pregnancy, but severe ankle edema or hand edema is likely to be preeclampsia.

2 If preeclampsia symptoms develop before the third trimester, think of hydatiform mole and/or choriocarcinoma.

3 Hypertension plus proteinuria in a pregnant patient is preeclampsia until proved otherwise.

4 Preeclampsia plus seizures = **eclampsia**. Eclampsia can be prevented by regular prenatal care. Catch it in preeclamptic stage, and treat appropriately.

5 Use magnesium sulfate for eclamptic seizures (also lowers blood pressure). Toxic magnesium effects include **hyporeflexia** (first sign of toxicity), respiratory depression, central nervous system depression, coma, and death.

6 Do *not* wait to follow-up and remeasure very high blood pressure in a pregnant patient (likely you would in nonpregnant patients with nonemergent elevated blood pressure levels). Err on the safe side; assume that it represents preeclampsia and start treatment.

7 Do *not* try to deliver the infant until the mother is stable (do *not* do a cesarean section while the mother is having a seizure!).

8 Preeclampsia and eclampsia cause uteroplacental insufficiency, IUGR, fetal demise, and increased maternal morbidity and mortality.

9 Preeclampsia and eclampsia are *not* risk factors for future development of hypertension or end-organ effects of hypertension.

PREMATURE RUPTURE OF MEMBRANES

Premature rupture of membranes (PROM) is rupture of the amniotic sac before the onset of labor. Diagnosis of rupture of the membranes (whether premature or not) is based on history and sterile speculum exam, which will show pooling of amniotic fluid, ferning pattern when the fluid is placed on a microscopic slide and allowed to dry, and/or positive nitrazine test (nitrazine paper turns blue in the presence of amniotic fluid). Ultrasound also should be done to assess amniotic fluid volume (as well as gestational age and any anomalies that may be present). Spontaneous labor often follows membrane rupture. If labor does not occur within 6 to 8 hours and the patient is at term, labor should be induced. If the cervix is highly unfavorable, you can wait 24 hours to attempt induction. PROM carries an increased risk of infection, both to the mother (chorioamnionitis) and infant (neonatal sepsis, pneumonia, meningitis), usually from group B streptococci, *Escherichia coli*, or *Listeria* spp.

Preterm premature rupture of membranes (PPROM) is PROM that occurs before 36 to 37 weeks' gestation. Risk of infection increases with the duration of ruptured membranes. Do a culture and Gram stain of amniotic fluid. If they are negative, treat with pelvic and bedrest and frequent follow-up. If positive for group B streptococci, treat the mother with a penicillin, even if she is asymptomatic.

PRETERM LABOR

Preterm labor is defined as labor between 20 and 37 weeks. Treat with lateral decubitus position, bed and pelvic rest, oral or IV fluids, and oxygen administration (all might stop the contractions). Then give a tocolytic (β_2 agonist or magnesium sulfate) if no contraindications are present (heart disease, hypertension, diabetes mellitus, hemorrhage, ruptured membranes, cervix dilated >4 cm). Patients may be discharged on oral tocolytic. Do *not* tocolyze the mother if it is dangerous to do so (preeclampsia, severe hemorrhage, chorioamnionitis, IUGR, fetal demise, or fetal anomalies incompatible with survival). Often steroids are given with tocolysis (if the infant is 24–34 weeks old) to hasten fetal lung maturity.

Fetal fibronectin may be detected in vaginal secretions of women presenting with signs and symptoms of preterm labor. Secretions negative for fibronectin (most useful value) indicates a low risk of delivering in the next few weeks (you can take a more conservative approach). If fetal fibronectin is positive, the risk of early delivery remains high and more aggressive treatment (e.g., tocolysis, hastening of fetal lung maturity) is employed.

Rh INCOMPATIBILITY AND HEMOLYTIC DISEASE OF THE NEWBORN

Rh incompatibility and hemolytic disease of the newborn occur when the mother is Rh-negative and the infant is Rh-positive. If both mother and father are Rh-negative, there is nothing to worry about—the infant will be Rh-negative. If the father is Rh-positive, the infant has a 50/50 chance of being Rh-positive. If the potential for hemolytic disease exists, check maternal Rh antibody titers every month, starting in the seventh month. Give RhoGAM automatically at 28 weeks and within 72 hours after delivery, as well as after any procedures that can cause transplacental hemorrhage (e.g., amniocentesis).

The development of disease requires previous **sensitization.** In other words, if a primiparous mother has never received blood products, her first Rh-positive infant will often not be affected by hemolytic disease (except in the rare case of sensitization during the first pregnancy from undetected fetomaternal bleeding, which usually occurs later in the pregnancy and can be prevented by RhoGAM administration at 28 weeks in most instances). The second Rh-positive infant, however, will be affected—unless you, the astute board taker/physician, administer RhoGAM appropriately. Any history of blood transfusion, abortion, ectopic pregnancy, stillbirth, or delivery can cause sensitization. If you check maternal Rh antibodies and they are strongly positive, RhoGAM is worthless, because sensitization has already occurred. RhoGAM administration is a good example of **primary prevention**.

RhoGAM Summary. Give RhoGAM only when the mother is Rh-negative and the father's blood type is unknown or Rh-positive. During routine prenatal care, check for Rh antibodies at the first visit. If the test is positive, do *not* give RhoGAM—you are too late. Otherwise, give RhoGAM routinely at 28 weeks and immediately after delivery. Also give RhoGAM after an abortion, stillbirth, ectopic pregnancy, amniocentesis, chorionic villus sampling, and any other invasive procedure during pregnancy that can cause transplacental bleeding.

 If fetal lungs are immature (lecithin-to-sphingomyelin ratio <2:1 or prostaglandin-negative) and the fetus is between 24 and 34 weeks' gestational age, corticosteroid administration can hasten lung maturity and thus reduce the risk of respiratory distress syndrome.

IMPORTANT POINTS

1 If not detected and prevented, Rh incompatibility can lead to fetal hydrops (edema, ascites, pleural and pericardial effusions) and death.

2 Amniotic fluid spectrophotometry gauges the severity of fetal hemolysis.

3 Treatment of hemolytic disease involves delivery if the fetus is mature. Check lung maturity with the lecithin-to-sphingomyelin ratio. Intrauterine transfusion is invasive but can be performed if needed; phenobarbital helps the fetal liver to break down bilirubin by inducing enzymes.

4 ABO blood group incompatibility also can cause hemolytic disease of the newborn when the mother is type O and the infant is type A, B, or AB. Previous sensitization is not required, because IgG antibodies, which can cross the placenta, occur naturally in patients with blood type O. Usually the disease is less severe than with Rh incompatibility, but treatment is the same. Other minor blood antigens also cause a reaction in rare cases.

SURGICAL CONDITIONS

Pregnant women can have the same surgical conditions as nonpregnant women. In general, treat the disease regardless of pregnancy. This general rule always works with acute surgical conditions (e.g., appendicitis, cholecystitis). With semi-urgent conditions (e.g., ovarian neoplasm), it is best to wait until the second trimester, when the patient is most stable. Purely elective cases are avoided. Appendicitis can manifest with right upper quadrant pain or tenderness due to displacement of the appendix by the uterus. Consider exploratory laparotomy if you are unsure and the patient has peritoneal signs.

THIRD-TRIMESTER BLEEDING

For third-trimester bleeding (very high yield), *always* do an ultrasound before a pelvic exam. Repeat: *Always* do an ultrasound before a pelvic exam. The differential diagnosis includes:

- **Abruptio placentae:** Predisposing factors include hypertension (with or without preeclampsia), trauma, polyhydramnios with rapid decompression after membrane rupture, cocaine or tobacco use, and PPROM. Do *not* forget that the patient can have this condition without visible bleeding (blood contained behind placenta). Patients have pain, uterine tenderness, and increased uterine tone with hyperactive contraction pattern. Fetal distress also is present. Abruptio placentae can cause disseminated intravascular coagulation if fetal products enter the maternal circulation. Ultrasound detects <5% of cases. Treat with IV fluids (and blood if needed) and rapid delivery (vaginal preferred).

- **Bleeding disorder:** Rarely manifests before delivery (more common after delivery).

- **"Bloody show":** With cervical effacement, a blood-tinged mucus plug may be released from the cervical canal and heralds the onset of labor. This event is *normal* and a diagnosis of exclusion.

- **Cervical cancer:** Can occur in pregnant patients too!

- **Cervical or vaginal lesions:** Examples include herpes simplex virus, gonorrhea, chlamydial or candidal infection.

- **Cervical or vaginal trauma:** Usually from intercourse.

- **Fetal bleeding:** Usually from vasa previa or velamentous insertion of the cord. The major risk factor is multiple gestation (the higher the number of fetuses, the higher the risk). Bleeding is *painless*, and the mother is completely stable while the fetus shows worsening distress (tachycardia initially, then bradycardia as the fetus decompensates). The Apt test is positive on uterine blood and differentiates fetal from maternal blood. Treat with immediate cesarean section.

- **Placenta previa** (Fig. 19-1): Predisposing factors include multiparity, increasing age, multiple gestation, and prior previa. This condition is why you *always* do an ultrasound before a pelvic exam. Bleeding is painless and may be profuse. Ultrasound is 95% to 100% accurate in diagnosis. Cesarean section is mandatory for delivery, but you may

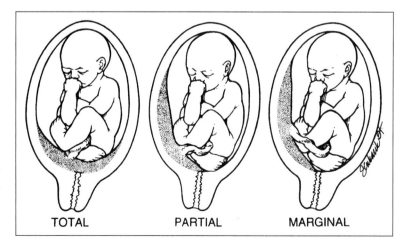

FIGURE 19-1. Three variations of placenta previa. (From Gabbe SG, Niebyl JR, Simpson JL (eds): Obstetrics: Normal & Problem Pregnancies. New York, Churchill Livingstone, 1986, p 495, with permission.)

TOTAL   PARTIAL   MARGINAL

try to admit with bed and pelvic rest and tocolysis if the patient is preterm and stable and the bleeding stops.

◆ **Uterine rupture:** Predisposing factors include previous uterine surgery, trauma, oxytocin, grand multiparity (several previous deliveries), excessive uterine distention (e.g., multiple gestation, polyhydramnios), abnormal fetal lie, cephalopelvic disproportion, and shoulder dystocia. Uterine rupture is characterized by *extreme pain* of sudden onset and often associated with maternal hypotension or shock. Fetal parts may be felt in the abdomen, or the abdominal contour might change. Treat with immediate laparotomy and usually hysterectomy after delivery.

In all patients with third-trimester bleeding, initiate **treatment** with IV fluids, and give blood if needed. Give oxygen, and get complete blood count, coagulation profiles, and ultrasound. Set up fetal and maternal monitoring. Do a drug screen if you are suspicious (cocaine causes placental abruption). Give RhoGAM if the mother is Rh-negative. The Kleihauer-Betke test quantifies fetal blood in maternal circulation and is sometimes used to calculate the dose of RhoGAM.

Evaluation of Fetal Well-Being

NONSTRESS TEST (NST)

With the mother resting, fetal heart rate tracing is obtained for 20 minutes. A normal strip has at least two accelerations of the heart rate, each of which is at least 15 bpm above baseline and lasts at least 15 seconds. This is the first screening test to evaluate fetal well-being; it is often done in the context of a biophysical profile.

BIOPHYSICAL PROFILE (BPP)

The BPP includes four measurements:

◆ **NST:** See above.

◆ **AF index:** Measures vertical pockets of amniotic fluid (in centimeters) in each of the four quadrants. The sum of the highest vertical pocket in each quadrant is used to determine whether oligohydramnios or polyhydramnios is present (AF index <5 cm = oligohydramnios, AF index >25 cm = polyhydramnios).

◆ **Fetal breathing movements:** Fetus should have at least 30 breathing movements in 10 minutes.

◆ **Fetal movements:** Fetus should have at least three body movements (e.g., flexion, body rotation) in 10 minutes.

If the fetus scores low on the BPP, the next test is the contraction stress test. With high-risk pregnancies (e.g., IUGR, diabetes mellitus, hypertension, alcohol or drug use, post-term pregnancy, history of problem pregnancies, maternal or physician concern), the BPP often is done once or even twice a week in the third trimester until delivery.

Contraction stress test (CST) (Fig. 19-2) is a test for uteroplacental dysfunction. Give oxytocin, and monitor the fetal heart strip. If late decelerations are seen on the fetal heart

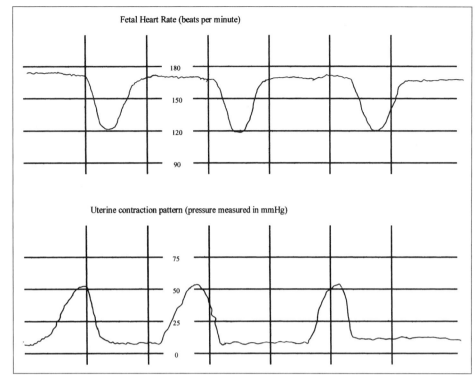

FIGURE 19-2. Positive contraction stress test with late decelerations. The nadir (i.e., valley or low point) of the fetal heart rate occurs just after the peak of each uterine contraction. This is a worrisome pattern and generally indicates uteroplacental insufficiency.

strip with each contraction, the test is positive, and usually a cesarean section is done if feasible.

Labor and Delivery

TRUE LABOR

Normal contractions occur at least every 3 minutes, are fairly regular, and are associated with cervical changes (effacement and dilation). **False labor** (Braxton–Hicks contractions) is characterized by irregular contractions with no cervical changes.

NORMAL LABOR

Characteristics of normal labor are shown in Table 19-2.

Signs of placental separation: fresh show of blood from vagina; umbilical cord lengthens; the fundus rises and becomes firm and globular.

Order of labor positions: descent, flexion, internal rotation, extension, external rotation, and expulsion

PROTRACTION AND ARREST

Protraction disorder occurs once true labor has begun if the mother takes longer than she should, according to Table 19-2. **Arrest disorder** occurs once true labor has begun if no

Table 19-2. CHARACTERISTICS OF NORMAL LABOR

Stage	Characteristics	Primigravida	Multigravida
First	Onset of true labor to full cervical dilation	<20 h	<14 h
Latent phase	From 0 to 3–4 cm dilation (slow, irregular)	Highly variable	Highly variable
Active phase	From 3–4 cm to full dilation (rapid, regular)	>1 cm/h dilation	>1.2 cm/h dilation
Second	From full dilation to birth of infant	30 min to 3 h	5–30 min
Third	From delivery of infant to delivery of placenta	0–30 min	0–30 min
Fourth	From placental delivery to maternal stabilization	Up to 48 h	Up to 48 h

change in dilation (as opposed to the slow change of protraction disorder) occurs over 2 hours *or* if no change occurs in descent over 1 hour. First, rule out abnormal lie or cephalopelvic disproportion. If everything is okay, treat with labor augmentation (oxytocin, prostaglandin gel, amniotomy). If this approach does not work, manage expectantly and do a cesarean section at the first sign of trouble.

The most common cause of failure to progress (protraction or arrest disorder), also known as dystocia (difficult birth), is cephalopelvic disproportion, defined as disparity between the size of the infant's head and the mother's pelvis. Labor augmentation is *contraindicated* in this setting.

When **shoulder dystocia** occurs, the first step is McRobert's maneuver (Fig. 19-3). Ask the mother to flex her thighs sharply against her abdomen. This maneuver might free the impacted shoulder. If it does not work, options are limited. A cesarean section is usually the procedure of choice (after pushing the infant's head back up into the birth canal).

HASTENING LABOR

Contraindications to labor induction and augmentation (similar to contraindications to vaginal delivery):

◆ Placenta or vasa previa

◆ Umbilical cord prolapse or presentation

◆ Transverse fetal lie

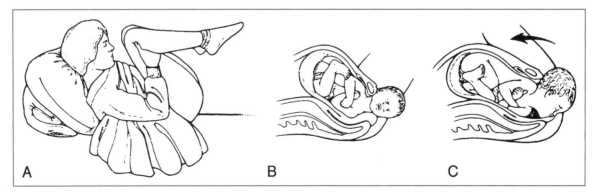

FIGURE 19-3. A, McRobert's maneuver with legs flexed on the maternal abdomen and chest. Compared to the angle with the legs extended in lithotomy **(B),** the angle of inclination of the pelvic area is increased when the legs are flexed **(C);** thus, the shoulder of the infant might become disengaged. (From Ratcliffe SD, Byrd JE, Sakornbut EL: Handbook of Pregnancy and Perinatal Care in Family Practice. Philadelphia, Hanley & Belfus, 1996, with permission.)

◆ Active genital herpes

◆ Known cervical cancer

◆ Known cephalopelvic disproportion

◆ Prior classic (vertical) uterine cesarean section incision (increased rate of uterine rupture). After a cesarean section with a lower (horizontal) uterine incision, the patient may deliver future pregnancies vaginally (but with slightly increased risk).

You may try oxytocin to augment ineffective uterine contractions. Watch out for uterine hyperstimulation (painful, overly frequent, and poorly coordinated uterine contractions), uterine rupture, fetal heart rate decelerations, and water intoxication (from the antidiuretic hormone–like effect of oxytocin). Treat all of these symptoms by first discontinuing oxytocin infusion (half-life is <10 min). Prostaglandin E_2 (dinoprostone) also may be used locally to induce (ripen) the cervix and is highly effective in combination with (often before) oxytocin. Prostaglandin E_2 also can cause uterine hyperstimulation. Amniotomy hastens labor but exposes the fetus and uterine cavity to possible infection if labor does not occur.

FETAL HEART MONITORING

Fetal heart monitoring is routinely done during labor and delivery, but its benefit is controversial. At term the normal heart rate is 110 to 160 bpm. Any value outside this range is worrisome. Know what a basic fetal heart strip with uterine contraction patterns looks like, and know the following abnormalities:

◆ **Early deceleration:** Peaks match up (fetal heart deceleration nadir and uterine contraction peak). Early deceleration signifies head compression (probable vagal response) and is *normal.*

◆ **Variable deceleration:** Variable with relation to uterine contractions. The most commonly encountered abnormality, variable deceleration signifies cord compression. Place the mother in a lateral decubitus position, administer oxygen by face mask, and stop any oxytocin infusion. If bradycardia is severe (<80–90 bpm) or does not resolve, measure fetal scalp pH.

◆ **Late deceleration:** Fetal heart deceleration comes after uterine contraction. Late deceleration signifies uteroplacental insufficiency and is the most worrisome pattern. First, place the mother in a lateral decubitus position, give oxygen by face mask, and stop oxytocin if it is being given. Next, give IV fluids if the mother is hypotensive (especially with epidural anesthesia). If late decelerations persist, measure fetal scalp pH.

◆ **Short-term variability (beat-to-beat variability):** Reflects the interval between successive heart beats. The normal value is 5 to 25 bpm. Variability consistently less than 5 bpm is worrisome, especially when combined with decelerations. Measure fetal scalp pH.

◆ **Long-term variability:** A 1-minute strip normally shows changes in the baseline heart rate. Fewer than three cycles per minute is worrisome, especially when combined with decelerations. Measure fetal scalp pH. *Special warning:* Long-term variability is decreased normally during fetal sleep.

◆ **Fetal tachycardia:** Heart rate >160 bpm. Poor indicator of fetal distress unless prolonged or marked. Often associated with oxytocin administration, maternal fever, or intrauterine infection.

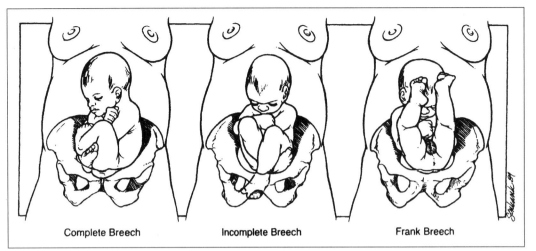

FIGURE 19-4. Three possible breech presentations. (From Gabbe SG, Niebyl JR, Simpson JL (eds): Obstetrics: Normal & Problem Pregnancies. New York, Churchill Livingstone, 1986, p 465, with permission.)

 Note   Any fetal scalp pH <7.2 is an indication for immediate cesarean delivery. If pH is >7.2, in general, continue to observe.

FETAL MALPRESENTATIONS

Although under specific guidelines babies in some frank and complete breeches may be delivered vaginally, it is acceptable to do a cesarean section for *any* breech presentation. With shoulder presentation or incomplete or footling breech, cesarean section is mandatory. For face and brow presentations, watchful waiting is best, as most convert to vertex presentations; if they do not convert, do a cesarean section. Breech presentations are shown in Figure 19-4.

ANESTHESIA

Epidural anesthesia is preferred in obstetric patients. General anesthesia involves a higher risk of aspiration and resulting pneumonia, because the gastroesophageal sphincter is relaxed in pregnancy and most patients have not been NPO. There are also concerns regarding the fetal effects of anesthesia. Spinal anesthesia can interfere with the mother's ability to push and has a higher incidence of hypotension than epidural anesthesia.

Postpartum

IMPORTANT POINTS

1 The top causes of maternal mortality are pulmonary embolism, pregnancy-induced hypertension, and hemorrhage (most texts say in that order).

2 When a postpartum mother develops shortness of breath, tachypnea, chest pain, hypotension, and/or disseminated intravascular coagulation, think of amniotic fluid pulmonary embolism.

3 If a postpartum patient goes into shock and you see no bleeding, think of amniotic fluid embolism, uterine inversion, or concealed hemorrhage (e.g., uterine rupture with bleeding into the peritoneal cavity)

BREAST-FEEDING

If a woman does not want to breast-feed, prescribe tight-fitting bras, ice packs, and analgesia. Bromocriptine and estrogens or oral contraceptives also may be used to suppress lactation.

If a woman does breast-feed, watch for **mastitis,** which usually develops in the first 2 months postpartum. Breasts are red, indurated, and painful, and nipple cracks or fissuring may be seen. *Staphylococcus aureus* is the usual cause. Treat with analgesics (e.g., acetaminophen, ibuprofen), warm and/or cold compresses, and continued breast-feeding with the affected breast(s) even though it is painful (use a breast pump to empty the breast if needed) to prevent further milk duct blockage and abscess formation. Antistaphylococcal antibiotic (e.g., cephalexin, dicloxacillin) is usually given for more than mild symptoms. If a fluctuant mass develops or there is no response to antibiotics within a few days, an abscess is likely present and must be drained.

Breast-feeding is *contraindicated* in patients with HIV or hepatitis B and in patients who use benzodiazepines, barbiturates, opiates, alcohol, caffeine or tobacco (in large amounts), antithyroid medications, lithium, chloramphenicol, anticancer agents, or ergot and its derivatives (e.g., methysergide).

CHORIOAMNIONITIS

Chorioamnionitis manifests with fever and tender, irritable uterus (usually postpartum but may be antepartum in patients with PROM or PPROM). Do a culture and Gram stain of amniotic fluid, and treat with ampicillin while awaiting culture results.

POSTPARTUM FEVER

Postpartum fever is defined as temperature >100.4° F (38° C) for at least two consecutive days. Postpartum fever usually is due to endometritis. Important predisposing factors are PROM or PPROM, prolonged labor, frequent vaginal exams during labor, and manual removal of placenta or retained placental fragments (good culture medium). Patients with endometritis have a tender uterus in addition to fever. Anaerobes usually are involved.

Treat with broad-spectrum penicillin or cephalosporin; add clindamycin, metronidazole, and gentamicin if the patient is doing poorly. Before antibiotics, do cultures of endometrium, vagina, blood, and urine. Do not forget the easy causes of postpartum fever, such as urinary tract infection or atelectasis and pneumonia, especially after cesarean section.

If a postpartum fever does not resolve with broad-spectrum antibiotics, there are two main possibilities: progression to *pelvic abscess* or **pelvic thrombophlebitis.** Get a computed tomography (CT) scan, which will show an abscess. If an abscess is present, it needs to be drained. If no abscess is seen on CT, think of pelvic thrombophlebitis, which manifests with persistent spiking fevers and lack of response to antibiotics. Give heparin for an easy cure (and retrospective diagnosis).

POSTPARTUM HEMORRHAGE

Postpartum hemorrhage is defined as estimated blood loss >500 mL during a vaginal delivery (>1000 mL during cesarean section). The most common cause is uterine atony (75%-80% of cases). Hemorrhage also may be caused by lacerations, retained placental tissue (placenta accreta, increta, or percreta), coagulation disorders (e.g,. disseminated intravascular coagulation, von Willebrand's disease), low placental implantation, and uterine inversion. The major risk factor for retained placental tissue is previous uterine surgery or cesarean section. Treatment might require a hysterectomy if conservative measures fail.

RETAINED PRODUCTS OF CONCEPTION

Retained products of conception is probably the most common cause of *delayed* postpartum hemorrhage. Remove the placenta manually to stop bleeding; then do curettage in the operating room under anesthesia. If placenta accreta, increta, or percreta is present (i.e., placental tissue grows abnormally into or through the myometrium), a hysterectomy is usually necessary to stop the bleeding.

UTERINE ATONY

Uterine atony is caused by overdistention of the uterus (multiple gestation, polyhydramnios, macrosomia), prolonged labor, oxytocin use, grandmultiparity (history of five or more deliveries), and precipitous labor (<3 h). Treat with dilute oxytocin infusion, and use bimanual compression and massage of the uterus while the infusion is running. If this approach fails, try ergonovine or another ergot drug (contraindicated with maternal hypertension) or prostaglandin F_{2a}. If this approach also fails, do a hysterectomy (can try ligating the uterine vessels if the patient strongly desires future fertility).

UTERINE INVERSION

The uterus inverts and can be seen outside the vagina, *usually as a result of pulling too hard on the cord.* Put the uterus back in place manually (anesthesia may be needed) and give IV fluids and oxytocin.

For the first several days after delivery, it is *normal* to have some vaginal discharge (lochia), which is red on the first few days and gradually turns to a white or yellowish-white color by day 10. If the lochia is foul smelling, or if there is associated uterine tenderness or fever, suspect endometritis.

20 GENERAL SURGERY

Common Disorders Requiring Surgery

ACUTE ABDOMEN

An inflamed peritoneum often leads to a laparotomy because it signifies a potentially life-threatening condition (important exceptions to laparotomy are pancreatitis, many cases of diverticulitis, and spontaneous bacterial peritonitis). The best physical confirmations of peritonitis are rebound tenderness and involuntary guarding. Voluntary guarding and tenderness to palpation are softer signs, because both are often present in more benign diseases. When you are in doubt about the diagnosis, and the patient is stable, *withhold pain medications* (do *not* mask symptoms before you have a diagnosis), get a computed tomography (CT) scan of the abdomen and pelvis, and do serial abdominal exams. If the patient is unstable or worsening, proceed to laparoscopy or laparotomy.

Localization of acute abdomen (Fig. 20-1):

◆ **Right upper quadrant:** Think of gallbladder (cholecystitis, cholangitis) or liver (abscess).

◆ **Left upper quadrant:** Think of spleen (rupture with blunt trauma).

◆ **Right lower quadrant:** Think of appendix (appendicitis), ileitis (e.g., Crohn's disease), or adnexal pathology in a reproductive-age female patient.

◆ **Left lower quadrant:** Think of sigmoid colon (diverticulitis) or adnexal pathology in a reproductive-age female patient.

◆ **Epigastric:** Think of stomach (penetrating ulcer) or pancreas (pancreatitis).

APPENDICITIS

Appendicitis peaks in 10- to 30-year-olds. The classic history is crampy, poorly localized periumbilical pain, followed by nausea and vomiting. Pain then localizes to the right lower quadrant, and patients develop peritoneal signs with worsening of nausea and vomiting. Leukocytosis is variable but classically is present. Patients who are hungry and ask for food do *not* have appendicitis. Remember positive Rovsing's sign (pushing on the left lower quadrant produces pain at McBurney's point) and McBurney's point tenderness (Fig. 20-2). CT scan of the abdomen and pelvis with oral and intravenous (IV) contrast (or ultrasound in pediatric and pregnant patients to spare radiation) can be used to

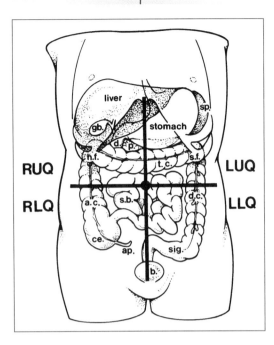

FIGURE 20-1. Topographic anatomy (four-quadrant construct) of the abdomen. ap, appendix; a.c., ascending colon; b, bladder; ce., cecum; d, duodenum; d.c., descending colon; gb, gallbladder; h.f., hepatic flexure; LLQ, left lower quadrant; LUQ, left upper quadrant; p, pancreas; RLQ, right lower quadrant; RUQ, right upper quadrant; s.b., small bowel; s.f., splenic flexure; sig., sigmoid colon; sp, spleen; t.c., transverse colon. (From James EC, Corry RJ, Perry JF: Principles of Basic Surgical Practice. Philadelphia, Hanley & Belfus, 1987, with permission.)

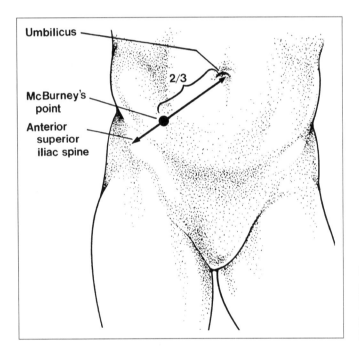

FIGURE 20-2. McBurney's point. This is the usual point of maximal tenderness in the right lower quadrant in appendicitis. (From James EC, Corry RJ, Perry JF: Principles of Basic Surgical Practice. Philadelphia, Hanley & Belfus, 1987, with permission.)

confirm the diagnosis, assess for complications such as perforation and abscess, and exclude other causes. Treatment is appendectomy.

BOWEL OBSTRUCTION

In *small bowel obstruction*, symptoms include bilious vomiting (seen early), abdominal distention, constipation, hyperactive bowel sounds (high-pitched, rushing sounds), and pain that usually is poorly localized. X-ray shows multiple air-fluid levels. Patients often have a history of previous surgery; the most common cause of small bowel obstructions in adults is adhesions, which usually develop from prior surgery. In children, think of intussusception, Meckel's diverticulum, or incarcerated hernia. Start treatment with nothing by mouth (NPO), nasogastric tube, and IV fluids. CT scan with IV contrast can help confirm the diagnosis, exclude complications, and assess the cause. If symptoms do not resolve or peritoneal signs occur, laparotomy is needed to relieve the obstruction.

Symptoms in *large bowel obstruction* include gradually increasing abdominal pain, abdominal distention, constipation, and feculent vomiting (seen late). In older patients, the most common causes are diverticulitis, colon cancer, and volvulus. Treat early with NPO and nasogastric tube. CT scan with IV contrast is used to confirm the diagnosis and assess the cause. A sigmoid volvulus (Fig. 20-3) often can be decompressed with an endoscope. Other causes or refractory cases require surgery to relieve the obstruction. In children, watch for Hirschsprung's disease. In adults, perform colon cancer screening after bout has resolved.

DIVERTICULITIS

Left lower quadrant pain in a patient older than 50 years is diverticulitis unless you have a good reason to think otherwise and is generally accompanied by a change in bowel habits, fever, and leukocytosis. The diagnosis is generally confirmed with a CT scan of the abdomen and pelvis using oral and IV contrast, which can also rule out a complicating abscess. Treat medically with avoidance of oral ingestion (NPO) and broad-spectrum antibiotics. If the disease is recurrent or refractory to medical therapy, consider sigmoid resection. Perform colon cancer screening (e.g., barium enema) after bout has resolved (not during active symptoms!) to exclude underlying colorectal carcinoma.

GALLBLADDER DISEASE

Ultrasound is the best first imaging study for suspected gallstones or gallbladder disease. For cholecystitis, a nuclear hepatobiliary or scintigraphy study (e.g., a hepato-iminodiacetic

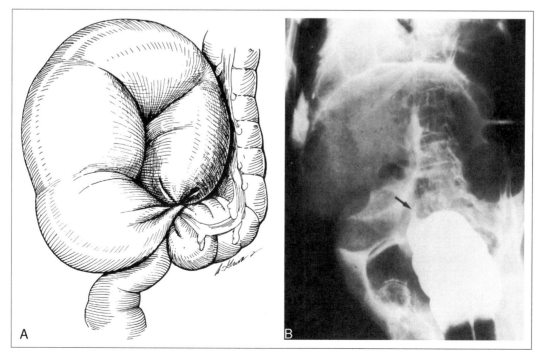

FIGURE 20-3. A, Sigmoid volvulus. **B,** Bird-beak sign (*arrow*) on meglumine (Gastrografin) enema in sigmoid volvulus.

acid [HIDA] scan) can be used to clinch a difficult diagnosis (nonvisualization of the gallbladder) if ultrasound is nondiagnostic.

◆ **Cholecystitis:** The classic patient is fat, forty, fertile, female, flatulent, and now febrile with right upper quadrant pain and tenderness. Gallstones are seen on ultrasound or the patient has a history of gallstones and/or gallstone-type symptoms, such as postprandial right upper quadrant colicky pain, bloating, and/or nausea and vomiting. Look for Murphy's sign. Give antibiotics to reduce inflammation, then perform cholecystectomy.

◆ **Cholangitis:** Right upper quadrant pain, fever and shaking chills, and jaundice. Patients often have a history of gallstones. Start antibiotics and do a cholecystectomy with intraoperative stone extraction (or preop endoscopic retrograde cholangiopancreatography [ERCP] stone extraction).

HERNIA

There are four common types (Fig. 20-4), and all can be treated with surgical repair:

◆ **Indirect:** *Most common type* in both sexes and all age groups. Hernia sac travels through the inner and outer inguinal rings (protrusion begins lateral to the inferior epigastric vessels) and *into the scrotum* or labial region because of a **patent** processus vaginalis (congenital defect).

◆ **Direct:** The hernia *(no sac)* protrudes medial to the inferior epigastric vessels because of weakness in the abdominal musculature of Hesselbach's triangle.

◆ **Femoral:** More common in women. Hernia (no sac) goes through the femoral ring onto the anterior thigh (located *below the inguinal ring*). This type is most susceptible to incarceration and strangulation.

◆ **Incisional:** After any wound (especially surgical), a hernia can occur through the site of the incision.

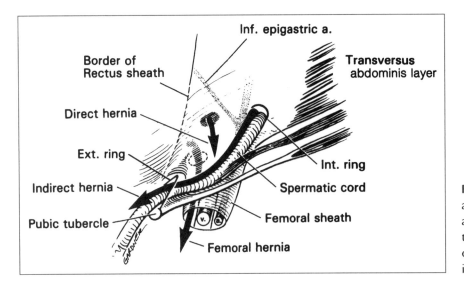

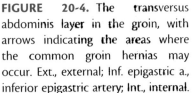

FIGURE 20-4. The transversus abdominis layer in the groin, with arrows indicating the areas where the common groin hernias may occur. Ext., external; Inf. epigastric a., inferior epigastric artery; Int., internal.

Complications:

◆ **Incarceration:** Herniated organs become trapped and swollen or edematous. Incarcerated hernias are the *most common* cause of small bowel obstruction in a patient who has never had abdominal surgery and the *second most common* cause in patients who have had abdominal surgery.

◆ **Strangulation:** The entrapment becomes so severe that the blood supply is cut off; necrosis can occur. Strangulation is a surgical emergency; the patient might present with symptoms of small bowel obstruction and shock.

PANCREATITIS

Look for epigastric pain in an alcohol abuser or patient with history of gallstones. Pain might radiate to the back. Serum amylase or lipase, if given, is elevated; if they have not been given, order them (generally ordered in all cases of abdominal pain of unknown etiology)! Common signs and symptoms include decreased bowel sounds, local ileus (sentinel loop of bowel on x-ray), and nausea and vomiting with anorexia. Treat with narcotics (meperidine, not morphine), NPO, nasogastric tube, IV fluids, and supportive care. Watch for complications of pseudocyst and pancreatic abscess, which can require surgical-type intervention.

PERFORATED ULCER

Patients often have no history of alcohol consumption or gallstones. X-ray classically shows free air under the diaphragm, and patients have a history of peptic ulcer disease. Amylase may be mildly elevated (Step 2 question might provide amylase value to trick you), but lipase is often normal, and free air doesn't occur in pancreatitis. Treat with surgery.

SPLENIC RUPTURE

History of blunt abdominal trauma, hypotension, tachycardia, shock, and Kerr's sign. CT confirms severity of injury, with observation and monitoring done for all but the most severe injuries. With active bleeding or complete rupture, endovascular embolization of the spleen or splenectomy are advised. Patients with Epstein–Barr virus infection (i.e., infectious mononucleosis) and splenomegaly should *not* play contact sports. Immunize all patients after splenectomy against encapsulated bacterial pathogens, if not already done (i.e., *H. influenzae*, pneumococcal and meningococcal vaccines).

Pulmonary Function, Cardiac History, and Surgery

A baseline chest x-ray is standard preoperative evaluation for patients older than 60 years and patients with known pulmonary or cardiovascular disease, but when to order pulmonary function tests is not as clear. The best indicator of possible **postoperative pulmonary complications** is preoperative pulmonary function. Overall, the best way to reduce pulmonary postoperative complications is to *stop smoking* preoperatively. Aggressive pulmonary toilet, incentive spirometry, minimal narcotics, and early ambulation help to prevent or minimize postoperative pulmonary complications. Spirometry and a good history are the best preoperative tests for assessment of pulmonary function. Spirometry evaluates forced vital capacity (FVC), forced expiratory volume in one second (FEV$_1$), FEV$_1$/FVC (%), and maximal voluntary ventilation.

IMPORTANT POINTS

1 Before surgery the patient should avoid oral ingestion for at least 8 hours to reduce the risk of aspiration. For this reason, general anesthesia is higher risk (usually avoided) in obstetrics, because patients have *not* been NPO when they go into labor.

2 Use compressive or elastic stockings, early ambulation, and/or low-molecular-weight heparin to help prevent deep vein thrombosis and pulmonary embolism. Warfarin is sometimes used for orthopedic procedures.

3 The most common cause of postoperative fever in the first 24 hours is atelectasis. Treat or prevent with early ambulation, chest physiotherapy and percussion, incentive spirometry, and proper pain control. Both too much pain and too many narcotics increase risk of atelectasis.

4 "Water, wind, walk, wound, and weird drugs" helps to recall causes of postoperative fever. Water = urinary tract infection, wind = atelectasis or pneumonia, walk = deep vein thrombosis, wound = surgical wound infection, and weird drugs = drug fever. If daily fever spikes occur, think about an intra-abdominal abscess—order a CT scan to locate. Drainage is required.

5 Perioperative β-blockers can reduce the risk of myocardial infarction in those at increased risk due to history of coronary artery disease or coronary disease risk factors.

6 Fascial or wound dehiscence classically occurs *5 to 10 days postoperatively*. Look for leakage of serosanguineous fluid from the wound, particularly after the patient coughs or strains, which is often associated with infection. Treat with antibiotics (if secondary to infection) and reclosure of the incision.

Trauma

If you spent your free time during your surgery rotation trying to catch up on lost sleep, go back and read a chapter about trauma from a general surgery text. Trauma and its management are high yield for Step 2.

ABCDEs are the key to management of patients with trauma. Always do them in order. For example, if the patient is bleeding to death and has a blocked airway, you must choose which problem to address first. The answer is airway management.

◆ **A = Airway:** Provide, protect, and maintain an adequate airway at all times. If the patient can answer questions, the airway is fine. You can use an oropharyngeal airway in uncomplicated cases and give supplemental oxygen. When you are in doubt or the patient's airway is blocked, intubate. If intubation fails, do a cricothyroidotomy.

◆ **B = Breathing:** Similar to airway, but even when the airway is patent, the patient might not be breathing spontaneously. The end result is the same: When you are in doubt or the patient is not breathing, intubate. If intubation fails, do a cricothyroidotomy.

◆ **C = Circulation:** If the patient seems hypovolemic (tachycardia, bleeding, weak pulse, paleness, diaphoresis, capillary refill >2 sec), give IV fluids and/or blood products. The initial procedure is to start two large-bore IV catheters and give a bolus of 10 to 20 mL/kg (roughly 1 L) of lactated Ringer's solution (IV fluid of choice in trauma). Reassess the patient after the bolus for improvement. Give another bolus if needed.

◆ **D = Disability:** Check neurologic function (Glasgow Coma Scale).

◆ **E = Exposure:** Strip the patient and "put a finger in every orifice" so that you do not miss any occult injuries.

IMPORTANT POINTS

1 All trauma patients generally get cervical spine, chest, and pelvic x-rays. CT scans of any affected areas are used liberally with significant injuries or symptoms.

2 Evaluate any head trauma with a noncontrast CT (better than magnetic resonance imaging [MRI] for acute trauma).

3 In **blunt abdominal trauma**, initial findings determine the course of action:
- If the patient is awake and stable, and your exam is benign, observe and repeat the abdominal exam later. Meanwhile, perform CT scan of the abdomen and pelvis with oral and IV contrast.
- If the patient is hemodynamically unstable (hypotension and/or shock that do not respond to a fluid challenge), proceed directly to laparotomy.
- If the patient has altered mental status, the abdomen cannot be examined, or an obvious source of blood loss explains the hemodynamic instability, order a CT scan of the abdomen and pelvis with oral and IV contrast (also get CT of the head and cervical spine with altered mental status). Diagnostic peritoneal lavage is no longer used because it is nonspecific and less sensitive than CT; it can also alter CT scan results.

4 In **penetrating abdominal trauma**, the type of injury and initial findings determine the course of action:
- With any gunshot wound, proceed directly to laparotomy.
- With a wound from a sharp instrument, management is more controversial. Either proceed directly to laparotomy (the better choice if the patient is unstable) or do CT scan of the abdomen and pelvis with oral and IV contrast. If the CT scan is positive, do a laparotomy; if it is negative, observe and repeat the abdominal exam later.

THORACIC TRAUMA

Six thoracic injuries that can be rapidly fatal and that you should be able to recognize:

◆ **Airway obstruction:** No audible breath sounds. Patients cannot answer questions even though they may be awake and gurgling. Treat with intubation. If intubation fails, do a cricothyroidotomy (or a tracheostomy in the operating room if time allows).

◆ **Open pneumothorax:** Open defect in the chest wall that causes poor ventilation and oxygenation. Treat with intubation, positive-pressure ventilation, and closure of the defect in the chest wall. You can use gauze and tape it *on three sides only* to allow excessive pressure to escape. Otherwise you could convert an open pneumothorax into a tension pneumothorax.

◆ **Tension pneumothorax:** Usually after blunt trauma. Air forced into pleural space cannot escape and collapses the affected lung, then shifts the mediastinum and trachea to the opposite side of the chest. You should be able to recognize this condition on a chest x-ray (Fig. 20-5). There are no breath sounds on the affected side, and chest percussion produces a hypertympanic sound. Hypotension and distended neck veins can result from impaired cardiac filling. Treat with needle thoracentesis followed by insertion of a chest tube.

◆ **Cardiac tamponade:** The classic history is penetrating trauma to the left chest (where the heart is located). Patients have hypotension (due to impaired cardiac filling), distended neck veins, muffled heart sounds, pulsus paradoxus (exaggerated fall in blood pressure on inspiration), and normal breath sounds. Treat with pericardiocentesis if the patient is unstable (put a catheter in the pericardial sac and aspirate the blood or fluid). If the patient is stable, you can do an echocardiogram or CT scan to confirm the diagnosis first.

◆ **Massive hemothorax:** Loss of more than 1 L of blood into the thoracic cavity. Patients have decreased (not absent) breath sounds in the affected area, dull note on percussion, hypotension or collapsed neck veins (from blood leaving the vascular tree), and tachycardia. Placement of a chest tube causes the blood to come out. Give IV fluids and/or blood before you place the chest tube. If bleeding stops after the initial outflow, get an x-ray and CT of chest to check for remaining blood or pathology and treat supportively. If bleeding does not stop, perform an emergent thoracotomy.

◆ **Flail chest:** When several adjacent ribs are broken in multiple places, the affected part of the chest wall can move paradoxically during respiration (in during inspiration, out during expiration). There is almost always an associated pulmonary contusion, which, combined with pain, can make respiration inadequate. When you are in doubt or the patient is not doing well, intubate and give positive pressure ventilation.

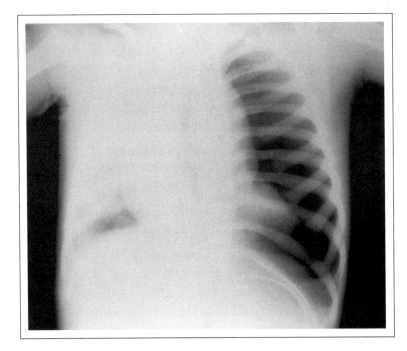

FIGURE 20-5. Left tension pneumothorax. (From James EC, Corry RJ, Perry JF: Principles of Basic Surgical Practice. Philadelphia, Hanley & Belfus, 1987, with permission.)

OTHER THORACIC INJURIES

- **Aortic rupture:** The most common cause of immediate death after an automobile accident or fall from a great height. Look for widened mediastinum on x-ray and appropriate trauma history. Get a CT scan of the chest with IV contrast if you are suspicious (second—less desirable—choice is conventional angiogram). Treat with surgical repair.

- **Liver lacerations and contusions:** Detected and graded by CT scan. Usually treated conservatively unless actively bleeding or shattered liver (endovascular embolization or surgical repair is needed in this setting).

- **Pulmonary contusion:** Lung "bruise" that causes immediate consolidation that can be detected on initial chest x-ray or CT. Main problem is difficulty in ventilation and oxygenation. Treat supportively with oxygen (use intubation if needed).

- **Diaphragm rupture:** Usually occurs on the left because the liver "protects" the right side. Look for bowel herniated into the chest. Can often be detected by CT scan if the diagnosis is in doubt. Fix surgically.

NECK TRAUMA

The neck is divided into three zones for trauma (Fig. 20-6):

- **Zone I:** Base of the neck (from 2 cm above the clavicles to the level of the clavicles)
- **Zone II:** Midcervical region (2 cm above the clavicle to the angle of the mandible)
- **Zone III:** The angle of the mandible to the base of the skull

With zone I and III injuries, do a CT angiogram before going to the operating room. With zone II injuries, the traditional and now outdated wisdom is to proceed to the operating room for surgical exploration without doing an arteriogram first, but CT angiogram (or carotid ultrasound) is now more commonly done before surgery to see if exploration is indicated. In the presence of obvious bleeding or a rapidly expanding hematoma, proceed to immediate surgical exploration.

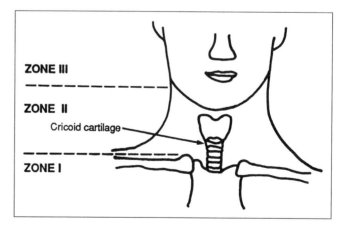

FIGURE 20-6. Neck zones for trauma. (From Markovchick V, Pons P: Emergency Medicine Secrets, 2nd ed. Philadelphia, Hanley & Belfus, 1999, with permission.)

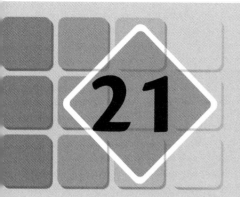

OPHTHALMOLOGY

Conjunctivitis

Conjunctivitis causes conjunctival vessel hyperemia. The three main causes are allergic (common), viral (common), and bacterial (rare) (Table 21-1). Conjunctivitis involves no loss of vision (other than transient blurriness due to tear film debris that resolves with blinking). If loss of vision is present, think of other, more serious conditions.

Neonatal conjunctivitis is usually due to one of three causes:

◆ **Chemical:** Silver nitrate (or erythromycin) drops are given prophylactically to all newborns to prevent gonorrheal conjunctivitis. The drops can cause a chemical conjunctivitis (with *no* purulent discharge) that develops within 12 hours of instilling the drops and resolves within 48 hours (pick this answer if conjunctivitis occurs in the *first 24 hours of life*).

◆ **Gonorrheal:** Look for symptoms of gonorrhea in the mother. The infant has an *extremely purulent* discharge at *2 to 5 days of age*. Treatment is topical (e.g., erythromycin ointment) plus intravenous (IV) or intramuscular (IM) third-generation cephalosporin (e.g., ceftriaxone). Infants who are given prophylactic drops should not get gonorrheal conjunctivitis.

◆ **Chlamydial (inclusion conjunctivitis):** The mother often reports no symptoms. The infant has mild to severe conjunctivitis beginning at *5 to 14 days of age*. Patients must be treated with systemic antibiotics (oral erythromycin usually is used) to prevent chlamydial pneumonia (a common complication). Prophylactic eyedrops do *not* effectively prevent chlamydial conjunctivitis.

Table 21-1. CONJUNCTIVITIS

Etiology	Unique Signs and Symptoms	Treatment
Allergic	Itching, bilateral, seasonal, long duration	Vasoconstrictors if needed
Viral*	Preauricular adenopathy, highly contagious (history of infected personal contacts); clear, watery discharge	Supportive, hand washing (prevents spread)
Bacterial	Purulent discharge; more common in neonates	Topical antibiotics

*Number-one cause is adenovirus.

IMPORTANT POINT

- If you forget everything else about neonatal conjunctivitis, remember the days after birth when the three causes occur.

Glaucoma

Glaucoma is best thought of as ocular hypertension with its resultant effects. Main risk factors are age older than 40 years, race (black), and family history. Glaucoma is the number-one cause of blindness in blacks of any age and the number-three overall cause of blindness. There are two types: open-angle glaucoma and closed-angle glaucoma.

- **Open-angle glaucoma:** Although it is traditional to talk about painful attacks, they are rare. Open-angle glaucoma causes 90% of cases of glaucoma, is *painless*, and does not involve acute attacks. The only signs are elevated intraocular pressure (usually 20–30 mm Hg), a gradually progressive visual field loss, and optic nerve changes (increased cup-to-disc ratio on funduscopic exam). Treat with several different types of medications (β-blockers, prostaglandin [latanoprost], acetazolamide, pilocarpine) or surgery if meds fail.

- **Closed-angle glaucoma:** Closed-angle glaucoma manifests with sudden ocular *pain*, haloes around lights, red eye, high intraocular pressure (>30 mm Hg), nausea and vomiting, sudden *decreased* vision, and a *fixed, mid-dilated pupil*. Treat *immediately* with pilocarpine drops and oral glycerin and acetazolamide to break the attack. Then use surgery to prevent further attacks (peripheral iridectomy).

In rare cases, **anticholinergic medications** can cause an attack of closed-angle glaucoma in a susceptible, previously untreated patient. Medications do not cause glaucoma attacks in open-angle glaucoma or patients previously treated surgically for closed-angle glaucoma.

Corticosteroids, whether applied directly to the eye (i.e. topical) or systemic, can cause glaucoma and cataracts. Topical steroids can worsen ocular herpes and fungal infections. For board purposes, do *not* give topical ocular steroids (especially if the patient has a dendritic corneal ulcer stained green by fluorescein).

Note The retinal and fundus changes seen in **diabetes** (dot-blot hemorrhages, microaneurysms, neovascularization; Fig. 21-1) and **hypertension** (arteriolar narrowing, copper/silver wiring, cotton wool spots, papilledema with severe hypertension) are fair game on Step 2. Make the diagnosis from the appearance of the fundus.

Loss Of Vision

SUDDEN UNILATERAL, *PAINLESS* VISION LOSS

A fairly short differential:

- **Central retinal artery occlusion:** Funduscopic appearance is classic. The most common cause is emboli (from carotid plaque or heart), and treatment is generally supportive unless the occlusion is due to temporal arteritis (discussed later).

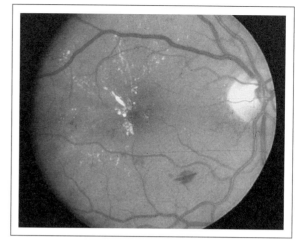

FIGURE 21-1. Background diabetic retinopathy with exudate, hemorrhages, and edema (dot and blot). (From Vander JF, Gault JA: Ophthalmology Secrets. Philadelphia, Hanley & Belfus, 1998, with permission.)

◆ **Central retinal vein occlusion:** Funduscopic appearance is also classic. No satisfactory treatment. Most common causes are hypertension, diabetes, glaucoma, and increased blood viscosity (e.g., leukemia). Complications are related to neovascularization (vision loss, glaucoma).

◆ **Optic neuritis or papillitis:** Usually takes at least a few hours to develop and is more often painful, but it can occur quickly and be painless. Is sometimes bilateral. If present in a 20- to 40-year-old woman, think multiple sclerosis. Worry about tumor if the patient is male, has signs of intracranial hypertension, or has other neurologic deficits. Lyme disease and syphilis are rare causes. Disc margins might appear blurred on funduscopic exam, just as in papilledema (intracranial pressure is generally normal with papillitis).

◆ **Retinal detachment:** History usually includes floaters and seeing flashes of light. Often described as a "curtain [or veil] coming down in front of my eye." This history should prompt immediate referral to an ophthalmologist, because surgery to reattach the retina can save the patient's sight.

◆ **Stroke or transient ischemic attack:** See the discussion of visual pathways.

◆ **Vitreous hemorrhage:** Usually due to bleeding from areas of neovascularization, classically in diabetic patients. It sometimes resolves or can improve after surgical vitrectomy.

SUDDEN, UNILATERAL *PAINFUL* VISION LOSS

Causes include:

◆ **Closed-angle glaucoma:** See the discussion earlier for presenting signs and symptoms and treatment.

◆ **Migraine headache:** Rare, but can occur. Look for nausea and vomiting and aura.

◆ **Optic neuritis:** More often painful than not, as mentioned earlier.

◆ **Trauma:** History gives it away. Encourage use of goggles or safety glasses during athletics and work. With chemical burns to the eye (acid or alkali), the key to management is copious irrigation with closest source of water (tap water is fine). The longer you wait, the worse the prognosis (don't get additional history in this instance). Alkali burns have a worse prognosis, because they tend to penetrate deeper into the eye.

SUDDEN *BILATERAL* VISION LOSS

This is rare. Consider:

◆ **Conversion reaction or hysteria**

◆ **Exposure to UV light:** Can cause keratitis (corneal inflammation) with resultant **pain**, foreign body sensation, red eyes, tearing, and decreased vision (usually some vision remains). Patient has a history of welding, using a tanning bed or sunlamp, or snow skiing (snow blindness). Treat with an eye patch (24 hours) and topical antibiotic, possibly also with an anticholinergic (cycloplegic agent, reduces pain).

◆ **Toxins:** Classic is methanol poisoning, usually seen in alcoholics.

GRADUAL-ONSET VISION LOSS, UNILATERAL OR BILATERAL

Longer differential, but more common than sudden-onset vision loss:

◆ **Cataracts:** The most common cause of a painless, slowly progressive loss of vision. Often bilateral, but one side may be worse than the other. Look for absent red reflex. Patient complains of "looking through a dirty windshield." Treatment is surgical. Can delay surgery until patient's daily activities are affected. Cataracts in a neonate should make you think of TORCH infections (toxoplasmosis, other agents, rubella, cytomegalovirus, herpes simplex virus) or an inherited metabolic disorder (e.g., galactosemia).

◆ **Diabetes:** Most common cause of blindness in adults younger than 50 years. Retinal and fundus changes in diabetes (dot-blot hemorrhages, microaneurysms, neovascularization). Treatment for proliferative diabetic retinopathy (neovascularization present) is laser applied to the periphery of the whole retina (panretinal photocoagulation). Focal laser treatment is often done for nonproliferative retinopathy with macular edema (laser applied only to the affected area).

◆ **Direct insult to brain:** Tumor or meningitis. See later section for visual pathway information.

◆ **Eye infection:** Cornea (herpes keratitis, corneal ulcer [Fig. 21-2]), retina (CMV retinitis in AIDS), orbital cellulitis (see later).

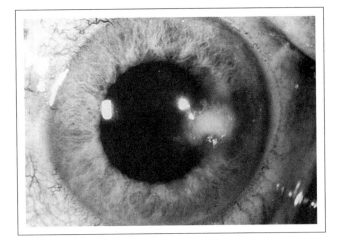

FIGURE 21-2. Infectious corneal ulcer caused by a filamentous fungus. Note the indistinct, feathery borders.

◆ **Glaucoma, open angle:** See earlier for specifics. Screen patients older than 40 years, especially if they are black or have diabetes or a positive family history. Most common cause of blindness in blacks.

◆ **Macular degeneration:** Most common cause of blindness in adults older than 55 years. Often bilateral, but one side may be worse than the other. Appearance of the fundus (macular drusen; Fig. 21-3) makes diagnosis. No good treatment for the most common (90% of cases) dry type (high doses of vitamins A, C, and E and mineral zinc can slow progression). The wet type can be treated with antiangiogenics (e.g., pegaptanib) and laser therapy with or without verteporfin.

◆ **Optic neuritis:** Classically from autoimmune-type conditions, infections (Lyme disease), or drugs (ethambutol).

◆ **Papilledema:** Classically from hypertension or other cause of increased intracranial pressure (brain tumor, pseudotumor cerebri) (Fig. 21-4).

◆ **Presbyopia:** Between ages 40 and 50 years, the lens loses its ability to accommodate, and people need bifocals or reading glasses for near vision. This is a normal part of aging and not a disease.

◆ **Uveitis:** Look for association with autoimmune-type diseases. Screen kids with juvenile rheumatoid arthritis regularly to detect uveitis (classic rheumatoid arthritis presentation in kids is uveitis, with or without joint symptoms). Usually treated with corticosteroids (by an ophthalmologist).

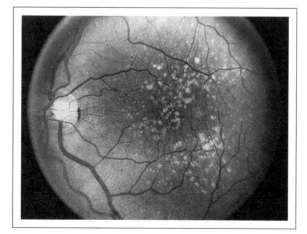

FIGURE 21-3. Drusen are the byproducts of retinal metabolism and manifest as focal yellow-white deposits deep to the retinal pigment epithelium. They serve as a marker of nonexudative age-related macular degeneration. (From Vander JF, Gault JA: Ophthalmology Secrets. Philadelphia, Hanley & Belfus, 1998, with permission.)

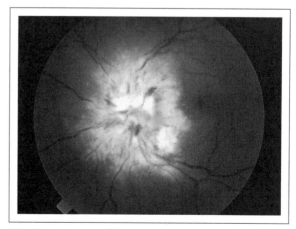

FIGURE 21-4. Papilledema, caused by cryptococcal meningitis in this case, is characterized by optic disc swelling and blurring of the disc margins.

Be able to differentiate **orbital cellulitis** from **preorbital cellulitis** (preseptal cellulitis). Both can involve swollen lids, fever, chemosis, and a history of facial laceration, trauma, insect bite, or sinusitis. Ophthalmoplegia, proptosis, severe eye pain, or decreased visual acuity indicates orbital cellulitis (a medical emergency). The most common bugs in both are *Streptococcus pneumoniae, Haemophilus influenzae* type b, and staphylococci or streptococci with a history of trauma. Complications of orbital cellulitis include extension into the skull, vein thromboses, and blindness. Treat either condition with blood cultures and administration of broad-spectrum antibiotics to cover the likely bugs until culture results are known. Computed tomography (CT) scan can exclude complications such as an abscess. Inpatient IV antibiotics are needed for orbital cellulitis.

Other Ophthalmologic Conditions and Complications

Hordeolum (stye) is a painful, red lump near the lid margin. Treat with warm compresses. **Chalazion** is a painless lump away from the lid margin. Treat with warm compresses. If the compresses don't work, use incision and drainage for both conditions.

Herpes simplex keratitis (Fig. 21-5) usually starts with conjunctivitis and a vesicular lid eruption, then progresses to the classic dendritic keratitis (seen with fluorescein). Treat with topical antivirals (e.g., idoxuridine, trifluridine). Corticosteroids are *contraindicated* with dendritic keratitis because they can make the condition worse.

Ophthalmic herpes zoster should be suspected with involvement of the tip of the nose and/or medial eyelid in a typical zoster dermatomal pattern (Fig. 21-6). Treat with oral famciclovir, valacyclovir, or acyclovir. Complications include uveitis, keratitis, and glaucoma.

Central retinal artery occlusion manifests with sudden (within a few minutes), painless, unilateral loss of vision. The funduscopic appearance is classic (pale fundus with

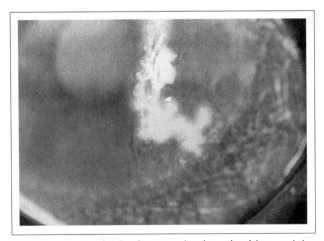

FIGURE 21-5. Classic herpes simplex dendrite staining brightly with fluorescein.

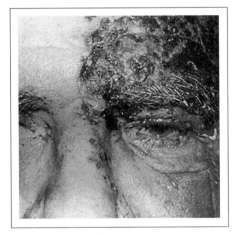

FIGURE 21-6. Characteristic appearance and location of herpes zoster skin lesions with involvement of the V1 distribution of the trigeminal nerve.

a red fovea [cherry-red spot in the macula]). No treatment is satisfactory. Look for coexisting symptoms of temporal arteritis: elderly patients with jaw claudication, tortuous temporal artery, markedly elevated erythrocyte sedimentation rate, and coexisting polymyalgia rheumatica symptoms of proximal muscle pain and stiffness. If temporal arteritis is suspected, start corticosteroids *immediately* before confirming the diagnosis with a temporal artery biopsy. The patient might lose vision in the other eye if you wait to confirm the diagnosis.

Children with a **lazy eye** or **strabismus** (deviation of the eye, usually inward) that persists beyond 3 months need ophthalmologic referral. The condition generally does not resolve on its own at this point and can cause blindness (amblyopia) in the affected eye. For this reason, visual screening must be done in pediatric patients; the visual system is still developing after birth until the age of 7 or 8 years. If one eye does not see well or is turned outward, the brain cannot fuse the two different images that it sees and suppresses the bad eye, which will not develop the proper neural connections. Thus, the eye will never see well and vision cannot be corrected with glasses (neural rather than refractive problem).

Ophthalmologic Cranial Nerve Palsies

Ophthalmologic cranial nerve (CN) palsies are usually due to vascular complications of diabetes and hypertension. Most cases resolve on their own within 2 months. In patients younger than 40 years, patients with other neurologic deficits or severe pain, and any patient who does not improve within 8 weeks, get a magnetic resonance (MR) image of the brain with contrast because benign causes are less likely.

- **Oculomotor (CN III):** The eye is down and out and can move only laterally. In cases due to hypertension or diabetes mellitus, the pupil is normal. Close observation is all that is needed; the condition resolves on its own in several weeks. A pupil that is ''blown'' (dilated, nonreactive) is a medical emergency; the most likely cause is an aneurysm or tumor. Get a brain MR image and MR angiogram.
- **Trochlear (CN IV):** When the gaze is medial, the patient cannot look down.
- **Abducens (CN VI):** The patient cannot look laterally with the affected eye.
- **CN V and VII:** These also affect the eye because of corneal drying (loss of corneal blink reflex).

Visual Pathways

The visual pathways (Fig. 21-7) make for classic board questions, just as on Step I. The most commonly tested example is bitemporal hemianopsia, which usually is due to a pituitary tumor. The visual field defects are listed in Table 21-2.

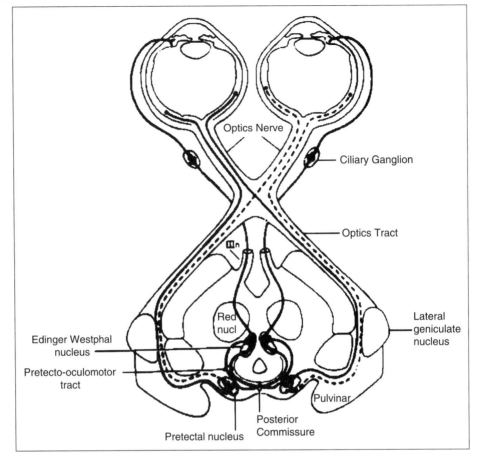

Optics Nerve

Ciliary Ganglion

Optics Tract

Lateral geniculate nucleus

Edinger Westphal nucleus

Pretecto-oculomotor tract

Red nucl

Pulvinar

Posterior Commissure

Pretectal nucleus

FIGURE 21-7. Light reflex pathway.

Table 21-2. LOCALIZATION OF VISUAL FIELD DEFECTS

Visual Field Defect	Location of Lesion
Right anopsia (monocular blindness)	Right optic nerve
Bitemporal hemianopsia	Optic chiasm (classically due to a pituitary tumor)
Left homonymous hemianopsia	Right optic tract
Left upper quadrant anopsia	Right optic radiations in the right temporal lobe
Left lower quadrant anopsia	Right optic radiations in the right parietal lobe
Left homonymous hemianopsia with macular sparing	Right occipital lobe (from posterior cerebral artery occlusion)

22 ORTHOPEDIC SURGERY

Fracture and Dislocation

FRACTURES

Pelvic fracture is the fracture with the *highest mortality rate*. Patients can bleed to death. If the patient is unstable, consider heroic measures such as military antishock trousers and external fixator.

For any fracture, always do a **neurologic and vascular exam** (Table 22-1) distal to the fracture site to see if there is neurologic or vascular compromise. Either may be an emergency. Also, get **two x-ray views** (usually anteroposterior and lateral) of the site, and consider x-rays of the joint above and below the fracture site.

In an **open fracture** (compound fracture), the skin is broken (lacerated) over the fracture site. Give antibiotics (cefazolin or cefazolin plus gentamicin if the laceration is large or contaminated), do surgical debridement, give tetanus vaccine, lavage fresh wounds (<8 hours old), and do an open reduction and internal fixation. The main complication in open fractures is infection.

In a **closed fracture,** the skin is intact over the fracture site.

Open versus closed reduction:

◆ Reasons to do open reduction include:

   ◆ Intraarticular fractures or articular surface malalignment

   ◆ Open (compound) fractures

   ◆ Nonunion or failed closed reduction

Table 22-1. PERIPHERAL NERVE EXAM

Nerve	Motor	Sensory	When Clinically Damaged
Radial	Wrist extension	Back of forearm, back of hand (first three fingers)	Humeral fracture (wrist drop)
Ulnar	Finger abduction	Front and back of last two fingers	Elbow dislocation (claw hand)
Median	Pronation, thumb opposition	Palmar surface (first three digits)	Carpal tunnel, humeral fracture
Axillary	Abduction, lateral rotation	Lateral shoulder	Upper humeral dislocation or fracture
Peroneal	Dorsiflexion/eversion	Dorsal foot and lateral leg	Knee dislocation (footdrop)

227

- ◆ Compromise of blood supply
- ◆ Multiple trauma (to allow mobilization at earliest possible point)
- ◆ Extremity function requiring perfect reduction (e.g., professional athlete)
- ◆ Closed reduction can be done for most other fractures (Table 22-1).

COMPARTMENT SYNDROME

Compartment syndrome usually occurs after fracture, crush injury, burn, or other trauma, or it can occur as a reperfusion injury (e.g., after revascularization procedure). The most common site is the calf. Symptoms and signs include pain on passive movement (out of proportion to injury), paresthesias, cyanosis or pallor, firm-feeling muscle compartment, hypesthesia or numbness (decreased sensation and two-point discrimination), paralysis (late, ominous sign), and elevated compartment pressure (>30–40 mm Hg). The diagnosis usually is made clinically without a need to measure pressure. Compartment syndrome is an *emergency*, and quick action can save an otherwise doomed limb. Pulses are *usually palpable* or detectable with Doppler ultrasound.

Treatment is an immediate fasciotomy; incising the fascial compartment relieves the pressure. Untreated, the condition progresses to permanent nerve damage and muscle necrosis.

The classic clinical scenarios associated with compartment syndrome are supracondylar elbow fractures in children, proximal or midshaft tibial fractures, electrical burns, arterial or venous disruption, and revascularization procedures.

Knee Ligament Injuries

Ligament injuries in the knee commonly cause pain, joint effusions, instability of the joint, and patient history of the joint "popping," "buckling," or "locking up."

- ◆ **Anterior cruciate ligament (ACL):** Most common. Perform the *anterior drawer test.* Place the knee in 90 degrees of flexion and pull forward (like opening a drawer). If the tibia pulls forward more than normal, the test is positive and the patient has an ACL tear.

- ◆ **Posterior cruciate ligament (PCL):** Perform the *posterior drawer test.* Push the tibia back with the knee in 90 degrees of flexion. If the tibia pushes back more than normal, the test is positive and the PCL is torn.

- ◆ **Medial collateral ligament (MCL):** Perform and *abduction or valgus stress test.* With the knee in 30 degrees of flexion, abduct the ankle while holding the knee. If the knee joint abducts abnormally far, the test is positive and the MCL is injured.

- ◆ **Lateral collateral ligament (LCL):** Perform an *adduction or varus stress test.* Adduct the ankle while holding the knee. If the knee joint adducts abnormally far, the test is positive and LCL injury is present.

 Magnetic resonance imaging (MRI) is routinely performed to evaluate and confirm suspected clinical injuries. Arthroscopy is used for injury repair or when an MRI is clinically suspected to be falsely negative.

Treatment for all ligament injuries can be nonsurgical (older patient, nonathlete, minor injury) or surgical (young patient, athlete, severe injury).

Degenerative Disk Disease

Lumbar disk disease and herniation is a common correctable cause of low back pain.

◆ The *most common site* is the **L5-S1 disk.** Herniation affects the S1 nerve root. Look for decreased ankle jerk, weakness of plantar flexors in the foot, pain from the midgluteal area to the posterior calf, and sciatica with the straight-leg raise test.

◆ The *second most common site* is **L4-L5** (Fig. 22-1). Herniation affects the L5 nerve root. Look for decreased biceps femoris reflex, weakness of foot extensors, and pain in the hip or groin.

The diagnosis is made by MRI, CT, or myelogram. Plain x-rays can show disk space narrowing, which is nonspecific, and can't visualize the disk itself, so they are rarely helpful. Conservative treatment consists of bedrest and analgesics. Surgery (diskectomy) is an option if conservative treatment fails.

Cervical disk disease (classic symptom = neck pain) is less common than lumbar disease. The C6-C7 disk is the most common site (C5-C6 is the second most common cervical disk). Herniation at the C6-C7 level affects the C7 nerve root. Look for decreased reflex and strength of the triceps and weakness of forearm extension.

Other Orthopedic Problems

Charcot's joints and neuropathic joints are seen most commonly in diabetes mellitus and other conditions causing peripheral neuropathy (e.g., B_{12} deficiency, tertiary syphilis). Lack of proprioception causes gradual arthritis and arthropathy and joint deformity.

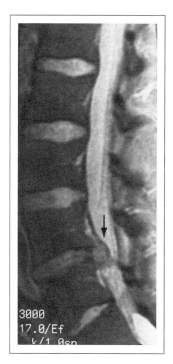

FIGURE 22-1. Large herniated disk at L4-L5. The gelatinous material from the nucleus pulposus becomes extruded from the disk, resulting in root compression and spinal stenosis (*arrow*).

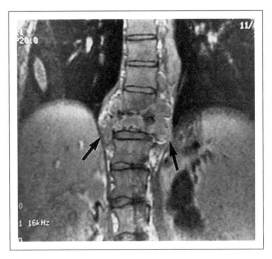

FIGURE 22-2. Septic spondylitis, lumbar spine. The pyogenic infection in this case results in narrowing and destruction of the involved disk space and osteomyelitis of the adjacent vertebral bodies. *Arrows* indicate the mass-like paraspinal extension of infectious spondylodiskitis.

Do x-rays for any (even minor) trauma in neuropathic patients, who might not feel even a severe fracture.

The most common cause of **osteomyelitis** is *Staphylococcus aureus*, but think of gram-negative organisms in immunocompromised patients and IV drug abusers, and think of *Salmonella* in sickle cell disease. Aspirate or biopsy the affected bone and do Gram stain, cultures and sensitivities, blood cultures, and complete blood cell count with differential if you are suspicious. MRI or bone scan can also help confirm the diagnosis (Figure 22-2).

Septic arthritis also is most commonly due to *S. aureus*, but in a sexually active adult (especially a promiscuous one), suspect gonococci. Aspirate the joint and do Gram stain, culture and sensitivities, blood cultures, and complete blood cell count with differential if you are suspicious.

IMPORTANT POINTS

1 With a true posterior knee dislocation, check pulses and perform CT angiogram (or MR or conventional angiogram) if pulses are asymmetric or decreased (vascular injury commonly associated).

2 The most common type of bone tumor is metastatic (from the breast, lung, or prostate).

3 The most common cause of a pathologic fracture is osteoporosis (Fig. 22-3), especially in elderly, thin women. Osteoporosis typically leads to hip or spine (compression) fractures, which are diagnosed with plain x-rays. Use CT or MRI if the diagnosis or age of the fracture is in doubt or if a nonosteoporotic pathologic cause of bone weakening is suspected.

4 A hip dislocation, fracture, or inflammation can cause referred pain to the knee (classic in children).

5 Pain in the anatomic snuff box after trauma (fall on an outstretched hand, especially in young adults) usually is due to a scaphoid bone fracture.

6 After a fall on an outstretched hand, the most likely fracture in older adults is a Colles' fracture (distal end of radius; Fig. 22-4).

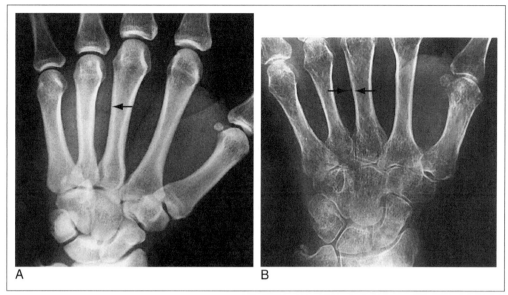

FIGURE 22-3. Osteoporosis. A, Note the normal cortical thickness at the third metacarpal shaft in this 30-year-old (*arrow*). **B,** The cortices of this elderly osteoporotic woman are markedly thinned (*arrows*).

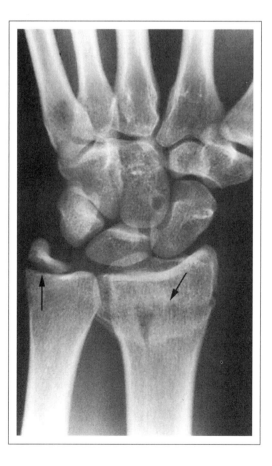

FIGURE 22-4. Colles' fracture (*arrow* on right side of figure) with associated ulnar styloid fracture (*arrow* on left side of figure).

Pediatric Orthopedics

Pediatric hip problems (Table 22-2) give referred pain to the knee, but the patient has no knee swelling or pain with palpation of the knee.

Congenital hip dysplasia, Legg–Calvé–Perthes disease, and slipped capital femoral epiphysis all may manifest in an adult as arthritis of the hip. Given the correct history (especially age of onset of symptoms!), you should be able to tell which disorder they had. X-rays may be taken, but history gives it away.

Osgood–Schlatter disease is osteochondritis of the tibial tubercle. It is often bilateral and usually manifests in boys 10 to 15 years old with pain, swelling, and tenderness in the knee. Treat with rest, activity restriction, and nonsteroidal antiinflammatory drugs (NSAIDs). The disease usually resolves on its own.

Scoliosis usually affects prepubertal girls and is idiopathic. Ask the patient to touch her toes, and look at the spine. With scoliosis, a lateral curvature is seen. X-rays are confirmatory and can be used to follow progression. Treat with a brace unless the deformity is severe (with rapid progression and/or respiratory compromise); then consider surgery.

Table 22-2. PEDIATRIC HIP PROBLEMS

Name	Age	Epidemiology	Symptoms and Signs	Treatment
CHD	At birth	Female, first-born, breech delivery	Barlow's and Ortolani's signs	Harness
LCP disease	4–10 y	Male, short with delayed bone age	Knee, thigh, and groin pain, limp	Orthoses
SCFE	9–13 y	Overweight, male, adolescent	Knee, thigh, and groin pain, limp	Surgical pinning

CHD, congenital hip dysplasia, LCP, Legg–Calvé–Perthes disease, SCFE, slipped capital femoral epiphysis.

23 NEUROSURGERY

Cranium and Skull

Whenever **intracranial hemorrhage** is suspected, order a computed tomographic (CT) head scan *without* contrast. Blood shows up as white and can cause a midline shift.

SUBDURAL HEMATOMA

Subdural hematoma (Fig. 23-1) is due to bleeding from veins that bridge the cortex and dural sinuses. The hematoma is *crescent-shaped*; it is common in alcoholics and after head trauma. Patients can present immediately after trauma or up to 1 to 2 months later. If the Step 2 question includes a history of head trauma, always consider the diagnosis of a subdural hematoma. Treat with surgical evacuation.

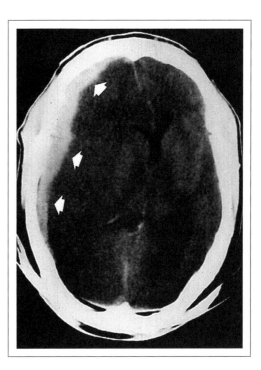

FIGURE 23-1. Subdural hematoma (*arrows*).

EPIDURAL HEMATOMA

Epidural hematoma is due to bleeding from meningeal arteries (classically, the middle meningeal artery). The hematoma is *lenticular-shaped* (i.e., lens or biconvex-shaped, Fig. 23-2). It is almost always associated with a skull fracture (classically, fracture of the temporal bone). More than 50% of patients have an ipsilateral blown pupil (see later). The classic history is a head trauma with loss of consciousness, followed by a lucid interval of minutes to hours, then neurologic deterioration. Treat with surgical evacuation.

SUBARACHNOID HEMORRHAGE

Subarachnoid hemorrhage is due to blood between the arachnoid and the pia mater. The most common cause is trauma, followed by ruptured berry aneurysms. Blood is seen in ventricles and around (but not in) the brain or brainstem. Patients classically present with the "worst headache of my life," although many die before they reach the hospital or may be unconscious. Awake patients have signs of meningitis (positive Kernig's and Brudzinski's signs). Remember the association between polycystic kidney disease and berry aneurysms. Although CT without contrast is always the test of choice, a lumbar tap shows *grossly bloody cerebrospinal fluid.*

Treat with support, anticonvulsants, and observation. In the absence of a trauma history, do a cerebral angiogram or MR angiogram to look for aneurysms and arteriovenous malformations, which can often be treated with open or endovascular surgery.

INTRACEREBRAL HEMORRHAGE

Intracerebral hemorrhage describes bleeding into the brain parenchyma. The most common cause is *hypertension;* other causes include arteriovenous malformations, coagulopathies, tumor, and trauma. Two thirds of hypertensive hemorrhages occur in the basal ganglia. Patients often present with coma; if awake, they have contralateral hemiplegia and hemisensory deficits. On CT, blood (white) is seen in brain parenchyma and

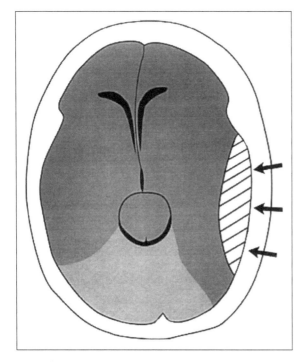

FIGURE 23-2. Biconvex epidural hematoma overlies the left temporal lobe (*arrows*).

sometimes extends into the ventricles. Surgery is reserved for large bleeds that are accessible (particularly cerebellar bleeds).

After a history of trauma, a **dilated, unreactive (blown) pupil on only one side** most likely represents impingement of the ipsilateral third cranial nerve and impending uncal herniation due to increased intracranial pressure. Of the different intracranial bleeds, this is most commonly seen with epidural hematomas. Do *not* do a lumbar tap on any patient with a blown pupil; you might precipitate uncal herniation and death. First do a noncontrast CT (second choice is magnetic resonance imaging [MRI]).

SKULL FRACTURES

Basilar skull fracture is diagnosed most confidently with CT of the head but is often suspected clinically based on one or more of four classic signs:

- **Battle's sign:** Postauricular ecchymosis
- **Cerebrospinal fluid otorrhea OR rhinorrhea:** Clear fluid from the ears or nose
- **Hemotympanum:** Blood behind the eardrum
- **Raccoon eyes:** Periorbital ecchymosis

IMPORTANT POINTS

1 Skull fractures of the calvarium are evaluated with noncontrast CT scan. Surgical indications are contamination (cleaning and debridement), impingement on brain parenchyma, or open fracture with cerebrospinal fluid leak. Otherwise, fractures may be observed and generally heal on their own.

2 Head trauma also may cause cerebral contusion or shear injury of the brain parenchyma, which might or might not show up on a CT scan, but both can cause temporary or permanent neurologic deficits.

INCREASED INTRACRANIAL PRESSURE

Normal intracranial pressure is 5 to 15 mm Hg. Increased pressure (intracranial hypertension) is suggested by bilaterally dilated and fixed pupils. Other symptoms include headache, papilledema, nausea and vomiting, and mental status changes. Look also for the classic Cushing's triad (increasing blood pressure, bradycardia, respiratory irregularity).

The first step is to put the patient in reverse Trendelenburg (head up) and intubate. Once intubated, the patient should be hyperventilated to rapidly lower the intracranial pressure. This approach decreases intracranial blood volume by causing cerebral vasoconstriction. If the decrease in pressure is not sufficient, mannitol diuresis can be tried to lessen cerebral edema. Furosemide is also used but is less effective. Barbiturate coma and decompressive craniotomy (bur holes) are last-ditch measures.

Cerebral perfusion pressure equals blood pressure minus intracranial pressure. In other words, do *not* treat hypertension initially in a patient with increased intracranial pressure; hypertension is the body's way of trying to increase cerebral perfusion.

Never do a lumbar tap on any patient with signs of increased intracranial pressure until a CT scan is done first. If the CT is negative, you can proceed to a tap, if one is needed or indicated.

HYDROCEPHALUS

In children, look for increasing head circumference, increased intracranial pressure, bulging fontanel, scalp vein engorgement, and paralysis of upward gaze. The most common causes include congenital malformations, tumors, and inflammation (hemorrhage, meningitis). Treat the underlying cause, if possible; otherwise, a surgical shunt is created to decompress the ventricles.

Spinal Cord

TRAUMA

Spinal cord trauma often manifests with spinal shock (loss of reflexes, loss of motor function, and hypotension). Get standard trauma x-rays (cervical spine, chest, pelvis) as well as additional spine x-rays and CT scans based on physical exam. MRI is the best noninvasive method to assess cord injury and compression. Give corticosteroids for spinal cord injuries (proved to improve outcome). Surgery is done for incomplete neurologic injury (some residual function is maintained) in the presence of correctable external compression (e.g., spine subluxation, bone chip).

COMPRESSION

Subacute spinal cord compression (vs. acute compression in trauma) is often due to metastatic cancer but also may be due to a primary neoplasm or subdural or epidural abscess or hematoma (especially after lumbar tap or after epidural or spinal anesthesia in a patient with a bleeding disorder or on anticoagulation). Patients present with local spinal pain (especially with bone metastases) and neurologic deficits below the lesion (hyperreflexia, positive Babinski's, weakness, sensory loss).

The first steps in the emergency department are to get a confirmatory CT or MRI, then give high-dose corticosteroids. Radiotherapy can be used for metastases from a known primary tumor that is radiosensitive. Alternatively, surgical decompression may be done.

◆ Prognosis is most closely related to pretreatment function; the longer you wait to treat, the worse the prognosis.

◆ For hematoma or for subdural or epidural abscess (seen especially in diabetic patients and usually due to *Staphylococcus aureus*), surgery is indicated for decompression and drainage.

SYRINGOMYELIA

Syringomyelia is a central pathologic cavitation of the spinal cord, usually in the cervical or upper thoracic region. Syringomyelia is sometimes idiopathic but classically occurs with Arnold–Chiari malformation or due to a tumor or past trauma. The classic presentation is a bilateral loss of pain and temperature sensation below the lesion in the distribution of a cape due to involvement of the lateral spinothalamic tracts. The cavitation in the cord gradually widens to involve other tracts, causing motor and sensory deficits. MRI is the imaging study of choice to confirm the diagnosis and exclude underlying Chiari malformation and tumor, and treatment is surgical (e.g., creation of a shunt, decompression of the skull base with a Chiari malformation, treat any causative tumor).

NEURAL TUBE DEFECTS

A triangular patch of hair over the lumbar spine indicates spina bifida occulta. Serious defects are obvious and occur most commonly in the lumbosacral region. Meningocele is defined as meninges outside the spinal canal; myelomenigocele is defined as central nervous system tissue plus meninges outside the spinal canal. Most importantly, giving folate to potential mothers reduces the incidence of neural tube defects. MRI is used to assess the extent of malformation if it is not obvious. No imaging or treatment is needed for spina bifida occulta, which occurs in up to 10% of the population.

24 EAR, NOSE, AND THROAT

Ears

HEARING LOSS

The most common cause is aging (presbycusis). A hearing aid can be used, if needed. History may suggest other causes:

- Exposure to prolonged or intense loud noise
- **Bacterial meningitis** is the most common cause of acquired hearing loss in children. Follow all children with hearing testing after a bout of meningitis.
- **Congenital TORCH infection** (toxoplasmosis, other agents, rubella, cytomegalovirus, herpes simplex virus)
- **Diabetes mellitus**
- **Drugs** (aminoglycosides, aspirin, quinine, loop diuretics, cisplatin)
- Hypothyroidism
- Labyrinthitis (may be viral or can follow or extend from meningitis or otitis media)
- Ménière's disease: accompanied by severe vertigo, tinnitus, nausea and vomiting; treated with anticholinergics, antihistamines (meclizine), or surgery (if refractory)
- Multiple sclerosis
- **Otosclerosis** is the most common cause of progressive conductive hearing loss in adults (vs. presbycusis, the most common cause of sensorineural hearing loss in adults). Otic bones become fixed together and impede hearing. Treat with hearing aid or surgery.
- Pseudotumor cerebri
- Sarcoidosis
- **Tumor** (usually acoustic neuroma, Fig. 24-1)

SUDDEN DEAFNESS

Sudden deafness develops over a few hours. It is most often due to a viral cause (endolymphatic labyrinthitis from mumps, measles, influenza, chickenpox, adenovirus). Hearing usually returns within 2 weeks, but loss may be permanent. No treatment has proved effective; empiric steroids often are used.

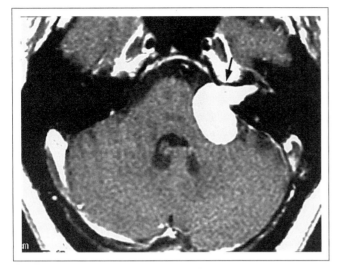

FIGURE 24-1. Magnetic resonance image reveals an acoustic neuroma (*arrow*).

VERTIGO

Vertigo may be due to the same eighth cranial nerve lesions that cause hearing loss (Ménière's disease, tumor, infection, multiple sclerosis). Another common cause is benign positional/paroxysmal vertigo, which is induced by certain head positions and may be accompanied by nystagmus without associated hearing loss. The condition often resolves spontaneously; treatment is not necessary.

OTITIS EXTERNA (SWIMMER'S EAR)

Otitis externa is most commonly due to *Pseudomonas aeruginosa*. Manipulation of the auricle produces pain; the skin of the auditory canal is erythematous and swollen. Patients might have foul-smelling discharge and conductive hearing loss. Treat with topical antibiotics (neomycin, polymyxin B). Steroids can reduce swelling.

OTITIS MEDIA

Otitis media is most commonly due to *Streptococcus pneumoniae*, *Haemophilus influenzae*, and *Moraxella catarrhalis*. Manipulation of the auricle produces no pain. Patients have earache, fever, erythematous and bulging tympanic membrane (light reflex and landmarks are difficult to see), and nausea and vomiting. Complications include tympanic membrane perforation (bloody or purulent discharge), mastoiditis (fluctuation and inflammation over the mastoid process 2 weeks after otitis), labyrinthitis, palsies of cranial nerves VII and VIII, meningitis, cerebral abscess, lateral sinus thrombosis, and chronic otitis media (permanent perforation of the tympanic membrane). Patients can get cholesteatomas with marginal perforations.

Treat cholesteatomas with surgical excision. Treat otitis with antibiotics to avoid complications (e.g., amoxicillin, second-generation cephalosporins such as cefuroxime, trimethoprim–sulfamethoxazole).

Recurrent otitis media is a common pediatric clinical problem (as well as prolonged secretory otitis, a result of incompletely resolved otitis) and can cause hearing loss with resultant developmental problems (speech, cognitive functions). Treatment consists of prophylactic antibiotics or tympanostomy tubes. Adenoidectomy is controversial but is thought to help in some cases by preventing blockage of the eustachian tubes.

Infectious myringitis (tympanic membrane inflammation) is caused by *Mycoplasma* spp., *Streptococcus pneumoniae*, or viruses. Otoscopy reveals vesicles on the tympanic membrane. Treat like otitis media (with antibiotics).

Nose and Sinuses

NOSEBLEED

The most common cause of nosebleed in children is nose-picking (trauma), but watch out for local tumor, leukemia, and other causes of thrombocytopenia (idiopathic thrombocytopenic purpura, hemolytic uremic syndrome). **Nasopharyngeal angiofibroma** should be suspected in adolescent boys with recurrent nosebleeds and/or obstruction but no history of trauma or blood dyscrasias. Leukemia **can** result in pancytopenia; look for associated fever and anemia.

RHINITIS

Rhinitis is edematous, vasodilated nasal mucosa and turbinates with clear nasal discharge. Causes:

Allergic (hay fever). Associated with seasonal flare-ups, boggy and bluish turbinates, early onset (<20 years old), nasal polyps, sneezing, pruritis, conjunctivitis, wheezing, asthma, eczema, positive family history, eosinophils in nasal mucus, and elevated immunoglobulin E (IgE). Skin tests might identify an allergen. Treat with avoidance when the antigen (e.g., pollen) is known; treat with antihistamines, cromolyn, and/or steroids for severe symptoms. Desensitization is also an option.

Bacterial infection. From *Streptococcus* A, *Pneumococcus*, or *Staphylococcus* spp. Do streptococcal throat culture, and treat with antibiotics if appropriate (sore throat, fever, tonsillar exudate).

Viral (common cold). From rhinovirus (most common), influenza, parainfluenza, coxsackievirus, adenovirus, respiratory syncytial virus, coronavirus, echovirus. Treatment is symptomatic; vasoconstrictors such as phenylephrine are used for short-term treatment but can cause rebound congestion.

SINUSITIS

Sinusitis is often caused by *S. pneumoniae, H. influenzae,* and other streptococci or staphylococci. Look for tenderness over affected sinus, headache, and purulent nasal discharge (yellow or green). X-ray or computed tomography (CT) shows opacification of the sinus (Fig. 24-2); CT is preferred to evaluate chronic sinusitis or suspected extension of infection outside the sinus (suggested by high fever and chills).

Treat with antibiotics (amoxicillin or cephalosporin for 2 weeks, up to 6 weeks for chronic cases). Operative intervention may be used for resistant cases (drainage procedure, sinus obliteration) or recurrent sinusitis from congenital defect (e.g., deviated nasal septum). Remember that the frontal sinuses are not well developed until after the age of 10 years.

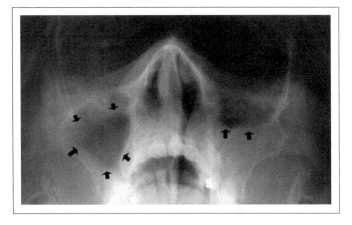

FIGURE 24-2. X-ray of sinusitis with mucosal thickening of the right maxillary sinus and an air-fluid level in the left maxillary sinus (*arrows*).

 After significant nasal bone fracture (which can be seen on x-ray or CT), watch for a septal hematoma, which must be removed to prevent pressure-induced septal necrosis.

Face, Neck, and Throat

BELL'S PALSY

Bell's palsy is the most common cause of facial paralysis. It has a sudden unilateral onset, usually after an upper respiratory infection. The most common identifiable cause is reactivation of a latent **herpes simplex I** virus infection in most cases. Nerve inflammation results in symptoms and signs of a *lower* motor neuron nerve lesion. Patients might have hyperacusis; everything sounds loud because the stapedius muscle in the ear is paralyzed. In severe cases, patients may be unable to close the affected eye; use saline drops to protect the eye.

Roughly 75% of patients recover completely without treatment, typically within 3 to 12 weeks. However, some have permanent symptoms, so antiherpes agents (e.g., valacyclovir, acyclovir) can be given to reduce the risk.

Other causes of unilateral facial paralysis:

◆ **Fracture (temporal bone):** Patients might have Battle's sign and/or bleeding from the ear.

◆ **Herpes zoster (Ramsay Hunt syndrome):** Eighth cranial nerve is commonly involved also. Look for vesicles on pinna and inside ear; encephalitis and meningitis may be present.

◆ **Lyme disease:** Can cause unilateral or bilateral facial nerve palsy.

◆ Meningitis

◆ Middle ear and mastoid infections

◆ **Tumor:** Especially in the cerebellopontine angle (acoustic neuroma [see Fig. 24-1]; consider neurofibromatosis) or glomus jugulare.

Get magnetic resonance imaging (MRI) scan (or CT scan as second choice) of the head to evaluate if the cause is not apparent or seems suspicious (especially if additional neurologic signs are present) after history and/or physical exam.

NECK MASS

In children, 75% of neck masses are benign. In patients older than 40 years, 75% are malignant. MRI and/or CT with contrast help evaluate.

Causes seen typically in children:

◆ **Branchial cleft cysts:** Lateral; often become infected.

◆ **Cystic hygroma:** A type of lymphangioma classically seen in the setting of Turner's syndrome. Treat with surgical resection.

◆ **Cervical lymphadenitis:** From streptococcal pharyngitis, Epstein–Barr virus (common in adolescents and adults in their 20s), cat-scratch disease, *Mycobacterium* spp. (scrofula). Can progress to an abscess (typically due to strep infection; Fig. 24-3), which often requires surgical drainage.

◆ **Thyroglossal duct cysts:** Midline; elevates with tongue protrusion.

In adults, think malignancy first when presented with a neck mass. It can be metastatic adenopathy from a mucosa-based malignancy (e.g., oral cavity, pharynx, or larynx), a lymphoma, or the tumor itself (e.g., thyroid malignancy). In kids, if the mass is malignant, the cause is likely leukemia or lymphoma or sometimes a sarcoma.

Work-up of unknown cancer in the neck in adults includes *random* biopsy of the nasopharynx, palatine tonsils, and base of the tongue as well as laryngoscopy, bronchoscopy,

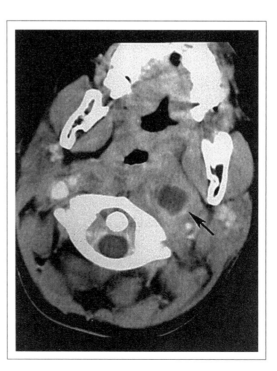

FIGURE 24-3. Computed tomographic scan reveals that cervical lymphadenitis has progressed to an abscess (*arrow*).

and esophagoscopy (with biopsies of any suspicious lesions)—the so-called triple endoscopy with triple biopsy. Positron emission tomography (PET) scan can also help identify primary malignancy in some cases.

PAROTID SWELLING

The classic but now rare cause is mumps. The best treatment for mumps and the complication of infertility is prevention through immunization. Parotid swelling also may be due to neoplasm (pleomorphic adenoma is the most common and is benign), alcoholism, Sjögren's syndrome, sialolithiasis (more common in the submandibular gland and is associated with significant pain), lymphadenopathy (there are lymph nodes in the parotid gland), and sarcoidosis.

VASCULAR SURGERY

Atherosclerosis

ABDOMINAL AORTIC ANEURYSM

Look for a pulsatile abdominal mass that can cause abdominal pain. If pain is present, suspect possible rupture of abdominal aortic aneurysm (AAA), although even an unruptured AAA may cause some pain. CT scan with intravenous (IV) contrast usually is used for initial evaluation in symptomatic patients (can use ultrasound in asymptomatic patients with pulsatile mass and suspected AAA). If the AAA is <5 cm and not leaking or ruptured, follow it with serial ultrasound to make sure that it is not enlarging. If the AAA is >5 cm (or you are told that it is rapidly enlarging) or there is evidence of leak or rupture, open or endovascular surgical correction should be done.

A pulsatile abdominal mass + hypotension = emergent laparotomy (means ruptured AAA, which has a mortality rate of roughly 90%). If there is time while the operating room staff is setting up, you can get CT or ultrasound, but don't delay laparotomy if imaging is not immediately available.

CAROTID STENOSIS

The classic presentation is a transient ischemic attack (TIA), especially amaurosis fugax, which is characterized by sudden-onset of transient unilateral blindness, sometimes described as a "shade pulled over one eye." Patients classically have a carotid bruit on exam. If a bruit is heard or the patient has a TIA, ultrasound or computed tomography (CT) angiogram or magnetic resonance (MR) angiogram of the carotid arteries (Fig. 25-1) should be done to determine the degree of stenosis.

◆ If stenosis is >70%, perform carotid endarterectomy (CEA) or endovascular carotid stenting whether the patient is asymptomatic or has had a TIA (or amaurosis fugax) or a small, nondisabling stroke. Clinical trials have shown that CEA provides the best long-term prognosis. Patients should *not* undergo CEA after a stroke that leaves them severely disabled (too late to make a difference), nor should they undergo CEA during a TIA or stroke in evolution. CEA is an *elective*, not emergent, procedure.

◆ If stenosis is <70% and the patient is asymptomatic, do *not* do CEA. Treat with daily aspirin instead. Stenoses in the 50% to 69% range are treated only in the setting of stuttering, recurrent TIAs that fail to respond to maximal medical management.

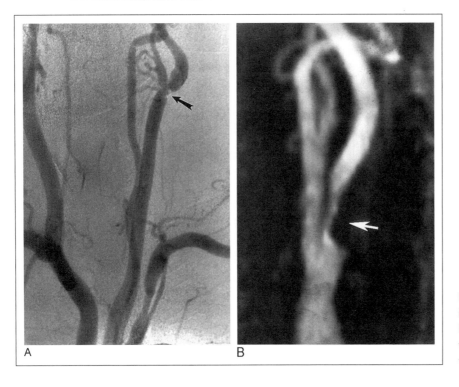

FIGURE 25-1. Atherosclerotic plaque involving the posterolateral wall of the left carotid bulb (*arrows*) on conventional angiogram **(A)** and magnetic resonance angiogram **(B)**.

◆ Carotid stenosis is a generalized marker for atherosclerosis. Virtually all patients have significant coronary artery disease; perioperative myocardial infarction is the most common cause of death in patients undergoing vascular surgery. Be sure to evaluate risk factors for atherosclerosis (cholesterol, hypertension, smoking, diabetes mellitus).

CLAUDICATION

Claudication is pain in the lower extremity brought on by exercise and relieved by rest. Claudication is an indicator of severe atherosclerotic disease and is the peripheral vascular equivalent of angina. Associated physical findings include cyanosis (with dependent rubor), atrophic changes (thickened nails, loss of hair, shiny skin), decreased temperature, and decreased (or absent) distal pulses. The best treatment is conservative: smoking cessation, exercise, and control of cholesterol, diabetes mellitus, and hypertension. β-Blockers theoretically can worsen claudication (due to β_2-receptor blockade) but are often indicated due to coexisting coronary/cardiac disease.

◆ If the patient progresses to rest pain in the forefoot that generally occurs at night and is relieved by hanging the foot over the edge of the bed, or if the patient cannot continue current lifestyle or work obligations, consider a revascularization procedure.

◆ Severe pain in the foot that has a sudden onset without previous history, trauma, or any associated chronic physical findings is generally more serious and might represent an embolus (Fig. 25-2) (look for atrial fibrillation) or compartment syndrome (commonly occurs after revascularization procedures).

◆ Claudication and peripheral vascular disease are generalized markers for atherosclerosis. Check patients for other atherosclerosis risk factors.

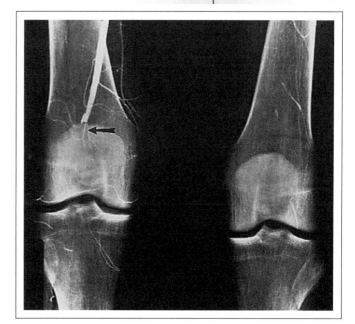

FIGURE 25-2. Right popliteal artery embolus (*arrow*).

LERICHE'S SYNDROME

Leriche's syndrome consists of claudication in the buttocks, buttock atrophy, and impotence in men. It is a classic marker for aortoiliac occlusive disease. Patients usually need an aortoiliac bypass graft or a stent or endograft.

MESENTERIC ISCHEMIA

The classic patient with mesenteric ischemia has a long history of postprandial abdominal pain (due to intestinal angina, similar to cardiac angina after exercising), which causes a fear of food and thus leads to extensive weight loss. This diagnosis is difficult because, like all atherosclerotic disease, it occurs in patients older than 40 years, who might have other disorders that cause the problem (e.g., peptic ulcer disease, pancreatic cancer, stomach cancer). Look for a history of extensive atherosclerosis (previous myocardial infarctions, cerebrovascular accidents, known coronary artery disease, or peripheral vascular disease with several risk factors), possible abdominal bruit, and a lack of jaundice (which would steer you toward pancreatic cancer). CT scan may be normal or show bowel wall thickening and atherosclerosis of the mesenteric arteries. Diagnose with CT, MR, or conventional angiogram and treat surgically with revascularization because of the risks of bowel infarction and malnutrition.

SUBCLAVIAN STEAL SYNDROME

Subclavian steal syndrome is usually caused by left subclavian artery obstruction proximal to the vertebral artery. To get blood to an exercising arm, blood is "stolen" from the vertebrobasilar system; it flows backward into the distal subclavian artery instead of forward into the brainstem. As a result, the patient develops *central nervous system (CNS) symptoms* (syncope, vertigo, confusion, ataxia, dysarthria) and *upper extremity claudication*. Treat with angioplasty or stent placement or, less commonly, surgical bypass.

Miscellaneous

AORTIC DISSECTION

Aortic dissection consists of aortic wall splits and blood dissecting in between layers of the media in the arterial wall. It classically causes a tearing or ripping type of chest pain that can radiate to the back and is generally seen in the setting of *hypertension* (whether essential or induced by cocaine, etc.) or *Marfan's syndrome*. When aortic dissection is suspected clinically, a CT scan of the chest (and possibly abdomen and pelvis) with IV contrast should be ordered.

Treatment depends on the type. A dissection involving the ascending aorta (Stanford type A and DeBakey types I and II) is treated with immediate surgery (5% of patients survive 1 year without surgery). A dissection that spares the ascending aorta (typically beginning just beyond the origin of the left subclavian artery in the isthmus of the aorta or proximal descending thoracic aorta and extending over a variable distance) is managed medically with antihypertensives (>70% of patients survive longer than 1 year without surgery), assuming there are no signs of impending rupture or end organ ischemia from vascular compromise.

An aortic dissection might or might not be associated with an aneurysm (the term "dissecting aneurysm" is not a good one).

CERVICAL RIB

A cervical rib can compromise subclavian vessel blood flow. Patients can develop upper extremity paresthesias, weakness, and cold temperature distention (arterial compromise) or edema or venous distention (venous compromise) *without* central nervous system symptoms. Treat with rib resection.

SUPERFICIAL THROMBOPHLEBITIS

Patients with varicose veins, localized leg pain with superficial cord-like induration or palpable clot, reddish discoloration, and mild fever have superficial thrombophlebitis (*not* deep vein thrombosis), which rarely leads to pulmonary embolism. Patients do not need anticoagulation. Treatment is often thrombectomy under local anesthesia; medical treatment (nonsteroidal antiinflammatory drugs [NSAIDs]) is used if pain is mild or the patient does not want surgery. Pain generally subsides in a few days on its own.

VENOUS INSUFFICIENCY

The term *venous insufficiency* generally refers to the lower extremities. Patients might have a history of deep vein thrombosis; swelling in the extremity with pain, fatigability, and heaviness, which are relieved by elevating the extremity; and/or varicose veins. Skin pigmentation can increase around the ankles, with possible skin breakdown and ulceration (Fig. 25-3). Initial treatment is conservative: elastic compression stockings, elevation with minimal standing, and treatment of any ulcers with cleaning, wet-to-dry dressings, and antibiotics (if cellulitis is present).

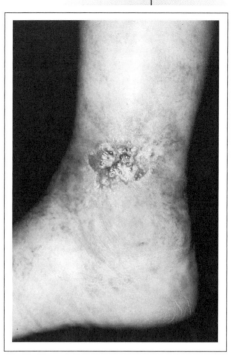

FIGURE 25-3. Venous stasis ulcer.

 After a penetrating trauma in an extremity (or iatrogenic catheter damage), an arteriovenous fistula or pseudoaneurysm can result. Look for bruits over the area or a palpable pulsatile mass. Such fistulas or pseudoaneurysms are generally treated with open or endovascular surgery.

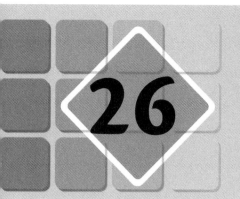

26 UROLOGY

Kidneys

NEPHROLITHIASIS

Signs and symptoms include severe flank pain, which often radiates to the groin and is colicky; hematuria; and stone on abdominal x-ray (85% of stones are radiopaque) or computed tomography (CT) (Fig. 26-1). Symptoms occur once the stone leaves the kidney and gets stuck in or irritates the renal pelvis or ureter, which can cause unilateral urinary obstruction and hydronephrosis and can lead to infection or kidney damage if not treated or if the stone doesn't pass.

◆ **Composition:** 75% of stones are composed of calcium (look for hypercalcemia and hyperparathyroidism; small bowel bypass also increases oxalate absorption and thus calcium stone formation), 15% are struvite or magnesium–ammonium–phosphate stones (think of infection, the cause of staghorn calculi), 7% are uric acid stones (look for history of gout or leukemia), and 2% are cystine stones (think of cystinuria).

◆ **Treat** stones with *lots of hydration*, narcotics for pain, and observation. Most stones pass by themselves. If not, do lithotripsy, uteroscopy with stone retrieval, or open surgery (if needed).

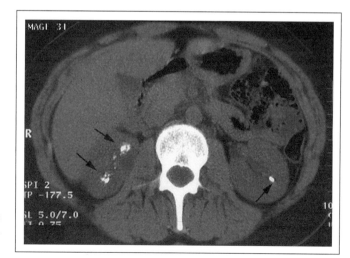

FIGURE 26-1. Unenhanced CT image demonstrates high-density areas in both kidneys (*arrows*), which represent renal calculi.

URINARY OBSTRUCTION

In addition to stones that obstruct the ureter, tumors are another potential cause of urinary obstruction. Either situation can lead to hydronephrosis and permanent damage if not addressed. Surgical intervention is indicated to relieve obstruction, whether via stone retrieval or lithotripsy, cancer surgery, or placement of a percutaneous nephrostomy tube (through the kidney into the renal collecting system to allow urine drainage), ureteral stent, or Foley or suprapubic catheter (for bladder outlet obstruction). In the setting of coexisting infection, prompt intravenous (IV) antibiotics are needed and emergent drainage is indicated.

POTTER'S SYNDROME

Bilateral renal agenesis causes oligohydramnios in utero (the fetus swallows fluid but cannot excrete it), limb deformities, abnormal facies, and hypoplasia of the lungs. It is generally incompatible with life.

RENAL TRANSPLANT

Transplant is an option for patients with end-stage renal disease, unless they have active infections or other life-threatening conditions (e.g., AIDS, malignancy). Lupus and diabetes mellitus are not contraindications to transplant. Living related donors are best (siblings or parents), especially when they are HLA-similar, but cadaveric kidneys are more common because of availability. Before the transplant, perform ABO and lymphocytotoxic (HLA) cross-matching.

◆ A transplanted kidney is placed in the iliac fossa (for easy biopsy access in case of problems as well as for technical reasons); usually the recipient's kidneys are left in place to reduce morbidity.

◆ Unacceptable kidney donors include newborns, persons older than 60 years, history of generalized or intra-abdominal sepsis, history of disease with possible renal involvement (e.g., diabetes mellitus, hypertension, lupus), and history of malignancy.

Types of renal rejection:

◆ **Hyperacute rejection:** Preformed cytotoxic antibodies (considered a type II hypersensitivity reaction) against donor kidney (happens with ABO mismatch as well as other preformed antibodies). Classic description: Surgery is complete, vascular clamps are released, and the kidney quickly turns bluish-black. Treat by removing the kidney.

◆ **Acute rejection:** T cell–mediated rejection that manifests during first several months with fever, oliguria, weight gain, tenderness and enlargement of the graft, hypertension, and/or renal function lab derangement. Treat by increasing corticosteroids, antithymocyte globulin, and/or other immunosuppressants.

◆ **Chronic rejection:** Mediated by T cells or antibodies. Late cause of renal deterioration manifesting with gradual decline in kidney function, proteinuria, and hypertension. Treatment is supportive and not effective, but the graft can last several years before it gives out completely. The patient may receive a new kidney transplant.

◆ **Asymptomatic rejection:** Follow creatinine to assess (more reliable than blood urea nitrogen).

Immunosuppressive medications used in transplant medicine:

◆ Antithymocyte globulin: Antibody against T cells

◆ Azathioprine: Antineoplastic that is cleaved into mercaptopurine and inhibits DNA and RNA synthesis, which decreases B-cell and T-cell production

◆ Cyclosporine: Inhibits interleukin-2 production

◆ OKT3: Antibody to CD3 receptor on T cells

◆ Steroids: Inhibit interleukin-1 production

Cyclosporine causes *nephrotoxicity*, which can be difficult to clinically distinguish from graft rejection. When in doubt, do a percutaneous needle biopsy of the graft, because histologic differentiation is usually possible. Renal ultrasound can also help to distinguish between nephrotoxicity and graft rejection. Practically speaking, if you increase the immunosuppressive dose, acute rejection should decrease, whereas cyclosporine toxicity stays the same or worsens.

Immunosuppression carries the risk of **infection** (with common as well as the strange bugs that infect patients with AIDS) and increased risk of **cancer** (especially lymphomas and epithelial cell cancers).

PROSTATE

Symptoms of **benign prostatic hypertrophy** (BPH) include urinary hesitancy, intermittency, terminal dribbling, decreased size and force of stream, sensation of incomplete emptying, nocturia, urgency, dysuria, and frequency.

◆ BPH can result in urinary retention, urinary tract infections, hydronephrosis, and even kidney damage or failure in severe cases.

◆ Drug therapy is started when the patient becomes symptomatic. Options include α_1-blockade (prazosin, terazosin, doxazosin) and antiandrogens (gonadotropin-releasing hormone analogues, flutamide, finasteride).

◆ Transurethral resection of the prostate (TURP) is used for more advanced cases, especially with repeated urinary tract infections, urinary retention, and hydronephrosis or kidney damage due to reflux. Prostatectomy also may be used but is a more complicated operation.

 With acute urinary retention (pain, palpation of full bladder on abdominal exam, history of BPH, no urination in past 24 hours), the first step is to empty the bladder. If you cannot pass a regular Foley catheter, do a suprapubic tap. Then address the underlying cause (surgery [TURP] is usually recommended for BPH in this setting).

SCROTUM AND TESTES

CRYPTORCHIDISM

Cryptorchidism is arrest of descent of the testicle(s) somewhere between the renal area and the scrotum. The more premature the infant, the greater the likelihood of cryptorchidism. Many arrested testes eventually descend on their own within the first year. After 1 year, surgical intervention (orchiopexy) is warranted to attempt to preserve fertility as well as facilitate future testicular exams (because of increased cancer risk). Cryptorchidism is a major risk factor for testicular cancer (40-fold increased risk), and bringing the testis into the scrotum does *not* alter the increased risk of testicular cancer. The higher the testicle is found (the farther away from the scrotum), the higher the risk of developing testicular cancer and the lower the likelihood of retaining fertility.

HYDROCELE AND VARICOCELE

Hydrocele represents a remnant of the processus vaginalis (remember embryology?) and transilluminates. It generally causes no symptoms and does not require treatment. A **varicocele** is a dilation of the pampiniform venous plexus ("bag of worms," usually on the left), does not transilluminate, *disappears in the supine position*, and occasionally is a cause of male infertility or pain (in which case it is surgically treated).

 The right testicular or ovarian vein drains into the inferior vena cava, whereas the left ovarian or testicular vein drains into the left renal vein.

TESTICULAR CANCER

Testicular cancer usually manifests as a painless mass in a young man (age 20–40 years). The main risk factor is cryptorchidism. Roughly 90% are germ cell tumors, the most common being seminoma. Treatment generally consists of orchiectomy and radiation. If disease is widespread, use chemotherapy. Alpha fetoprotein is a tumor marker for yolk sac tumors, whereas human chorionic gonadotropin (hCG) is a marker for choriocarcinoma. Leydig cell tumors can secrete androgens and cause precocious puberty.

 Remember mumps as a cause of orchitis (painful, swollen testis, usually unilateral, in a postpubertal male patient). The best treatment is prophylactic (immunization). Mumps rarely causes sterility because it is usually unilateral.

TESTICULAR TORSION AND EPIDIDYMITIS

Testicular torsion and epididymitis are compared in Table 26-1.

Table 26-1. DIFFERENTIAL DIAGNOSIS OF TESTICULAR TORSION AND EPIDIDYMITIS

Feature	Testicular Torsion	Epididymitis
Age (y)	<30 (usually prepubertal)	>30
Appearance	Testes may be elevated into the inguinal canal; swelling	Swollen testis, overlying erythema, positive urinalysis, urethral discharge, urethritis, prostatitis
Prehn's sign	Pain stays the same or worsens with testicular elevation	*Pain decreases with testicular elevation*
Treatment	*Immediate* surgery to salvage testis; orchiopexy of *both* testes	Antibiotics*

*In men <40 years, epididymitis is commonly due to a sexually transmitted disease (chlamydial infection, gonorrhea); treat accordingly. In men >40, it is commonly due to urinary tract infection bugs; treat with trimethoprim–sulfamethoxazole or ciprofloxacin.

Penis

IMPOTENCE

Impotence is most commonly caused by vascular or neurologic problems. Medications are also a common culprit (especially antihypertensives and antidepressants). Diabetes mellitus may be a vascular (increased atherosclerosis) or neurogenic cause of impotence. Remember "Point and Shoot": parasympathetics mediate erection; sympathetics mediate ejaculation. Patients undergoing dialysis also are commonly impotent.

The history often gives you a clue if the cause of impotence is *psychogenic*. Look for a normal pattern of nocturnal erections, selective dysfunction (a patient who has normal erections when masturbating but not with his wife), and stress, anxiety, or fear when the cause is psychological.

PENILE ANOMALIES

Hypospadias occurs when the urethra opens on the ventral side (undersurface when flaccid) of the penis; **epispadias,** when the urethra opens on the dorsal side (top) of the penis (associated with extrophy of the bladder). Treat both surgically. **Chordee** is a bending of the penis most evident during erection that can occur in either condition but is classic in hypospadias (when it is a downward bending).

Miscellaneous

TRAUMA

In patients with trauma, especially when pelvic fractures are present, look for signs of urethral injury (high-riding, ballottable prostate, blood at the urethral meatus, ecchymosis) *before* trying to pass a Foley catheter. If any of these signs are present or pelvic fractures are severe, do *not* try to pass a Foley catheter until you have gotten a retrograde urethrogram to rule out urethral injury. Urethral injury is a contraindication to a Foley catheter.

HEMATURIA

Worry about cancer on boards (kidney > bladder > ureteral > urethral) when hematuria is painless. Hematuria is classically due to urolithiasis when painful. Get a CT scan without contrast for suspected urinary tract stones, and get a CT with and without contrast for painless hematuria to assess for malignancy (i.e., CT urogram) or with trauma. If imaging work-up is negative, endoscopy via a urethral approach is generally indicated in adults. If red blood cell casts are present, think glomerulonephritis. In reproductive-age women, watch for false positives from menstrual bleeding due to improper specimen collection.

27 EMERGENCY MEDICINE

Burns

Burns may be thermal, chemical, or electrical. Initial management of all burns includes *lots of intravenous (IV) fluids* (use lactated Ringer's solution, or use normal saline if Ringer's solution is not a choice), removal of all clothes and other smoldering items on the body, copious irrigation of chemical burns, and, of course, the ABCs (airway, breathing, circulation). You should have a very low threshold for intubation; use 100% oxygen until significant carboxyhemoglobin from carbon monoxide inhalation is ruled out.

CHEMICAL BURNS

Alkali burns are worse than acidic burns, because alkali penetrates more deeply. Treat all chemical burns with copious irrigation from the nearest source (e.g., tap water).

ELECTRICAL BURNS

With electrical burns, most of the destruction is internal and can lead to myoglobinuria, acidosis, and renal failure. Use *lots* of IV fluids to prevent such complications. The immediate, life-threatening risk with electricity exposure or burns (including lightning and putting a finger in an electrical outlet) is cardiac arrhythmias. Get an electrocardiogram (EKG).

THERMAL BURNS

Severity classification:

◆ **First-degree** burns involve epidermis only (painful, dry, red areas with *no* blisters). Keep clean.

◆ **Second-degree** burns involve epidermis and some dermis (painful and swollen, with blisters and open, weeping surfaces). Remove blisters; apply antibiotic ointment (e.g., silver nitrate, silver sulfadiazine, neomycin) and dressing.

◆ **Third-degree** burns involve all layers of the skin, including nerve endings (*painless*, dry, and charred). Surgical excision of eschar and skin grafting are required. Watch for compartment syndrome; treat with escharotomy.

INFECTION

Burned skin is much more prone to infection, usually by *Staphylococcus aureus* or *Pseudomonas* spp. (with *Pseudomonas* infection, look for a fruity smell and/or blue-green color). Prophylactic antibiotics are given topically only. Give a tetanus booster to all burn patients unless they received it recently (within the past 5 years).

Body Temperature

HYPOTHERMIA

Hypothermia is defined as body temperature <95° F (35° C), usually accompanied by mental status changes and generalized neurologic deficits. If the patient is conscious, use slow rewarming with blankets. If the patient is unconscious, consider immersion in a tub of warm water. It is most important to monitor the EKG for arrhythmias, which are common with hypothermia. You also may see the classic J wave, a small, positive deflection following the QRS complex. Also monitor electrolytes, renal function, and acid–base status.

- With frostnip (cold, painful areas of skin; mild) and frostbite (cold, anesthetic areas of skin; more severe), treat with warming of affected areas using warm water (not scalding hot) and generalized warming (e.g., blankets).

- A patient is not considered dead until he or she is *warm and dead*; in other words, do *not* give up resuscitation efforts until the patient has been warmed.

HYPERTHERMIA

Hyperthermia may be due to heat stroke. Look for a history of heat exposure and high temperature (>104° F). Treat with immediate cooling (wet blankets, ice, cold water). The immediate threats to life are convulsions (which should be treated with diazepam) and cardiovascular collapse. Rule out infection and other classic culprits:

- **Malignant hyperthermia:** Look for succinylcholine or halothane exposure. Treat with **dantrolene**.

- **Neuroleptic malignant syndrome:** Caused by taking an antipsychotic. First, stop the medication. Second, treat with support (especially lots of IV fluids to prevent renal shutdown from rhabdomyolysis), and consider giving dantrolene.

- **Drug fever:** Idiosyncratic reaction to a medication that usually was started within the past week.

Other Emergencies

NEAR DROWNING

Fresh water is classically thought to be worse than sea water (though many dispute this claim), because fresh water, if aspirated, can cause hypervolemia, electrolyte disturbances, and hemolysis. Intubate such patients if they are unconscious, and monitor arterial blood gases if they are conscious. Patients who drown in cold water often do better than those who drown in warm water because of decreased metabolic needs. Death usually results from hypoxia and/or cardiac arrest.

CHOKING

Leave choking patients alone if they are speaking, coughing, or breathing. If they stop doing all three, perform the Heimlich maneuver.

TOOTH AVULSION

Put the tooth back in place with no cleaning (or rinse it only in saline), and stabilize as soon as possible. The sooner this procedure is done, the better the prognosis for salvage of the tooth.

28 PEDIATRICS

Milestones

There are a million milestones during an infant's development, but concentrate on the common ones listed in Table 28-1. Rough average ages are given; the exact age is not as important as the overall pattern when you are looking for dysfunctional development. When in doubt, use a formal developmental test.

Screening and Preventive Care

Screening and preventive care are important parts of well-baby exams that also can help answer parents' questions. For example, a mother complains that her 4-year-old child sleeps 11 hours every night (this is normal). The answer to the question, "What should you do next?" may be to get an objective hearing exam, which is a routine screening procedure in a 4-year-old child. Height, weight, blood pressure, developmental and behavioral assessment, history and physical exam, and anticipatory guidance (counseling and discussion about age-appropriate concerns) should be done at every visit.

ANEMIA

Routine screening (hemoglobin and hematocrit) is somewhat controversial; traditionally screening was done once in the first year (8–12 months), once between ages 4 and 6 years, and once during adolescence. If any risk factors for iron deficiency are present during infancy (prematurity, low birth weight, ingestion of cow's milk before 12 months, low dietary intake, low socioeconomic status), definitely screen the hemoglobin and hematocrit if given the option. Give all infants prophylactic iron supplements (already in formula); start full-term infants at 4 to 6 months and preterm infants at 2 months.

ANTICIPATORY GUIDANCE
Tell parents to

◆ Keep the water heater <110° F to 120° F.
◆ Use car restraints.
◆ Put baby to sleep on the side or back to help prevent sudden infant death syndrome (most common cause of death in children aged 1–12 months).

Table 28-1. DEVELOPMENTAL MILESTONES

Milestone	Age*
Social smile	1–2 mo
Cooing	2–4 mo
While prone, lifts head up 90°	3–4 mo
Rolls front to back	4–5 mo
Voluntary grasp (no release)	5 mo
Stranger anxiety	6–9 mo
Sits with no support	7 mo
Pulls to stand	9 mo
Plays pat-a-cake	9–10 mo
First words	9–12 mo
Imitates others' sounds	9–12 mo
Voluntary grasp with voluntary release	10 mo
Waves "bye-bye"	10 mo
Separation anxiety	12–15 mo
Walks without help	13 mo
Can build tower of 2 cubes	13–15 mo
Good use of cup and spoon	15–18 mo
Understands 1-step commands (no gesture)	15 mo
Can build tower of 6 cubes	2 y
Runs well	2 y
Ties shoelaces	5 y

*When the development of a premature infant is assessed, the infant's age is reduced in the first 2 years. For example, subtract 3 months from the chronologic age of an infant born prematurely after 6 months' gestation; therefore, the infant is expected to perform at the 6-month-old interval at the age of 9 months.

◆ Do not use infant walkers (which cause injuries).

◆ Watch out for small objects (risk of aspiration).

◆ Do not give cow's milk before 1 year of age.

◆ Introduce solid foods gradually, starting at 6 months.

◆ Supervise children in a bathtub or swimming pool.

APGAR SCORE

The Apgar score is commonly done at 1 and 5 minutes after birth. Do *not* wait until the 1-minute mark to evaluate the newborn; you may have to suction or intubate the infant 3 seconds after delivery. The Apgar score includes five categories with a maximum score of 2 points per category and a total maximum of 10 points.

◆ **Heart rate:** 0 = absent; 1 = rate <100 bpm; 2 = rate >100 bpm

◆ **Respiratory effort:** 0 = none; 1 = slow, weak cry; 2 = good, strong cry

◆ **Muscle tone:** 0 = limp; 1 = some flexion of extremities; 2 = active motion

◆ **Reflex irritability** (response to stimulation of sole of foot or catheter put in nose): 0 = none; 1 = grimace; 2 = grimace and strong cry, cough, or sneeze

◆ **Color:** 0 = pale, blue; 1 = body pink and extremities blue; 2 = completely pink

Continue to score every 5 minutes until the infant reaches a score of 7 or more (while resuscitating).

FLUORIDE

Start supplementation in the first few years of life if water is inadequately fluoridated (rare) or if the patient is fed exclusively from a premixed, ready-to-eat formula (non-fluoridated water is used in such products). Most children need no supplementation.

HEARING AND VISION

Hearing and vision should be measured objectively once by or at 4 years old. Measure every few years until adulthood, more often if history dictates.

After a bout of meningitis, all children should be screened objectively for hearing loss (the most common neurologic complication of meningitis). Hearing screening is also important after congenital TORCH infections, measles and mumps, and chronic middle ear effusions and otitis media.

Check the red reflex at birth and routinely thereafter to detect congenital cataracts (usually due to congenital rubella, other TORCH infections, or galactosemia) or retinoblastoma (look for leukocoria).

It is normal for children to have occasional ocular misalignment (strabismus) until 3 months; after that, strabismus should be evaluated further to prevent possible blindness in the affected eye.

HEIGHT, WEIGHT, AND HEAD CIRCUMFERENCE

Head circumference should be measured routinely in the first 2 years, height and weight routinely until adulthood. All are markers of general well-being. The pattern of growth along plotted growth curves (which you need to know how to read) tells you more than any raw number. If a patient has always been low or high compared with peers, this pattern is generally benign. Parents commonly bring in a child with delayed physical growth or delayed puberty, and you must know when to reassure and follow-up and when to do further testing and questioning. If a patient goes from a normal curve to an abnormal curve, this is a much more worrisome pattern.

- **Failure to thrive** (<5th percentile for age) is most commonly due to psychosocial or functional problems. Watch for child abuse. Organic causes usually have specific clues to trigger your suspicion.
- **Obesity** is usually due to overeating; less than 5% of cases are due to organic causes (Cushing's or Prader–Willi syndrome).
- Increased **head circumference** can mean hydrocephalus or tumor, whereas decreased head circumference can mean microcephaly (e.g., from congenital TORCH infection [toxoplasmosis, other agents, rubella, cytomegalovirus, herpes simplex virus]).

IMMUNIZATIONS

When to give normal immunizations (Table 28-2) is constantly being updated, so the administration schedule for common vaccines is often given, but of course, this material is still fair game on Step 2. High yield: special patient populations (pneumococcal vaccine for patients with sickle cell disease or splenectomy) and vaccine contraindications (no measles, mumps, and rubella or influenza vaccine for egg-allergic patients, no live vaccines to pregnant women or immunocompromised patients) (Table 28-3).

Table 28-2. PEDIATRIC VACCINE RECOMMENDATIONS

Vaccine	When to Give in Routine Cases
Hepatitis B	0–1, 1–4, and 6–18 months (3 doses)
Diphtheria, tetanus, pertussis (DTP)	2, 4, 6, 15–18 months and 4–6 years (5 doses) plus tetanus booster (Td) every 10 years
Haemophilus influenzae type b	2, 4, 6, 12–15 months (4 doses)
Pneumococcus spp. (heptavalent)	2, 4, 6, 12–15 months (4 doses)
Polio, inactivated (IPV)	2, 4, 6–18 months and 4–6 years (4 doses)
Measles, mumps, rubella (MMR)	12–15 months and 4–6 years (2 doses)
Hepatitis A	12–18 months, second dose 6 months after first (2 doses)
Varicella	12–18 months (1 dose)
Meningococcal	11–12 years old (or at high school entry)

Table 28-3. WHO SHOULD RECEIVE PEDIATRIC VACCINATIONS

Vaccine	Indications and Contraindications
Hepatitis B	Give first dose at birth with hepatitis B immune globulin if mother has active hepatitis B
Influenza	Give to children >6 months with immunodeficiency, heart or lung disease (including asthma), or on chronic aspirin therapy (to prevent Reye's syndrome)
Measles, mumps, rubella (MMR)	Avoid in children with anaphylactic reaction to eggs or neomycin; avoid in those with immunodeficiency other than HIV/AIDS
Meningococcal	Give to children >2 years with terminal complement deficiencies or functional or anatomic asplenia
Pneumococcus spp.	Give to children >2 years who have not been vaccinated if they have immunodeficiency of any kind, are asplenic, or lack splenic function (sickle cell disease)
Polio, inactivated (IPV)	Avoid in children with anaphylaxis to neomycin or streptomycin
Varicella	Avoid in children with immunodeficiency or anaphylaxis to neomycin

LEAD

Initial screen at 12 months if risk is low, at 6 months if risk is high (residence in old building, paint chip eater, home near battery-recycling plant). Screening asymptomatic children for serum lead level is important because chronic low-level lead exposure can lead to permanent neurologic sequelae. If the level is <10 µg/dL, rescreen at 24 months if risk is low or at 12 months if risk is high. After 2 years old, screen annually only in high-risk patients. If level >10 µg/dL, closer follow-up and intervention are needed. Treat with decreased lead exposure (best and first treatment) as well as as-needed lead chelation therapy (succimer preferred in children, dimercaprol used in more severe cases).

METABOLIC AND CONGENITAL DISORDERS

All states mandate screening for hypothyroidism and phenylketonuria at birth (within the first month). Most mandate screening for galactosemia and sickle cell disease. If any of the screens are positive, the first step is a confirmatory test to make sure that the screen gave you a true positive.

TUBERCULOSIS

Screen for tuberculosis immediately if it is suggested by history; screen annually at any age if risk factors are present (HIV, incarceration). If the only risk factor is living in a high-risk area or immigrant parents, screen once at 4 to 6 years old and once at 11 to 16 years old. If no risk factors are present, do not screen.

URINALYSIS

Universal screening is not recommended. However, do screen for renal disease when a boy younger than 6 years develops a urinary tract infection or a girl younger than 6 years has more than one urinary tract infection or develops pyelonephritis. Get a *voiding cystoure-throgram* and a *renal ultrasound*.

VITAMIN D

Some authorities still recommend that all breast-fed infants receive vitamin D; most recommend it only for high-risk patients (inadequate maternal vitamin D intake, little sunlight exposure and/or dark skin, exclusively breast-fed beyond 6 months of age). Start supplements by 6 months. Formula-fed infants do not require vitamin D supplements, because formula contains vitamin D.

OTHER

Give sexually active adolescents an annual Pap smear and screen for sexually transmitted diseases. The first dental referral should be made around 2 to 3 years old.

 Children have different normal laboratory and physiology values (normal values usually are given): lower blood pressure, higher heart and respiratory rates, and different hemoglobin and hematocrit values (higher at birth, lower throughout childhood). The renal, pulmonary, hepatic, and central nervous systems are still not fully mature and functional at birth.

Preadolescence and Puberty

TANNER STAGES

Stage 1 is preadolescent, stage 5 is adult. Increasing stages are assigned for testicular and penile growth in boys and breast growth in girls; pubic hair development is used for both sexes. Puberty = changes from stage 1 status.

- **Boys:** Average age of puberty is 11.5 years. The first event usually is testicular enlargement.
- **Girls:** Average age of puberty is 10.5 years. The first event usually is breast development.

DELAYED PUBERTY

Delayed puberty is defined as no testicular enlargement in boys by age 14, no breast development or pubic hair in girls by age 13. The usual cause is *constitutional delay*. Parents often have a similar history. In this normal variant, the growth curve lags behind others of the same age but is consistent. Delayed puberty is rarely due to primary testicular failure (Klinefelter's syndrome, cryptorchidism, history of chemotherapy, gonadal dysgenesis) or ovarian failure (Turner's syndrome, gonadal dysgenesis). Other rare causes include hypothalamic or pituitary defects, such as Kallmann's syndrome or tumor.

PRECOCIOUS PUBERTY

Precocious puberty is usually idiopathic, but it can be caused by McCune–Albright syndrome (in girls), ovarian tumors (granulosa, theca cell, or gonadoblastoma), testicular tumors (Leydig cell), central nervous system disease or trauma, adrenal neoplasm, or congenital adrenal hyperplasia (boys only; usually 21-hydroxylase [21-OH] deficiency). Most patients with an uncorrectable idiopathic precocious puberty are given long-acting gonadotropin-releasing hormone agonists (e.g., leuprolide) to suppress progression of puberty and thus prevent premature epiphyseal closure.

Child Abuse

Watch for failure to thrive; multiple fractures, bruises, or injuries in different stages of healing; shaken baby syndrome (subdural hematomas and retinal hemorrhages with no external trauma signs); behavioral, emotional, and interaction problems; sexually transmitted diseases; and multiple personality disorder (sexual abuse). Metaphyseal "bucket handle" and metaphyseal "corner" fractures on x-ray (Fig. 28-1) are essentially pathognomonic of child abuse. Consider abuse whenever the injury does not fit the story.

 Reporting any child abuse suspicion is mandatory. You do not need proof and cannot be sued.

Other Pediatric Disorders

Cavernous hemangioma is first noticed a few days after birth. Lesions increase in size after birth and gradually resolve within the first 2 to 5 years of life in at least 50% of patients. The best treatment in most cases is to do nothing but observe and follow up.

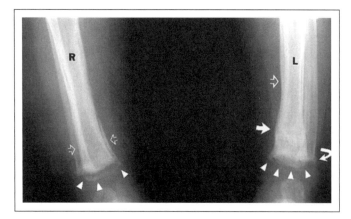

FIGURE 28-1. Metaphyseal bucket handle fractures of the distal tibias (*arrowheads*). Note the periosteal reaction extending proximally along both tibial shafts (*open arrows*). In addition, there is a corner fracture of the left distal fibula (*curved arrow*) and a healing transverse fracture of the left distal tibia (*heavy arrow*).

Caput succedaneum: Diffuse swelling or edema of the scalp that crosses the midline and is benign. **Cephalhematomas** are subperiosteal hemorrhages that are sharply limited by sutures and do not cross the midline. Cephalhematomas are usually benign and self-resolving, but rarely they indicate an underlying skull fracture; get a CT scan to rule it out.

Large anterior fontanel can indicate hypothyroidism, hydrocephalus, rickets, or intra-uterine growth retardation. The anterior fontanel usually is closed by 18 months; delayed closure may be due to the same factors.

IMPORTANT POINTS

1 Reye's syndrome can cause encephalopathy and/or liver failure in children taking aspirin. The syndrome usually develops after influenza or varicella infection. Avoid aspirin in children; use acetaminophen instead.

2 The Moro and palmar grasp reflex should disappear by 6 months.

3 Check the umbilical cord at birth for two arteries, one vein, and the absence of the urachus. If there is only one artery, consider the possibility of congenital renal malformations (get a renal ultrasound to check).

4 Female infants might have a milky-white (and possibly blood-tinged) vaginal discharge in the first week of life. This discharge is physiologic and caused by maternal hormone withdrawal.

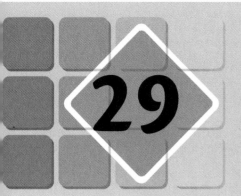

29 PHARMACOLOGY

General Pharmacology

SIDE EFFECTS

Bizarre, unique, and fatal side effects are tested as well as common side effects of common drugs (Table 29-1).

The **side effects of diuretics** are high yield. Thiazides cause hyperglycemia, hyperuricemia, hyperlipidemia, hyponatremia, hypokalemic metabolic alkalosis, and hypovolemia. Thiazides also cause *calcium retention* and, because they are sulfa drugs, should be avoided in patients with sulfa allergy. Loop diuretics cause hypokalemic metabolic alkalosis, hypovolemia, ototoxicity, and *calcium excretion*. All loop diuretics except ethacrynic acid are also sulfa drugs. Carbonic anhydrase inhibitors cause *metabolic acidosis*.

Antihypertensives are notorious for causing sedation, depression (the worst is methyldopa), and sexual dysfunction. β-Blockers also cause bradycardia, heart block, and congestive heart failure in susceptible patients. Calcium channel blockers also should be avoided in some cardiac patients for the same reason. Because β-blockers can precipitate asthmatic attacks and mask the symptoms of hypoglycemia, they should be avoided in asthmatics and used with caution in diabetics (benefits often outweigh risks, such as with a prior myocardial infarction). α_1-Antagonists are notorious for severe first-dose orthostatic hypotension.

The side effects of **psychiatric medications** are also high yield. See Chapter 17, Psychiatry.

ANTIDOTES

Antidotes to drug poisoning or overdose are listed in Table 29-2.

DRUG INTERACTIONS

A few drug–drug interactions are high yield. Do *not* give the following drugs together:

- Monoamine oxidase inhibitors and meperidine (can cause coma)
- Monoamine oxidase inhibitors and selective serotonin reuptake inhibitors (can cause the serotonin syndrome: hyperthermia, rigidity, myoclonus, autonomic instability)
- Aminoglycosides and loop diuretics (enhanced ototoxicity)
- Thiazides and lithium (lithium toxicity)

Table 29-1. SIDE EFFECTS

Drug	Side Effect(s)
Anesthesia and Pain Management	
Acetaminophen	Liver toxicity (in high doses)
Aspirin	GI bleeding, hypersensitivity
Halogen anesthetics	Malignant hyperthermia
Halothane	Liver necrosis
Local anesthetics	Seizures
Methoxyflurane	Diabetes insipidus
Morphine	Sphincter of Oddi spasm
Opiates	SIADH
Succinylcholine	Malignant hyperthermia
Infectious Diseases	
Aminoglycosides	Hearing loss, renal toxicity
Chloramphenicol	Aplastic anemia, gray baby syndrome
Clindamycin	Pseudomembranous colitis (may be caused by any broad-spectrum antibiotic)
Dideoxyinosine (DDI)	Pancreatitis, peripheral neuropathy
Ethambutol	Optic neuritis
Isoniazid	Vitamin B_6 deficiency, lupus, liver toxicity
Metronidazole	Disulfiram-like reaction with alcohol
Penicillins	Anaphylaxis, rash with Epstein–Barr virus
Quinolones	Teratogens (cartilage damage)
Tetracyclines	Photosensitivity, teeth staining in children
Vancomycin	Red man syndrome
Zidovudine (AZT)	Bone marrow suppression
Internal Medicine	
Acetazolamide	Metabolic acidosis
Amiodarone	Thyroid dysfunction, pulmonary fibrosis
Angiotensin-converting enzyme inhibitors	Cough; can damage fetal kidneys
Chlorpropamide	SIADH
Clofibrate	Increased GI neoplasms
Demeclocycline	Diabetes insipidus
Digitalis	Gastrointestinal disorders, vision changes, arrhythmias
Heparin	Thrombocytopenia, thrombosis
HMG CoA reductase inhibitors	Liver and muscle toxicity
Hydralazine	Lupus erythematosus
Methyldopa	Hemolytic anemia (Coombs' positive)
Niacin	Skin flushing, pruritus
Phenytoin	Folate deficiency, teratogen, hirsutism
Procainamide	Lupus erythematosus
Quinine	Cinchonism (e.g., tinnitus, vertigo)
Trimethadione	Terrible teratogen

Valproic acid	Neural tube defects in offspring
Warfarin	Necrosis, teratogen

Oncology

Bleomycin	Pulmonary fibrosis
Busulfan	Pulmonary fibrosis, adrenal failure
Cisplatin	Nephrotoxicity
Cyclophosphamide	Hemorrhagic cystitis
Doxorubicin	Cardiomyopathy
Vincristine	Peripheral neuropathy

Psychiatry

Bupropion	Seizures
Clozapine	Agranulocytosis
Lithium	Diabetes insipidus, thyroid dysfunction
Monoamine oxidase inhibitors	Tyramine crisis (cheese, wine)
Selective serotonin reuptake inhibitors (SSRIs)	Anxiety, agitation, insomnia
Thioridazine	Retinal deposits, cardiac toxicity
Trazodone	Priapism

Miscellaneous

Cyclosporine	Renal toxicity
Isotretinoin	Terrible teratogen
Minoxidil	Hirsutism
Oxytocin	SIADH
Sulfa drugs	Allergies, kernicterus in neonates

GI, gastrointestinal; HMG CoA, 3-Hydroxy-3-methylglutaryl-coenzyme A; SIADH, syndrome of inappropriate secretion of antidiuretic hormone

Table 29-2. ANTIDOTES

Poisoning or Overdose	Antidote
Acetaminophen	Acetylcysteine
Benzodiazepines	Flumazenil
β-Blockers	Glucagon
Carbon monoxide	Oxygen (hyperbaric if severe)
Cholinesterase inhibitors	Atropine, pralidoxime
Copper or gold	Penicillamine
Digoxin	Normalize potassium and other electrolytes, digoxin antibodies
Iron	Deferoxamine
Lead	Edetate
Methanol or ethylene glycol	Ethanol
Muscarinic receptor blockers	Physostigmine
Opioids	Naloxone
Quinidine or tricyclic antidepressants	Sodium bicarbonate (cardioprotective)

IMPORTANT POINTS

1 Barbiturates, antiepileptics, isoniazid, alcohol, and rifampin induce hepatic enzymes; cimetidine, amiodarone, macrolide antibiotics (e.g., erythromycin), metronidazole, cyclosporine, and ketoconazole and other azole antifungals inhibit hepatic enzymes (important for drug–drug interactions).

2 If a patient responds to placebo, it does *not* mean that the disease is psychosomatic; it means simply that the patient responded to placebo! Normal people with real diseases often have an improvement in symptoms with placebo. Never give placebo to patients as an experiment.

Hormone Replacement Therapy and Oral Contraceptives

HORMONE REPLACEMENT THERAPY

Hormone replacement therapy (HRT) is no longer thought to be beneficial for women other than for symptom relief. Observation during therapy is necessary, because estrogen and progesterone are not harmless. Every patient should make the decision on her own after weighing the risks and benefits.

◆ **Known benefits:** Decreased osteoporosis, decreased fractures (especially hip fractures), reduced hot flushes, and reduced genitourinary symptoms (dryness, urgency, atrophy-induced incontinence, frequency)

◆ **Known risks:** Increased risk of endometrial cancer (eliminated by coadministration of progesterones), increased risk of venous thromboembolism, and increased risk of gall-bladder disease. The risk of breast cancer might increase after 10 or more years of use, but this risk is controversial.

◆ **Other side effects:** Endometrial bleeding, breast tenderness, nausea, bloating, and headaches

◆ **Absolute contraindications:** Unexplained vaginal bleeding, active liver disease, history of thrombophlebitis or thromboembolism, history of endometrial or breast cancer

◆ **Relative contraindications:** Seizure disorder, hypertension, uterine leiomyomas, familial hyperlipidemia, migraines, thrombophlebitis, endometriosis, gallbladder disease

IMPORTANT POINTS

1 Women who take estrogen therapy need an endometrial biopsy and dilation and curettage (D&C) at the onset of treatment to rule out hyperplasia and cancer and an evaluation of any unexplained bleeding, even while on therapy, unless they have had a normal evaluation in the past 6 months.

2 The main reason to give progesterone with estrogen is to eliminate the increased risk of endometrial cancer. If a women has no uterus, do *not* give progesterone.

ORAL CONTRACEPTIVES

Oral contraceptives should not be given to women older than 35 years who smoke or have other cardiovascular risk factors (hypercholesterolemia or untreated hypertension) because of an increased risk of sudden death. Oral contraceptives are the most common cause of secondary hypertension in women, and any woman who is noted to have increased blood pressure should discontinue oral contraceptives and have her blood pressure rechecked at a later date.

◆ **Absolute contraindications:** Smoking after age 35 years, pregnancy (do pregnancy test before prescribing), breast-feeding, active liver disease, hyperlipidemia, uncontrolled hypertension, diabetes mellitus with vascular changes, prolonged immobilization of an extremity, history of thromboembolism or thrombophlebitis, coronary artery disease, stroke, sickle cell disease, estrogen-dependent neoplasm (breast, endometrium), liver adenoma, and history of cholestatic jaundice of pregnancy

◆ **Relative contraindications:** Depression, migraine headaches (can trigger attacks), oligomenorrhea, undiagnosed amenorrhea, gallbladder disease, and cigarette smoking before age 35.

◆ **Side effects:** Glucose intolerance (check for diabetes mellitus annually in patients at high risk), depression, edema (bloating), weight gain, cholelithiasis, benign **liver adenomas** (Fig. 29-1), melasma ("the mask of pregnancy"), nausea, vomiting, headache, hypertension, and drug interactions (drugs such as rifampin and antiepileptics can induce metabolism of oral contraceptives and reduce their effectiveness).

◆ **Benefits:** A *50% reduction in ovarian cancer*; decrease in the incidence of menorrhagia, dysmenorrhea, benign breast disease, functional ovarian cysts (*often prescribed for the previous four effects*), premenstrual tension, iron-deficiency anemia, ectopic pregnancy, and salpingitis

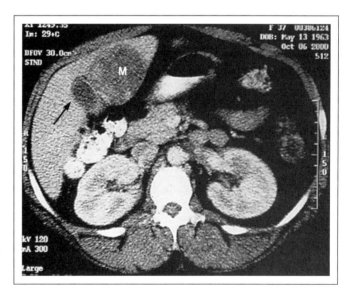

FIGURE 29-1. Contrasted computed tomography (CT) image demonstrating a nonspecific solid mass (M) in the left hepatic lobe adjacent to the gallbladder (*arrow*). The gallbladder is darker than the mass due to lower density of normal fluid in the gallbladder. Given a history of birth control pill use, this would be a slam dunk diagnosis for a hepatic adenoma on the boards (even without the CT image), but in the real world it would likely have to be biopsied to exclude other tumor histology.

IMPORTANT POINTS

1 Because of the risks of thromboembolism, oral contraceptives should be stopped 1 month before elective surgery and not restarted until 1 month after surgery.

2 The risk of breast cancer does *not* seem to be increased with oral contraceptives, except in long-term users (controversial; unlikely to be asked on boards). Cervical neoplasia may be increased, possibly because of the confounding factor of increased sexual relations and number of partners; nonetheless, oral contraceptive users should have at least annual Pap smears.

Analgesics and Antiinflammatories

EFFECTS

Aspirin and nonsteroidal antiinflammatory drugs (NSAIDs) inhibit cyclooxygenase (COX) centrally and peripherally, giving them antiinflammatory, antipyretic, analgesic, and antiplatelet properties. Aspirin inhibits COX irreversibly and thus for the life of the platelet, whereas other NSAIDs inhibit COX reversibly. COX-2 inhibitors only inhibit the COX-2 isozyme and thus *have no antiplatelet effects*. Acetaminophen is mostly central acting; thus, it is only an analgesic and antipyretic with no platelet or antiinflammatory effects.

Toxicity and side-effect issues:

◆ Aspirin and other NSAIDs can cause gastrointestinal (GI) upset, GI bleeding, and gastric ulcers; aspirin can aggravate gout. Always consider GI bleeding and ulcer in any patient taking aspirin or NSAIDs. COX-2 inhibitors (e.g. celecoxib), or an NSAID–prostaglandin E_1 combination can help prevent GI damage.

◆ NSAIDs also can cause renal damage (interstitial nephritis and papillary necrosis), especially in patients who take them chronically and have preexisting renal disease. Renal insufficiency can be seen with long-term use of NSAIDs and can occur acutely in patients with significant renal artery stenosis.

◆ Higher aspirin doses cause tinnitus, vertigo, respiratory alkalosis and metabolic acidosis, hyperthermia, coma, and death.

◆ Aspirin can be removed by dialysis in severe overdose.

◆ Do *not* give aspirin to people with asthma and nasal polyps. Hypersensitivity reactions are extremely common in this group; look for nasal polyps in anyone with an asthmatic-type reaction to aspirin (people with asthma can have an asthma attack after taking aspirin—even those without nasal polyps).

◆ Do *not* give aspirin to children younger than 8 years who have fever or viral infection; it can cause Reye's syndrome (look for encephalopathy and liver dysfunction).

◆ Phenylbutazone can cause fatal aplastic anemia and agranulocytosis and should not be used chronically.

◆ Acetaminophen causes liver toxicity in high doses due to depletion of glutathione. Treat with acetylcysteine.

Low-dose aspirin has been proved to be of benefit in reducing the risk of stroke in patients with a transient ischemic attack or previous stroke. Aspirin also is proven to reduce the risk of myocardial infarction (MI) in patients who have had a previous MI, in patients with stable or unstable angina who have not had an MI, and in those with coronary artery disease or its equivalent (e.g., peripheral vascular disease). Generally, use of aspirin for primary prevention of MI or stroke in a patient with no definite history of MI, angina, or coronary artery disease is not appropriate. Studies have not shown a clear benefit, and there may be an increased risk of hemorrhagic stroke and/or sudden death. If the patient has a history of liver or kidney disease, peptic ulcer disease, GI bleeding, poorly controlled hypertension, or bleeding disorder, the risks of aspirin prophylaxis can outweigh the benefits.

IMPORTANT POINTS

1 Give aspirin to any patient in the emergency department who has unstable angina, myocardial infarction, or transient ischemic attack (if CT scan of brain shows no hemorrhage).

2 Stop aspirin 1 week before surgery; stop other NSAIDs on the day before surgery.

# RADIOLOGY

Table 30-1 lists radiologic screening and confirmatory tests.

Table 30-1. SCREENING AND/OR CONFIRMATORY RADIOLOGIC TESTS FOR DIFFERENT DISEASES

Condition	Screening (or Only) Test to Order	Confirmatory Test	Comments
Cardiovascular			
Aortic aneurysm/ dissection	CT with contrast	MRA with contrast (rarely needed)	
Aortic tear (trauma)	CT with contrast		
Carotid stenosis	Duplex US, MRA or CTA	Conventional angiogram	
Gastrointestinal			
Abdominal abscess	CT scan with contrast		
Abdominal trauma	CT scan with contrast	Laparoscopy (rarely indicated for diagnosis)	
Appendicitis	US (pediatrics and pregnant) or CT with contrast	Laparoscopy (rarely indicated for diagnosis)	
Bowel perforation	Abdominal x-ray	CT scan with contrast	Laparoscopy only for uncertain cases and treatment
Cholecystitis	US	Nuclear hepatobiliary study (HIDA scan)	
Choledocholithiasis	US	ERCP or MRCP (CT sometimes helpful)	
Cholelithiasis	US	CT or MRCP sometimes helpful	
Diverticulitis	CT scan with contrast		No endoscopy or barium enema acutely
Esophageal obstruction	Barium x-ray or endoscopy	Endoscopy	
Esophageal tear	Chest x-ray followed by Gastrografin x-ray	Endoscopy or surgery	
Hematemesis	Endoscopy		

Table continued on following page

Table 30-1. SCREENING AND/OR CONFIRMATORY RADIOLOGIC TESTS FOR DIFFERENT DISEASES (Continued)

Condition	Screening (or Only) Test to Order	Confirmatory Test	Comments
Intestinal obstruction	Abdominal x-ray	CT scan with contrast	
Lower GI bleeding*	Barium enema or endoscopy	Endoscopy	
Meckel's diverticulum	Meckel's scan (nuclear medicine)		
Peptic ulcer disease	Upper GI series or endoscopy	Endoscopy	
Pyloric stenosis	US; upper GI series second choice		
Unknown GI bleeding*	Nuclear medicine bleeding study		For brisk bleed, angiography or laparotomy
Upper GI bleeding*	Upper GI series or endoscopy	Endoscopy	
Gynecologic			
Fibroid uterus	US	MRI	
Ovarian pathology	US	MRI or laparoscopy (CT sometimes helpful)	
Pelvic mass (female)	US	MRI or CT with contrast or laparoscopy	
Pregnancy evaluation	US (transvaginal detects sooner than transabdominal)		First get β-hCG
Neurologic			
Acute stroke	CT without contrast	MRI of brain without contrast	
Brain tumor	CT or MRI with contrast		
Head trauma	CT without contrast		
Intracranial hemorrhage	CT without contrast		
Multiple sclerosis	MRI of brain with contrast		
Skull fracture	CT without contrast		
Orthopedic			
Arthritis	X-ray	MRI if more detailed evaluation is needed	
Bone metastases	Bone scan	PET scan	Plain x-rays for multiple myeloma
Fracture	X-ray		CT scan without contrast can help evaluate complex fractures
Osteomyelitis	X-ray	Bone scan, tagged white blood cell nuclear scan, or MRI with contrast	

Respiratory

Chest mass	Chest x-ray	CT scan with contrast	
Chest trauma	Chest x-ray	CT scan with contrast	
Hemoptysis	Chest x-ray	Bronchoscopy and/or CT scan with contrast	
Pneumonia	Chest x-ray		
Pulmonary embolism	CT with contrast	Conventional pulmonary arteriogram (rarely indicated)	Ventilation/perfusion nuclear scan if can't give contrast
Pulmonary nodule	Chest x-ray followed by chest CT with contrast	PET scan	

Urologic

Hematuria (persistent)	CT scan with contrast (without contrast if *painful* hematuria)	Cystoscopy	
Hydronephrosis	US or CT scan		
Nephrolithiasis	CT scan without contrast	Intravenous pyelography rarely indicated or used	

Note: With suspected GI perforation, do not use barium (it can cause a chemical peritonitis); use water-soluble contrast (e.g., Gastrografin).

*For brisk bleeds, endoscopy is preferred. For occult bleeding, barium study or endoscopy may be used. An "unknown" GI bleed means that initial tests failed to localize the bleed and that the patient is still actively bleeding.

CT, computed tomography; CTA, computed tomographic angiogram; ERCP, endoscopic retrograde cholangiopancreatography; GI, gastrointestinal; hCG, human chorionic gonadotropin; HIDA, hepato-iminodiacetic acid; MRA, magnetic resonance angiogram (an MRI test); MRCP, magnetic resonance cholangiopancreatography; MRI, magnetic resonance imaging; PET, positron emission tomography; US, ultrasound

31 LABORATORY MEDICINE

Electrolytes

- Hyperkalemia may be caused by a hemolyzed blood sample (consider rechecking the lab if it doesn't make sense) or rhabdomyolysis (due to high intracellular potassium concentration).

- Alkalosis can cause hypokalemia and symptoms of hypocalcemia (perioral numbness, tetany) due to cellular shift; acidosis can cause hyperkalemia by the same mechanism.

- Hyponatremia may be caused by hyperglycemia, hyperproteinemia, or hyperlipidemia; these forms of secondary hyponatremia will correct with correction of the glucose, lipid, or protein levels.

- Correcting hyponatremia aggressively (especially with hypertonic saline [3%]) can cause brainstem damage (osmotic myelinolysis, aka central pontine myelinolysis).

- Hypokalemia and/or hypocalcemia may be due to hypomagnesemia. You cannot correct the hypokalemia until you correct the hypomagnesemia.

- Watch for hypophosphatemia in diabetic ketoacidosis.

Enzymes

- Increased levels of amylase and lipase may be due to sources other than the pancreas (salivary glands, gastrointestinal [GI] tract, renal failure, ruptured tubal pregnancy), but elevation of both in the same patient with abdominal pain is almost always due to pancreatitis.

- Alkaline phosphatase can be elevated by biliary disease, bone disease, or pregnancy. If the elevation is due to biliary disease, γ-glutamyltranspeptidase (GGT) and/or 5-nucleotidase (5-NT) also should be elevated.

- Elevated creatine kinase (CK) may be due to muscle injury (striated or myocardial), drugs (3-hydroxy-3-methylglutaryl-coenzyme A [HMG-CoA] reductase inhibitors), or burns (CK-MB is more specific for cardiac muscle).

Other

- Hypothyroidism can cause elevated cholesterol.
- Blood urea nitrogen-to-creatinine ratio >15 usually implies dehydration.
- Positive results on the rapid plasma reagin or Venereal Disease Research Laboratory (VDRL) test for syphilis may be due to systemic lupus erythematosus.
- In patients with isosthenuria and hyposthenuria—the inability to concentrate urine—think of diabetes insipidus or sickle cell disease or trait.
- The erythrocyte sedimentation rate (ESR) is a worthless test in pregnancy; ESR is elevated by pregnancy itself. A high-normal blood urea nitrogen (BUN) or creatinine level can mean renal disease in pregnancy.
- Elevated levels of the binding protein can cause elevation of the total concentration of a substance without elevating the free or active portion of that substance, which is rarely important clinically and doesn't need treatment (e.g., elevated thyroid hormone with elevation of thyroid-binding globulin levels, decrease in calcium levels due to decreased albumin levels). Check the free/unbound/active portion of the substance of interest or notice or order the associated carrier or binding protein level to make sure you don't fall for this one.

32 ETHICS AND PATIENT ENCOUNTERS

Consent

- Do *not* force adult Jehovah's Witness patients to accept blood products (or force any competent adults to accept any treatment they don't want!), and don't give a treatment behind a competent patient's back without consent because it's "in their best interest."

- If a child has a life-threatening condition and the parents refuse a simple, curative treatment (e.g., antibiotics for meningitis), first try to persuade the parents to change their minds. If they will not, your second option is to get a court order to give the treatment and get hospital support services involved. Don't give the treatment until you talk to the courts if you can avoid it.

- Let competent people die if they want to do so. *Never* force treatments on adults of sound mind. Respect wishes for passive euthanasia, but avoid active euthanasia.

- Informed consent involves giving the patient information about the *diagnosis* (his or her condition and what it means), the *prognosis* (the natural course of the condition without treatment), the *proposed treatment* (description of the procedure and what the patient will experience), the *risks and benefits* of the treatment, and the *alternative treatments*. The patient then can choose what he or she wants to do. The documents seen on hospital wards that patients are made to sign are *neither required nor sufficient* for informed consent; they are used for documentation and medicolegal purposes (i.e., lawsuit paranoia).

- Living wills and do-not-resuscitate (DNR) orders should be respected and followed if done correctly. For example, if in a living will the patient says that a ventilator should not be used if he or she is unable to breathe independently, do not put the patient on a ventilator, even if the spouse, son, or daughter makes the request.

Confidentiality

- Do not tell anyone how your patient is doing unless he or she is directly involved with care and needs to know or is an authorized family member. If a colleague asks about a friend who happens to be your patient, refuse to answer.

- Break confidentiality only in the following situations:

- The patient asks you to do so.
- Child abuse is suspected.
- The courts mandate you to tell.
- You have a duty to protect life. (If the patient says that he or she is going to kill someone or him- or herself, tell the intended victim and the authorities.)
- The patient has a reportable disease. You must report it to the authorities. They will deal with it.
- The patient is a danger to others. If the patient is blind or has seizures, let the proper authorities know so that they can take away the patient's license to drive. If the patient is an airplane pilot and a paranoid, hallucinating schizophrenic, authorities need to know.

Competence

- When the patient is incompetent, a guardian (surrogate decision maker or health care power of attorney) should be appointed by the court.
- Depression always should be evaluated as a reason for the patient's "incompetence." Patients who are suicidal might refuse all treatment; this decision should not be respected until the depression is treated.
- Patients can be hospitalized against their will in psychiatry (if they are a danger to self or others) for a limited time. After 1 to 3 days, patients usually get a hearing to determine whether they have to remain in custody. This practice is based on the principle of beneficence (a principle of doing good for the patient and avoiding harm).
- Restraints can be used on an incompetent or violent patient (delirious, psychotic) if needed, but their use should be brief and reevaluated often. Restraints have caused injuries and even death in some cases and can do more harm than good.
- Patients younger than 18 years do *not* require parental consent in the following situations:
  - If they are emancipated (married, living on their own and financially independent, parents of children, serving in the armed forces)
  - If they have a sexually transmitted disease, want contraception, or are pregnant
  - If they want drug treatment or counseling
  - Some states have exceptions to these rules, but for boards let such minors make their own decisions.
- If a patient is comatose and no surrogate decision maker has been appointed, the wishes of the family generally should be respected. If there is a family disagreement or ulterior motives are evident, talk to your hospital ethics committee. Use courts as a last resort.
- In a pediatric emergency when parents and other family members are not available, treat the patient as you see fit. In incompetent or comatose adults, the same principle is followed if no responsible parties, caregivers, or relatives can be located.

Communication

◆ Do *not* hide a diagnosis from patients (including pediatric patients) if they want to know the diagnosis—even if the family asks you do so. Do *not* lie to any patient because the family asks you to do so. The flip side also applies: Do *not* force patients to receive information against their will. If they don't want to know the diagnosis, don't tell them.

◆ If a patient cannot communicate, give any required emergency care unless you know that the patient does not want it.

◆ Ask patients open-ended questions (cannot be answered "yes" or "no"), and always ask "why" if a patient's actions, words, or requests puzzle you.

◆ Don't get mad at patients and yell at them, even if they deserve it.

◆ Parents might ask you to test their child for drugs or sexually transmitted diseases, etc., without telling the child. Don't do it.

◆ Be a patient advocate, always.

◆ When confronting patients, don't be harsh or judgmental.

◆ Always try to get more history and information from the patient when given the option, unless the patient is unstable and needs immediate intervention.

Care

◆ Patients might refuse your treatment and instead choose to use a wild Tanzanian root they read about on the Internet for their condition. Support their decision and agree to help however you can.

◆ "Withdrawing" and "withholding" care are no different in a legal sense. Just because the patient is on a respirator does not mean that you cannot stop it.

◆ In terminally ill patients, give enough medication to relieve pain. Don't be afraid to give narcotics if needed, and don't worry about addiction in this setting.

◆ Consultation of a subspecialist is appropriate in many settings. For example, if a patient has a thoracic aortic dissection, a vascular or cardiothoracic surgical consult is not only reasonable but expected. The boards want you to know the treatment options, but they might ask a question or two to make sure you are not too cocky in your abilities.

PHOTOS AND FIGURES

Although some questions with photos can be answered without looking at the photo, this is not always the case. The entities listed below are fair game for Step 2. See your nearest clinical atlas or textbook for images not included here or elsewhere in the book.

Blood Smears

ANEMIA

- Folate/B_{12} anemia (macrocytic, hypersegmented neutrophils)
- Iron deficiency anemia
- Sideroblastic anemia

CANCER

- Acute lymphoblastic leukemia
- Acute myeloid leukemia (Auer rods)
- Chronic lymphocytic leukemia (smudge cell)
- Chronic myelocytic leukemia
- Hairy cell leukemia
- Multiple myeloma
- Reed–Sternberg cell (Hodgkin's lymphoma)

OTHER

- Acanthocytes (abetalipoproteinemia)
- Basophilic stippling (lead poisoning, thalassemia)
- Döhle bodies (toxic lymphocytes; for boards, think of Epstein–Barr virus)
- Heinz bodies and ''bite cells'' (glucose-6-phosphate dehydrogenase [G6PD] deficiency)
- Howell–Jolly bodies (asplenia or splenic dysfunction)
- Malaria
- Reticulocytes

◆ Schistocytes and helmet cells (disseminated intravascular coagulation, thrombotic thrombocytopenic purpura, microangiopathic hemolysis)

◆ Sickle cell disease

◆ Spherocytosis

◆ Target cells (thalassemia, severe liver disease)

◆ Teardrop cells (myelofibrosis, myelodysplasia)

Ophthalmology

OPHTHALMOLOGIC PROBLEMS

◆ Bacterial conjunctivitis (especially in neonates)

◆ Cataracts (bad enough to notice with the naked eye)

◆ Central retinal artery occlusion (fundus)

◆ Central retinal vein occlusion (fundus)

◆ Glaucoma (closed-angle attack or acute)

◆ Herpes simplex keratitis (dendritic ulcer seen with fluorescein; avoid steroids)

◆ Orbital cellulitis (gross picure of a patient's face)

◆ Retinoblastoma (leukocoria; white reflex instead of red)

OPHTHALMOLOGIC SIGNS OF OTHER PROBLEMS

◆ Diabetic fundus

◆ Graves' disease (exophthalmos)

◆ Hypertensive fundus

◆ Kayser–Fleischer ring (Wilson's disease)

◆ Papilledema

◆ Roth's spots (think of endocarditis)

◆ Xanthelasma

Dermatology and Skin Findings

DERMATOLOGY

◆ Acne

◆ Actinic keratosis

◆ Allergic contact dermatitis

◆ Basal cell skin cancer

◆ Cavernous hemangiomas (in children, most lesions resolve on their own)

◆ Condyloma acuminata

◆ Erythema infectiosum (slapped cheek rash with fever resolution just before rash appears)

- Erythema multiforme (target lesion)
- Heliotrope rash (dermatomyositis)
- Henoch–Schönlein purpura (rash)
- Impetigo
- Keloids (usually in blacks)
- Melanoma of the skin
- Molluscum contagiosum
- Pityriasis rosea
- Psoriasis (skin findings and nail pitting)
- Scabies
- Squamous cell skin cancer
- Temporal arteritis (patient's face reveals a tortuous-looking temporal artery)
- Tinea capitis
- Tinea corporis and tinea cruris
- Vitiligo (associated with pernicious anemia and hypothyroidism)

SKIN FINDINGS

- Abdominal striae (Cushing's syndrome)
- Acanthosis nigricans (marker for visceral malignancy)
- Adenoma sebaceum (i.e., angiofibromas, marker for tuberous sclerosis)
- Arterial insufficiency (skin changes)
- Café-au-lait patches (neurofibromatosis in patients with normal IQ, McCune–Albright syndrome with mental retardation)
- Cheilitis or stomatitis (think of B vitamin deficiencies)
- Clubbing of the fingers
- Cullen's sign (blue periumbilical area, marker for severe pancreatitis)
- Diabetic foot ulcers (similar in appearance to arterial insufficiency ulcers but usually *painless*)
- Erythema marginatum (rheumatic fever)
- Erythema nodosum (think of inflammatory bowel disease, infections [the classic example is *Coccidioides immitis* or tuberculosis], or sarcoidosis)
- Grey Turner's sign (blue flank, marker for severe pancreatitis)
- Herpes (1 and 2)
- Hirsutism (know conditions associated with it)
- Janeway's and Osler's lesions (endocarditis)
- Lyme disease (erythema chronicum migrans)
- Malar rash (lupus)
- *Neisseria* spp. septicemia (severe purpura)
- Neurofibromatosis (skin neurofibromas)

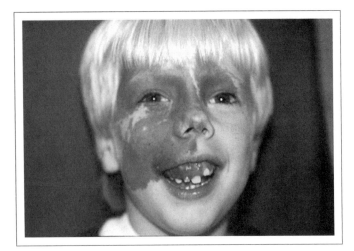

FIGURE 33-1. Sturge–Weber syndrome.

- Oral hairy leukoplakia (caused by Epstein–Barr virus; seen in HIV-positive patients)
- Pretibial myxedema (Graves' disease)
- Pyoderma gangrenosum (think of inflammatory bowel disease)
- Raynaud's phenomenon (finger autoamputation; often seen in scleroderma)
- Rocky Mountain spotted fever rash
- Stasis dermatitis or venous insufficiency (skin changes, ulcers)
- Sturge–Weber syndrome (hemangioma; port-wine stain on one side of face, Fig. 33-1)
- Syphilis (chancre, condyloma lata, secondary syphilis rash)
- Toxic shock syndrome, scalded skin syndrome (blisters and skin peeling off in large sheets)
- Varicella zoster virus (chickenpox, shingles, trigeminal and ophthalmic involvement)

Microscopic Findings

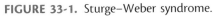

- Caseating granulomas (tuberculosis, fungi)
- Clue cells (*Gardnerella* spp. vaginitis)
- *Giardia* spp.
- Goodpasture's disease (linear immunofluorescence in kidney)
- Gout (rhomboid-shaped crystals from a joint with no birefringence)
- Gram stain (gram-negative = red; gram-positive = blue) plus morphology and clustering tendencies (see Chapter 10, Infectious Disease, for classic examples)
- Koilocytosis (think of human papillomavirus or cytomegalovirus)
- Noncaseating granulomas (sarcoidosis)
- Positive India ink preparation for *Cryptococcus* meningitis (Fig. 33-2)
- Pseudogout (rhomboid-shaped crystals with weakly positive birefringence)
- *Trichomonas* spp.

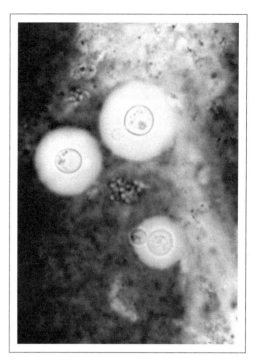

FIGURE 33-2. A positive India ink preparation revealing the classic budding yeasts with a wide capsule indicating *Cryptococcus neoformans.*

Radiologic Findings

CARDIOVASCULAR

- Abdominal aortic aneurysm on computed tomography (CT) scan or angiogram
- Congestive heart failure on chest x-ray
- Severe carotid artery stenosis on angiogram

GASTROINTESTINAL AND ABDOMINAL

- Achalasia (esophagus on barium swallow x-ray)
- Colon cancer on barium enema (apple-core and napkin-ring lesions)
- Congenital diaphragmatic hernia (Fig. 33-3)
- Duodenal atresia ("double-bubble" sign)
- Esophageal atresia (barium x-ray or nasogastric tube coiled in neck on chest x-ray)
- Liver tumor on CT scan (metastasis 20 times more likely than primary tumor)
- Sigmoid volvulus on barium enema (bird's beak appearance)
- Small bowel obstruction (air-fluid levels) on abdominal x-ray
- Staghorn urinary calculus on abdominal x-ray
- Toxic megacolon (Hirschsprung's disease or inflammatory bowel disease, infection) on abdominal x-ray (dilated air-filled colon with wall thickening)

HEAD AND NECK

- Appearance of a large cerebrovascular accident (stroke) on CT or magnetic resonance image (MRI)

- Epidural hematoma (on a CT scan)
- Sinusitis (maxillary or frontal sinus opacification)
- Subdural hematoma (on a CT scan)

PULMONARY

- Classic chest x-ray of tuberculosis (upper lobe scarring and cavitary changes)
- Grossly abnormal ventilation–perfusion lung scan ($\dot{V}/\dot{Q}$ mismatch)
- Lobar pneumonia
- Lung abscess on chest x-ray (air-fluid level in a mass)
- Pancoast's tumor on chest x-ray (large upper lobe lung cancer or mass; can cause Horner's syndrome)
- Pleural effusion
- Pneumothorax and tension pneumothorax
- Sarcoidosis (bilateral hilar adenopathy, Fig. 33-4)

SKELETAL

- Lytic lesions of bone on x-ray (consider possible malignancy)
- Multiple myeloma (multiple, rounded, punched-out lesions on skull x-ray)
- Osteoarthritis (osteophytes, interphalangeal joint changes)
- Osteosarcoma (sunray or sunburst pattern on an extremity x-ray)
- Shoulder dislocation on x-ray
- Slipped capital femoral epiphysis (x-ray)

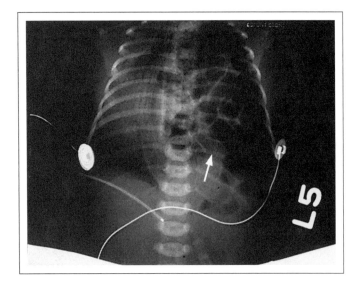

FIGURE 33-3. Frontal chest radiograph reveals multiple bowel loops (*arrow*) in the left hemithorax with shift of mediastinal structures to the right causing some compression of the right lung.

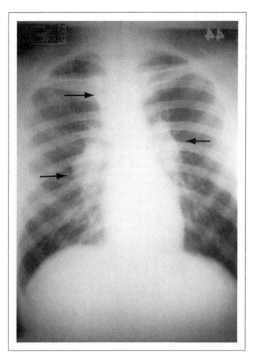

FIGURE 33-4. Sarcoidosis. Frontal chest radiograph reveals bilateral hilar adenopathy (*lower right and left arrows*), right paratracheal adenopathy (*upper left arrow*), and difficult-to-visualize central interstitial-type infiltrates.

General Clinical Photos and Figures

FACE
- Bell's palsy (facial asymmetry)
- Congenital syphilis (Hutchinson's teeth, saddle nose deformity)
- Fetal alcohol syndrome (facies)
- Graves' disease (exophthalmos)
- Horner's syndrome (unilateral ptosis and miosis and history of hemianhydrosis)
- Peutz–Jeghers syndrome (freckling pattern on face)
- Scleroderma (late-stage facies)

GROSS APPEARANCE
- Achondroplasia (overall appearance; usually autosomal dominant)
- Acute pharyngitis (viral or streptococcal)
- Acute tonsillitis (*Streptococcus* spp. or Epstein–Barr virus; rarely diphtheria in unimmunized patient)
- Cushing's syndrome (facies, striae)
- Dactylitis (sickle cell disease)
- Decubitus ulcers (best prevention is frequent turning of patient)
- Down's syndrome (facies, simian crease)
- Erb's palsy (waiter's tip)

◆ Gynecomastia (normal finding in pubertal boys)

◆ Pseudohermaphrotidism (picture of ambiguous genitalia; look for 21-hydroxylase deficiency)

◆ Rheumatoid arthritis (swan-neck deformity, boutonnière deformity, ulnar deviation, rheumatoid nodules)

◆ Spina bifida (gross appearance; encephalocele, meningoceleocele, meningomyelocele, patch of hair in spina bifida occulta)

◆ Strawberry tongue (scarlet fever and Kawasaki's disease)

◆ Tanner stages (male and female)

◆ Turner's syndrome (body habitus, widely spaced nipples, webbed neck, cubitus valgus)

◆ Varicose veins

PATHOLOGY

◆ Candidal infection (vaginal, thrush)

◆ Dilated cardiomyopathy (gross specimen; severe disease)

◆ Fetal heart strips (normal, short-term, and long-term variability; early, variable, and late decelerations)

◆ Gonorrhea (yellowish discharge)

◆ Gout (podagra, tophi)

◆ Hypertrophy of the heart (gross specimen; severe disease)

◆ Karyotype showing Down's (trisomy 21), Turner's (XO), or Klinefelter's (XXY) syndrome

◆ Osteoarthritis (Heberden's and Bouchard's nodes)

◆ Osteomyelitis extending to the skin (think of *Staphylococcus* or *Salmonella* spp. in sickle cell disease)

◆ Polycystic kidneys (gross pathologic specimen appearance)

34 SIGNS, SYMPTOMS, AND SYNDROMES

Signs and Syndromes

- **Babinski's sign:** Stroking the foot yields extension of the big toe and fanning of other toes in patients with upper motor neuron disease.
- **Beck's triad:** Jugular vein distention, muffled heart sounds, and hypotension in cardiac tamponade; do pericardiocentesis.
- **Brudzinski's sign:** Pain on neck flexion with meningeal irritation.
- **Charcot's triad:** Fever and chills, jaundice, and right upper quadrant pain in patients with cholangitis.
- **Courvoisier's sign:** A painless, palpable gallbladder should make you think of pancreatic cancer.
- **Chvostek's sign:** Tapping on the facial nerve elicits tetany in hypocalcemia.
- **Cullen's sign:** Bluish discoloration of periumbilical area due to retroperitoneal hemorrhage (pancreatitis).
- **Cushing's reflex:** Hypertension, bradycardia, and irregular respirations with very high intracranial pressure.
- **Grey Turner's sign:** Bluish discoloration of flank from retroperitoneal hemorrhage (think of pancreatitis).
- **Homan's sign:** Calf pain on forced dorsiflexion of the foot in patients with deep vein thrombosis (insensitive and unreliable but classic).
- **Kehr's sign:** Pain referred to the left shoulder with a ruptured spleen.
- **Leriche's syndrome:** Claudication and atrophy of the buttocks with impotence (seen with aortoiliac occlusive disease).
- **McBurney's sign:** Tenderness at McBurney's point with appendicitis.
- **Murphy's sign:** Arrest of inspiration when palpating right upper quadrant under the rib cage in patients with cholecystitis.
- **Ortolani's sign/test:** A palpable or audible click with abduction of an infant's flexed hip means congenital hip dysplasia.
- **Prehn's sign:** Elevation of a painful testicle relieves pain in epididymitis (vs. torsion).

◆ **Rovsing's sign:** Pushing on the left lower quadrant produces pain at McBurney's point in patients with appendicitis.

◆ **Tinel's sign:** Tapping on the volar surface of the wrist elicits paresthesias in carpal tunnel syndrome.

◆ **Trousseau's sign:** Pumping up a blood pressure cuff causes carpopedal spasm (tetany) in hypocalcemia.

◆ **Trousseau's syndrome:** Migratory thrombophlebitis (i.e., pops up in one site, goes away, then appears in a different part of the body) as a sign of visceral malignancy.

◆ **Verner–Morrison syndrome:** Watery diarrhea, achlorhydria, and hypokalemia due to a pancreatic islet cell tumor oversecreting vasoactive intestinal peptide (i.e. VIPoma)

◆ **Virchow's triad:** Stasis, endothelial damage, and hypercoagulability (three broad categories of risk factors for deep vein thrombosis).

Word Associations

Word associations are not 100% accurate, but they are useful in board exam emergencies.

◆ **Abdominal striae:** Cushing's syndrome (or possible pregnancy)

◆ **Ambiguous genitalia and hypotension:** Female patient with 21-hydroxylase deficiency (give corticosteroids and IV fluids)

◆ **Anaphylaxis from immunoglobulin therapy:** Immunoglobulin A (IgA) deficiency

◆ **Baby >10 pounds:** Maternal diabetes

◆ **Bilateral hilar adenopathy in a black female patient:** Sarcoidosis

◆ **Bitot's spots:** Vitamin A deficiency

◆ **Bronze (skin) diabetes:** Hemochromatosis (look also for cardiac and liver dysfunction)

◆ **Cat-like cry in children:** Cri-du-chat syndrome

◆ **Café-au-lait spots:** Neurofibromatosis (if mental retardation is present, think of McCune–Albright syndrome or tuberous sclerosis)

◆ **Cherry-red spot on the macula:** Tay–Sachs disease (no hepatosplenomegaly) or Niemann–Pick disease (hepatosplenomegaly)

◆ **Children who torture animals:** Conduct disorder (may be antisocial as adults)

◆ **Clue cells:** *Gardnerella* sp. infection

◆ **Constant clearing of throat (children):** Tourette's syndrome

◆ **Currant jelly stools in children:** Intussusception

◆ **Daytime sleepiness and occasional falling down (cataplexy):** Narcolepsy

◆ **Decreased breath sounds in a trauma patient:** Pneumothorax

◆ **Dendritic corneal ulcers:** Herpes keratitis (seen best with fluorescein; avoid steroids)

◆ **Fractures or bruises in different stages of healing (children):** Child abuse

◆ **Friction rub:** Pericarditis (Fig. 34-1)

◆ **Heavy young woman with papilledema and negative radiology:** Pseudotumor cerebri

◆ **Heliotrope rash:** Dermatomyositis

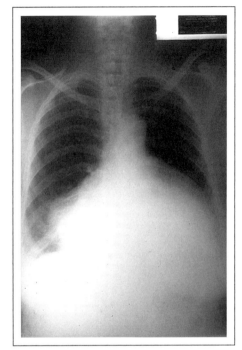

FIGURE 34-1. Enlarged globular cardiac silhouette is statistically more likely to be related to chronic cardiomegaly from heart disease, but keep in mind that an enlarged cardiac silhouette on chest x-ray can be due to cardiomegaly, pericardial effusion, and/or cardiac or paracardiac mass. The globular "water bottle" configuration is suggestive, and if a friction rub is heard in the chest or if a recent prior chest x-ray showed a normal cardiac size, the chest radiographic findings would be highly suggestive. In this case, the patient had a large pericardial effusion.

- **Honey or home-canned goods:** Infant botulism
- **Increased hemoglobin A2 and anemia:** Thalassemia
- **Intermittent bursts of swearing or repetitive grunting:** Tourette's syndrome
- **Kayser–Fleischer ring:** Wilson's disease
- **Koilocytosis:** Human papillomavirus or cytomegalovirus
- **Kussmaul's breathing:** Deep, rapid breathing seen in metabolic acidosis (think of diabetic ketoacidosis)
- **Left lower quadrant tenderness or rebound:** Diverticulitis
- **Low-grade fever in first 24 hours after surgery:** Atelectasis
- **Malar rash:** Lupus erythematosus
- **Meconium ileus:** Cystic fibrosis
- **Postpartum fever unresponsive to broad-spectrum antibiotics:** Septic pelvic thrombophlebitis (give heparin for a cure and retrospective diagnosis)
- **Rash after ampicillin or amoxicillin for a sore throat:** Epstein–Barr virus infection
- **Rectal prolapse:** Cystic fibrosis
- **Salty-tasting baby:** Cystic fibrosis
- **Shopping sprees:** Mania
- **Sudden death in a young athlete:** Hypertrophic obstructive cardiomyopathy
- **Vietnam or Iraq war veteran:** Posttraumatic stress disorder
- **Worst headache of patient's life:** Subarachnoid hemorrhage

ABBREVIATIONS

AAA	abdominal aortic aneurysm
Ab	antibody
ABC, ABCD, ABCDE	**a**irway, **b**reathing, **c**irculation, **d**isability, **e**xposure (trauma protocol)
ABG	arterial blood gas
ABO	blood types (A, B, AB or O)
ACE	angiotensin-converting enzyme
ACEI	angiotensin-converting enzyme inhibitor
ACL	anterior cruciate ligament
ACTH	adrenocorticotropic hormone
ADH	antidiuretic hormone
ADHD	attention-deficit/hyperactivity disorder
AFP	alpha fetoprotein
AIDS	acquired immunodeficiency syndrome
ALL	acute lymphoblastic leukemia
ALS	amyotrophic lateral sclerosis (aka Lou Gehrig's disease)
ALT	alanine aminotransferase
AML	acute myeloid leukemia
ANA	antinuclear antibody
ANCA	antineutrophil cytoplasmic antibody
ANOVA	analysis of variance
ARB	angiotensin receptor blocker
ARDS	acute respiratory distress syndrome
ARF	acute renal failure
ASA	acetylsalicylic acid (aspirin)
ASD	atrial septal defect
AST	aspartate aminotransferase
ATG	antithymocyte globulin
AVM	arteriovenous malformation
AXR	abdominal x-ray
AZT	azidothymidine (zidovudine)
B, β	beta
BP	blood pressure

BPH	benign prostatic hyperplasia, benign prostatic hypertrophy
BPP	biophysical profile
BT	bleeding time
BUN	blood urea nitrogen
C	Celsius, centigrade (e.g., 37° C); complement (e.g., C1, C3, C4); cervical (e.g., C5 vertebral body)
c-section	cesarean section
CA	cancer antigen (e.g., CA-125)
CAD	coronary artery disease
CBC	complete blood count
CD	cluster of differentiation (e.g., CD4, CD8)
CEA	carcinoembryonic antigen
CHD	coronary heart disease; congenital hip dysplasia
CHF	congestive heart failure
CK	creatine kinase
CLL	chronic lymphocytic leukemia
cm	centimeter
CML	chronic myelocytic (or myelogenous) leukemia
CMV	cytomegalovirus
CN	cranial nerve
CNS	central nervous system
CO	carbon monoxide or cardiac output
CO_2	carbon dioxide
COPD	chronic obstructive pulmonary disease
COX	cyclooxygenase
CPD	cephalopelvic disproportion
CPK	creatine phosphokinase
Cr	creatinine
CRF	chronic renal failure
CSF	cerebrospinal fluid
CT	computed tomography scan
CVA	cerebrovascular accident (stroke)
CXR	chest x-ray
D_5W	5% dextrose in water
D&C	dilation and curettage
DDI	dideoxyinosine (antiretroviral medication)
DES	diethylstilbestrol
DI	diabetes insipidus
DIC	disseminated intravascular coagulation
DIP	distal interphalangeal (joint)
DKA	diabetic ketoacidosis
dL	deciliter
DM	diabetes mellitus
DMSA	2,3-dimercaptosuccinic acid, succimer
DNA	deoxyribonucleic acid
DTP	diphtheria, tetanus, pertussis (trivalent vaccine)
DUB	dysfunctional uterine bleeding

DVT	deep venous thrombosis
EBV	Epstein–Barr virus
ECG	electrocardiogram
EDTA	edetate (ethylenediaminetetraacetic acid)
EEG	electroencephalogram
EKG	electrocardiogram
ELISA	enzyme-linked immunosorbent assay
EMG	electromyogram
ERCP	endoscopic retrograde cholangiopancreatography
ESR	erythrocyte sedimentation rate
FDP	fibrin degradation product
Fe	iron
FEV	forced expiratory volume
FEV_1	forced expiratory volume in 1 second
FFP	fresh frozen plasma
FSH	follicle-stimulating hormone
FTA-ABS	fluorescent treponemal antibody-absorption test (for syphilis)
FVC	forced vital capacity
g	gram
G6PD	glucose-6-phosphate dehydrogenase
GERD	gastroesophageal reflux disease
GGT	γ-glutamyltranspeptidase
GI	gastrointestinal
GnRH	gonadotropin-releasing hormone
GU	genitourinary
GYN	gynecology or gynecologic
H_2	histamine type 2 receptor
H&P	history and physical examination
HAV	hepatitis A virus
Hb_{A1c}	glycosylated hemoglobin
HBcAb/Ag	hepatitis B core antibody/antigen
HBeAb/Ag	hepatitis B e antibody/antigen
HBsAb/Ag	hepatitis B surface antibody/antigen
HBV	hepatitis B virus
HC	head circumference
hCG	human chorionic gonadotropin
HCV	hepatitis C virus
HDL	high-density lipoprotein
HELLP	**h**emolysis, **e**levated **l**iver enzymes, **l**ow **p**latelets (syndrome)
5-HIAA	5-hydroxyindoleacetic acid
HIV	human immunodeficiency virus
HLA	human leukocyte antigen
HPV	human papillomavirus
h	hour(s)
HRT	hormone replacement therapy
HSP	Henoch–Schönlein purpura
HSV	herpes simplex virus

HTN	hypertension
HUS	hemolytic uremic syndrome
IBD	inflammatory bowel disease
IBS	irritable bowel syndrome
ICP	intracranial pressure
ICU	intensive care unit
Ig	immunoglobulin (e.g., IgA, IgM, IgG, IgE)
IL	interleukin (e.g., IL-2)
IM	intramuscular
IPV	inactivated poliovirus vaccine
IQ	intelligence quotient
IU	international units
IUD	intrauterine device
IUGR	intrauterine growth retardation, intrauterine growth restriction
ITP	idiopathic thrombocytopenic purpura
IV	intravenous
IVC	inferior vena cava
IVDA	intravenous drug abuse
IVF	intravenous fluids; in vitro fertilization
IVP	intravenous pyelogram
K	potassium
kg	kilogram
KOH	potassium hydroxide
L	liter or lumbar (e.g., L5 nerve root)
LA	left atrium
LAE	left atrial enlargement
lb	pound
LCP	Legg–Calvé–Perthes disease
LDH	lactate dehydrogenase
LDL	low-density lipoproteins
LES	lower esophageal sphincter
LFT(s)	liver function test(s)
LGI	lower gastrointestinal (below the ligament of Treitz)
LH	luteinizing hormone
LLQ	left lower quadrant
LMN	lower motor neuron
LMP	last menstrual period
LR	lactated Ringer's solution
L/S	lecithin/sphingomyelin ratio
LSD	lysergic acid diethylamide
LUQ	left upper quadrant
LV	left ventricle
LVH	left ventricular hypertrophy
MAI	*Mycobacterium avium–intracellulare* complex
MAOI	monoamine oxidase inhibitor
MCHC	mean corpuscular hemoglobin concentration
MCL	medial collateral ligament

MCP	metacarpophalangeal (hand joint)
MCV	mean corpuscular volume
MEN	multiple endocrine neoplasia
mg	milligram
MG	myasthenia gravis
MgSO$_4$	magnesium sulfate
MHA-TP	microhemagglutination assay for antibodies to *Treponema pallidum* (for syphilis)
MI	myocardial infarction
mL	milliliter
mm	millimeter
MMR	measles, mumps, rubella (vaccine)
mo	month(s)
MRA	magnetic resonance angiogram
MRCP	magnetic resonance cholangiopancreatography
MRI	magnetic resonance imaging scan
MRSA	methicillin-resistant *Staphylococcus aureus*
Na	sodium
NPH	isophane insulin suspension (neutral protamine Hagedorn)
NPO	nothing by mouth
NPV	negative predictive value
NS	normal saline
NSAID	nonsteroidal antiinflammatory drug
O$_2$	oxygen
OA	osteoarthritis
OCP	oral contraceptive pill
OPV	oral poliovirus vaccine
P$_1$, P$_2$	heart sounds made by the pulmonary valve
PCN	penicillin
PCOS	polycystic ovary syndrome
PCP	phencyclidine; *Pneumocystis* pneumonia
PCWP	pulmonary capillary wedge pressure
PDA	patent ductus arteriosus
PE	pulmonary embolus
PEEP	positive end-expiratory pressure
PG	prostaglandin (e.g., PGE2, PGF); phosphatidylglycerol
pH	hydrogen ion concentration scale (measures acidity)
PH	pulmonary hypertension
PID	pelvic inflammatory disease
PIP	proximal interphalangeal (joint)
PMN	polymorphonuclear leukocyte
PMS	premenstrual syndrome
PO$_4$	phosphate
PPD	purified protein derivative (tuberculosis skin test)
PPV	positive predictive value
prn	as needed (pro re nata)
PPROM	preterm premature rupture of the membranes

PROM	premature rupture of the membranes
PSA	prostate-specific antigen
PT	prothrombin time
PTH	parathyroid hormone
PTT	partial thromboplastin time
PUD	peptic ulcer disease
PVC	premature ventricular contraction
PVD	peripheral vascular disease
RA	right atrium; rheumatoid arthritis
RAE	right atrial enlargement
RAI	radioactive iodine
RBC	red blood cell
RDW	red blood cell distribution width
REM	rapid eye movement (dream sleep)
RF	rheumatic fever
Rh	Rhesus blood group antigen
RI	reticulocyte index
RLQ	right lower quadrant
RNA	ribonucleic acid
RPR	rapid plasma reagin test (for syphilis)
RSV	respiratory syncytial virus
RUQ	right upper quadrant
RV	right ventricle
RVH	right ventricular hypertrophy
S	sacral (e.g., S1 nerve root)
S_1, S_2, S_3, S_4	heart sounds 1 to 4
SBO	small bowel obstruction
SCD	sickle cell disease
SCFE	slipped capital femoral epiphysis
SD	standard deviation
SIADH	syndrome of inappropriate antidiuretic hormone secretion
SIDS	sudden infant death syndrome
spp.	species
SSRI	selective serotonin reuptake inhibitors
STD	sexually transmitted disease
SVC	superior vena cava
Svo_2	systemic venous oxygen saturation
SVR	systemic vascular resistance
T1DM	type 1 diabetes mellitus
T2DM	type 2 diabetes mellitus
T_3	triiodothyronine
T_4	thyroxine
TB	tuberculosis
TCA	tricyclic antidepressant
Td	tetanus–diphtheria booster vaccine
TE	tracheoesophageal
TIA	transient ischemic attack

TIBC	total iron-binding capacity
TIPS	transjugular intrahepatic portosystemic shunt
TMP-SMX	trimethoprim–sulfamethoxazole
TOF	tetralogy of Fallot
TORCH	toxoplasmosis, other infections, rubella, cytomegalovirus, herpes simplex
tPA	tissue plasminogen activator
TRH	thyroid-releasing hormone
TSH	thyroid-stimulating hormone
TTP	thrombotic thrombocytopenic purpura
TURP	transurethral resection of the prostate
UGI	upper gastrointestinal (proximal to the ligament of Treitz)
UMN	upper motor neuron
URI	upper respiratory infection
US	ultrasound
UTI	urinary tract infection
VACTERL	vertebral, anal, cardiac, tracheoesophageal, renal, limb (malformations)
VDRL	Venereal Disease Research Laboratory test (for syphilis)
VFib, Vfib	ventricular fibrillation
VIPoma	pancreatic tumor that secretes vasoactive intestinal peptide
VMA	vanillylmandelic acid
$\dot{V}/\dot{Q}$	ventilation–perfusion (ratio)
VSD	ventricular septal defect
VTach, Vtach	ventricular tachycardia
vWF	von Willebrand's factor
WBC	white blood cells
WPW	Wolff–Parkinson–White syndrome
yr	year(s)

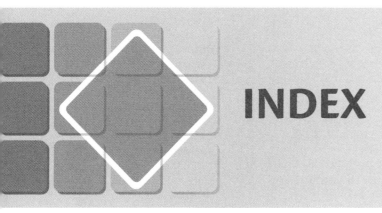

INDEX

Note: Page numbers followed by the letter f refer to figures; those followed by t refer to tables; and those followed by b refer to boxed material. Page numbers in **boldface type** indicate complete chapters.

Contraceptives, 180, 185, 187
oral. *See* Oral contraceptives.
Contraction stress test (CST), 202–203, 203f
Contractions, in labor and delivery, 203–205, 204t
fetal heart rate and, 205
Contrast agents
barium as. *See* Barium contrast studies.
in disease-specific screening and confirmatory tests, 277t–279t
renal failure caused by, 7, 68
Contusion(s)
liver, 217
lung, 217
Conversion disorder, 173
Conversion reaction, vision loss with, 222
Cooling measurements, for hyperthermia, 258
Coombs test, 82, 148
Copper
deficiency *vs.* toxicity of, 22t
excessive accumulation of, 54, 76
Cor pulmonale, 34, 43
Corneal disorders, vision loss from, 222, 223f
Coronary artery disease (CAD), 27, 30
low-dose aspirin for, 275
Coronary heart disease (CHD)
cholesterol risk for, 11
hypertension risk for, 5
MI risk with, 27
smoking risk for, 11, 12
Correlation coefficient, 163
Corticosteroids
for IBD, 50, 51
for rheumatologic disorders, 74, 75, 77
glaucoma and, 220
Corynebacterium diphtheriae, 118
Court mandates, for treatment, 284
Courvoisier's sign, 97, 295
Cow's milk, 261, 262
Cranial nerves
lesions of, 137–138, 138f
stroke localization and, 137t
palsies of, 8, 225, 240
Craniotomy
decompressive, 235
trauma indications for, 233–235

Creatine kinase (CK), 27, 142, 281
Creatine phosphokinase (CPK), 68, 168
Creatinine
blood urea nitrogen ratio to, 282
in pregnant patient, 190, 282
in renal disease, 67, 68
CREST syndrome, 56, 77
Cretinism, 62
Cri-du-chat, 156, 296
Cricothyrotomy, 147, 214
Crigler-Najjar syndrome, 59
Crohn's disease, 49, 50, 51f, 51t
Cromolyn, for asthma, 40
Cross-sectional survey, 165
Croup, 118
Crush Step 2
Step 1 *vs.*, 1
tips for, 1–2
Crying
cat-like, 156, 296
high-pitched, 156
Cryoprecipitate, 85
Cryptococcal infection, in HIV, 149
Cryptococcus neoformans 107, 149
in meningitis, 290, 291f
Cryptorchidism, 104, 253–254
Cryptosporidium spp., 150
Crystals, in gout, 74
Cullen's sign, 56, 295
Culture(s)
blood, 70, 230
in arthritis, 74, 75
in osteomyelitis, 230
of pleural effusion, 44
urine, 69, 70
Culture and sensitivity, in infectious disease, 107, 108t, 109t
Cushing's disease, 64, 100
Cushing's reflex, 295
Cushing's syndrome, 5, 64
tumors associated with, 91, 100
Cushing's triad, 235
Cyclooxygenase (COX) inhibitors, 274
Cyclophosphamide, for rheumatologic disorders, 77
Cyclosporine, use in transplants, 253
Cyclothymia, 169
Cyst(s)
breast, 181

Cyst(s) (*continued*)
dermoid, 98
neck, 243
ovarian, 180, 186
renal, 5, 68–69, 154
skin, 125t
unicameral bone, 105
Cystadenocarcinoma, 98
Cystic fibrosis (CF)
genetics of, 154
miscellaneous presentations of, 297
neonatal jaundice related to, 59
pulmonary manifestations of, 41, 43
Cystic hygroma, 243
Cysticercosis, 145
AIDS-associated, 149
Cystinuria, renal stones related to, 71
Cystocele, 186
Cystourethrogram, voiding, 69–70
Cytomegalovirus (CMV), 297
in pneumonia, 41, 112
in pregnant patient, 195
retinitis associated with, 149, 222
Cytopenias, 148
Cytotoxic reaction, 148

D

D dimer, in coagulopathies, 86
Danazol, 183
Dandy–Walker syndrome, 141
Danger to others, 284
Danger to self, 284
Dantrolene, 168, 258
Data comparisons, in biostatistics, 163
Dawn phenomenon, in diabetes mellitus, 9
Deafness, sudden, 239
Death. *See* Mortality rates.
sudden. *See* Sudden death.
Death rate, 161
Decelerations, of fetal heart rate, 205
Decompression surgery
craniotomy as, 235
for spinal cord metastases, 89
Decubitus ulcers, 127, 157
Deep vein thrombosis (DVT), 32–33, 248
coagulopathies associated with, 87
postoperative, 214

Lymphoma(s), 90t, 93f
  AIDS-associated, 149

M

Macrocytic anemia, 84–85
  diagnosis of, 79, 80b
Macrosomia, 189, 193
Macula
  cherry-red spot on, 296
  degeneration of, 223, 223f
Macule, 124t
Magnesium deficiency, 14
  toxicity vs., 21, 22t
Magnesium disturbances, 17,
  19, 20, 281
Magnesium sulfate
  for preeclampsia, 4, 198
  toxicity of, 20
Magnetic resonance (MR)
    angiogram
  disease-specific screening and
      confirmatory tests, 277t
  for renovascular
      hypertension, 5
  in neurosurgery, 234
  in rheumatologic disorders, 77
  in vascular surgery, 245,
      246f, 247
Magnetic resonance imaging
    (MRI)
  disease-specific screening and
      confirmatory tests,
      278t–279t
  for cancer detection, 95, 100,
      101f, 103
  in ear, nose, and throat
      disorders, 240f, 243
  in gynecological disorders,
      179, 180, 182, 183
  in neurology, 135, 140, 142,
      145, 145f, 146
  surgical applications,
      235–237
  in orthopedics, 228, 229, 230
  of spinal cord metastases, 89
Magnetic resonance (MR)
    venography, 32
Malabsorption syndrome, 21,
  22t, 49
Malignancies. See also
    Cancer(s).
  metastatic, 89, 97, 100, 101f,
      102f, 230
Malignant hyperthermia, 258
Malignant melanoma, 104,
  104f, 130
Malingering, 173
Mallory-Weiss tears, 56

Mammography, 95, 160t,
  181, 182
Mandible, in neck trauma,
  217, 217f
Manganese, deficiency vs.
  toxicity of, 22t
Mania, 169, 297
Manometry, esophageal, 29,
  55, 56
Marfan's syndrome, 154, 248
Marijuana, abuse of, 177
Mass(es)
  abdominal, 245
  breast, 94–95, 181–182
  CNS, 140
  neck, 243–244
  pulsatile, 245, 249
Mastectomy, 95
Mastitis, 181, 182, 207
Mastoiditis, 240
Maternal mortality rate, 161
Maturation, secondary
    characteristics of, 179, 188
MB isoenzyme, in MI, 27
McBurney's point, 209, 210f
McBurney's sign, 295
McCune–Albright
    syndrome, 296
McRobert's maneuver, 204,
    204f
Mean corpuscular volume
    (MCV), in anemias, 79, 83
Measles, 115
  German, 116
  mumps, and rubella (MMR)
      vaccine, 149, 264t
Mechanical ventilation
  for ARDS, 41
  withdrawal of, 283, 285
Meckel's diverticulum, 58t
Meconium aspiration, 43
Meconium ileus, 58t, 297
Medial collateral ligament
    (MCL), 228
Mediastinal shift, 292f
Medicaid, 161
Medicare, 161
Medullary thyroid nodule, 105
Medulloblastoma, 100, 141
Megaloblastic anemia, 22t
Meigs' syndrome, 98
Melanocyte-stimulating
    hormone (MSH), 64
Melanoma, malignant, 104,
    104f, 130
Menarche, disorders associated
    with, 182, 188
Ménière's disease, 239, 240
Meningiomas, 100

Meningitis, 116–117
  bacterial, 239
  C. neoformans, 149, 222f,
      290, 291f
  CSF findings in, 135t, 140
  empiric treatment of, 108t
  herpes encephalitis
      and, 117, 117f
  pediatric complications
      of, 263
Meningocele, 237
Meningococcal vaccine, 264
Meningococcus, 109t
Menopause, 182, 185
Menorrhagia, 182
Menstrual cycle/menstruation
  absence of. See Amenorrhea.
  breast cancer and, 95
  in DUB, 182
Mental retardation, 175
  genetics of, 155–156, 156f
Mesenteric ischemia, 247
Metabolic acidosis, 14–15
  chronic renal failure and, 69
Metabolic alkalosis, 14–15
Metabolic disturbances
  alcohol causing, 20, 21
  chronic renal failure and, 69
  liver failure and, 54
  neonatal jaundice related
      to, 59
  pediatric screening for, 264
Metabolism, in geriatric
    patients, 157
Metacarpophalangeal (MCP)
    joints, rheumatoid arthritis
    of, 74, 74f
Metanephrines, 64, 100
Metaphyseal fractures, in child
    abuse, 266, 266f
Metaplasia, Barrett's, 45, 55
Metastatic malignancies, 89,
    97, 100, 101f, 102f, 230
Metered dose inhalers, for
    emphysema, 39
Metformin, for diabetes, 8
Methadone, 177
Methanol poisoning, 222
Methimazole, for
    hyperthyroidism, 62
Methotrexate, for arthritis,
    74, 75
Methyldopa, anemia caused
    by, 79
α-Methyldopa, for
    hypertension, 4
Metronidazole, for C. difficile, 50
Microcytic anemia, 81–82
  diagnosis of, 79, 80b